W9-CBA-895

Complications in Endovascular Therapy

Complications in Endovascular Therapy

edited by

Kenneth Ouriel

The Cleveland Clinic Foundation
Cleveland, Ohio, U.S.A.

Barry T. Katzen

Baptist Cardiac & Vascular Institute
University of Miami School of Medicine
Miami, Florida, U.S.A

Kenneth Rosenfield

Massachusetts General Hospital
Boston, Massachusetts, U.S.A.

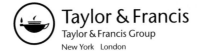

Taylor & Francis
Taylor & Francis Group
New York   London

Published in 2006 by
Taylor & Francis Group
270 Madison Avenue
New York, NY 10016

© 2006 by Taylor & Francis Group, LLC

No claim to original U.S. Government works
Printed in the United States of America on acid-free paper
10 9 8 7 6 5 4 3 2 1

International Standard Book Number-10: 0-8247-5420-4 (Hardcover)
International Standard Book Number-13: 978-0-8247-5420-4 (Hardcover)

Library of Congress Cataloging-in-Publication Data

Catalog record is available from the Library of Congress

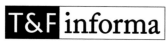

Taylor & Francis Group
is the Academic Division of T&F Informa plc.

Visit the Taylor & Francis Web site at
http://www.taylorandfrancis.com

Preface

In his well-known oratory "The Strenuous Life," Theodore Roosevelt said, "Far better it is to dare mighty things, to win glorious triumphs, even though checkered by failure, than to take rank with those poor spirits who neither enjoy much nor suffer much, because they live in the gray twilight that knows not victory nor defeat."*

Roosevelt's thoughts exemplify the successful interventionalist. At a time when the field of percutaneous interventional therapy is exploding, successful clinicians must be innovators—explorers in the area of new technology, not afraid to attempt novel innovations in an effort to enhance the well-being of a patient too old, too frail, or otherwise unwilling to undergo a standard surgical procedure. The interventionalist must sometimes design treatment strategies without the availability or comfort of long-term clinical outcome data. He or she must be willing to risk failure when piecing together bits of anecdotal information to arrive at a rational treatment for a particular patient with a specific clinical problem.

It is easy to achieve acceptable clinical outcome if one limits the scope of procedures to those that are straightforward, well defined, and without technical challenge. At this point in the evolution of interventional therapies, however, few procedures fill this bill. Endovascular complications may occur quickly and without warning. With this in mind, the key to success for any interventionalist centers on an appreciation of the myriad complications that can occur during the course of a procedure. In this manner, the complications can be anticipated, avoided preemptively or, when they do occur, be handled quickly and efficiently.

This book was developed to provide the practicing endovascular practitioner with a compendium that outlines the diagnosis and treatment of complications that occur during the course of interventional procedures. The chapter authors have been chosen for their particular expertise in a given technique or disease. Each author is a high-volume clinical operator, an innovator with vast endovascular experience. And the highest volume, most technically proficient clinicians are also the very same individuals who have experience in the gamut of complications that develop as the result of these interventions. When speaking about his own medical problems, a wise

---

* "The Strenuous Life" delivered to the Hamilton Club by Theodore Roosevelt, Chicago, IL, April 10th, 1899. http://www.theodoreroosevelt.org/research/speech%20strenuous.htm

clinician once stated, "I never want to be treated by a doctor who hasn't personally experienced every potential complication. This is the doctor who will be the best at avoiding and treating problems when they occur." While it is neither desirable nor possible for each of us to experience every potential complication associated with a specific procedure, the study of the experience of others will accelerate our learning process. Careful scrutiny of the chapters of this text will aid in the recognition and avoidance of complications of interventional procedures. Studying the errors of others will allow us to avoid identical errors, to attain a similar level of expertise without traveling the longer and more arduous path of experiential learning.

Roosevelt encouraged us to "boldly face the life of strife, resolute to do our duty well... resolute to be both honest and brave, to serve high ideals, yet to use practical methods." We must recognize and analyze our own mistakes and the mistakes of others, carefully evaluating the actions that led to an untoward event. Only then we will be able to avoid these complications in the future. Ultimately, the study of complications will be followed by an improvement in the results of interventional treatment to the point where the long-term outcome of a minimally invasive procedure achieves or exceeds that of traditional open surgery.

Kenneth Ouriel
Barry T. Katzen
Kenneth Rosenfield

Acknowledgment

A special acknowledgment goes to Lisa Bodzin, Coordinating Editor in the Department of Vascular Surgery at The Cleveland Clinic Foundation for careful review of the manuscripts, and for her assistance and guidance with this book. Her editorial contributions and valuable administrative data collection were assets in carrying out this project.

Contents

Contributors

Alex Abou-Chebl Interventional Neurology, Section of Stroke and Neurological Intensive Care, The Cleveland Clinic Foundation, Cleveland, Ohio, U.S.A.

Julie E. Adams Department of Vascular Surgery, The Cleveland Clinic Foundation, Cleveland, Ohio, U.S.A.

Gary M. Ansel Peripheral Vascular Intervention, Section of Cardiology, Riverside Methodist Hospital, MidOhio Cardiology and Vascular Consultants, Columbus, Ohio and Department of Internal Medicine, Medical College of Ohio, Toledo, Ohio, U.S.A.

Christopher Bajzer Department of Cardiovascular Medicine, The Cleveland Clinic Foundation, Cleveland, Ohio, U.S.A.

Curtis W. Bakal Department of Radiology, University of Medicine and Dentistry of New Jersey—New Jersey Medical School, Newark, New Jersey, U.S.A.

Deepak L. Bhatt Department of Cardiovascular Medicine, The Cleveland Clinic Foundation, Cleveland, Ohio, U.S.A.

Mark W. Burket Medical University of Ohio–Toledo, Toledo, Ohio, U.S.A.

Ruth L. Bush Division of Vascular Surgery and Endovascular Therapy, Michael E. DeBakey Department of Surgery, Baylor College of Medicine, and The Methodist Hospital, Houston, Texas, U.S.A.

Daniel G. Clair Department of Vascular Surgery, The Cleveland Clinic Foundation, Cleveland, Ohio, U.S.A.

Frank J. Criado Center for Vascular Intervention and Division of Vascular Surgery, Union Memorial Hospital-MedStar Health, Baltimore, Maryland, U.S.A.

Gregory S. Domer Center for Vascular Intervention and Division of Vascular Surgery, Union Memorial Hospital-MedStar Health, Baltimore, Maryland, U.S.A.

Matthew J. Eagleton Section of Vascular Surgery, University of Michigan, Ann Arbor, Michigan, U.S.A.

Andrew C. Eisenhauer Interventional Cardiovascular Medicine, Cardiovascular Division, Brigham and Women's Hospital and Harvard Medical School, Boston, Massachusetts, U.S.A.

Pamela Flick Department of Radiology, Concentrated Care Center, Georgetown University Hospital, Washington, D.C., U.S.A.

Roy Greenberg Department of Vascular Surgery, The Cleveland Clinic Foundation, Cleveland, Ohio, U.S.A.

Lazar J. Greenfield Section of Vascular Surgery, University of Michigan, Ann Arbor, Michigan, U.S.A.

Ziv J. Haskal Division of Vascular and Interventional Radiology, College of Physicians and Surgeons, New York Presbyterian Hospital, Columbia University, New York, New York, U.S.A.

L. Nelson Hopkins Department of Neurosurgery and Toshiba Stroke Research Center (JUH, LNH), School of Medicine and Biomedical Sciences, University at Buffalo, State University of New York, Buffalo, New York, U.S.A.

Jay U. Howington Department of Neurosurgery and Toshiba Stroke Research Center (JUH, LNH), School of Medicine and Biomedical Sciences, University at Buffalo, State University of New York, Buffalo, New York, U.S.A.

Michael R. Jaff Vascular Medicine, Vascular Diagnostic Laboratory, Lenox Hill Hospital, New York, New York, U.S.A.

Hilde Jerius Center for Vascular Intervention and Division of Vascular Surgery, Union Memorial Hospital-MedStar Health, Baltimore, Maryland, U.S.A.

Krishna Kandarpa Department of Radiology, UMass Memorial Health Care, University Campus, North Worcester, Massachusetts, U.S.A.

Vikram S. Kashyap Department of Vascular Surgery, The Cleveland Clinic Foundation, Cleveland, Ohio, U.S.A.

K. Kasirajan Department of Vascular Surgery, Emory University, Atlanta, Georgia, U.S.A.

Tulsidas S. Kuruvanka Department of Cardiovascular Medicine, The Cleveland Clinic Foundation, Cleveland, Ohio, U.S.A.

John Carlos Lantis II Division of Vascular Surgery, College of Physicians and Surgeons, St. Luke's-Roosevelt Hospital Center, Columbia University, New York, New York, U.S.A.

Peter H. Lin Division of Vascular Surgery and Endovascular Therapy, Michael E. DeBakey Department of Surgery, Baylor College of Medicine, and The Methodist Hospital, Houston, Texas, U.S.A.

Alan B. Lumsden Division of Vascular Surgery and Endovascular Therapy, Michael E. DeBakey Department of Surgery, Baylor College of Medicine, and The Methodist Hospital, Houston, Texas, U.S.A.

Sean P. Lyden Department of Vascular Surgery, The Cleveland Clinic Foundation, Cleveland, Ohio, U.S.A.

Kenneth Ouriel Department of Vascular Surgery, The Cleveland Clinic Foundation, Cleveland, Ohio, U.S.A.

Eric K. Peden Division of Vascular Surgery and Endovascular Therapy, Michael E. DeBakey Department of Surgery, Baylor College of Medicine, and The Methodist Hospital, Houston, Texas, U.S.A.

David A. Phillips Department of Radiology, UMass Memorial Health Care, University Campus, North Worcester, Massachusetts, U.S.A.

Mary C. Proctor Section of Vascular Surgery, University of Michigan, Ann Arbor, Michigan, U.S.A.

Krishna Rocha-Singh Vascular Medicine Program, Prairie Heart Institute, Springfield, Illinois, U.S.A.

Wael E. A. Saad Mallinckrodt Institute of Radiology, St. Louis, Missouri, U.S.A.

David Sacks Section of Interventional Radiology, Reading Hospital and Medical Center, West Reading, Pennsylvania, U.S.A.

Mark J. Sands Section of Vascular and Interventional Radiology, The Cleveland Clinic Foundation, Cleveland, Ohio, U.S.A.

Timur P. Sarac Department of Vascular Surgery, The Cleveland Clinic Foundation, Cleveland, Ohio, U.S.A.

Jacqueline Saw Cardiac Catheterization Laboratory, Vancouver General Hospital, University of British Columbia, Vancouver, British Columbia, Canada and Department of Cardiovascular Medicine, The Cleveland Clinic Foundation, Cleveland, Ohio, U.S.A.

Piotr S. Sobieszczyk Interventional Cardiovascular Medicine, Cardiovascular Division, Brigham and Women's Hospital and Harvard Medical School, Boston, Massachusetts, U.S.A.

David L. Waldman Department of Radiology, University of Rochester Medical Center, Rochester, New York, U.S.A.

Michael Wholey Cardiovascular and Interventional Radiology, University of Texas Health Science Center at San Antonio, San Antonio, Texas, U.S.A.

Jay S. Yadav Department of Cardiovascular Medicine, The Cleveland Clinic Foundation, Cleveland, Ohio, U.S.A.

1

Quality Improvement for Endovascular Procedures

David Sacks
Section of Interventional Radiology, Reading Hospital and Medical Center, West Reading, Pennsylvania, U.S.A.

Curtis W. Bakal
Department of Radiology, University of Medicine and Dentistry of New Jersey—New Jersey Medical School, Newark, New Jersey, U.S.A.

INTRODUCTION

Quality improvement (QI) is not usually a popular topic for discussion. It brings images of a bureaucratic "big brother" watching and punishing human errors with no benefit to patients. On the other hand, QI is ideally intended to document the quality of care one provides in clinically relevant ways with opportunities to improve. It is the purpose of this chapter to describe the latter, including specific ways to set up a QI program using useful and relevant criteria.

QI has always been important, but more recently has become increasingly so for several reasons. First, for endovascular procedures there are now multiple specialties performing identical procedures in the angiography suite, the cardiac catheterization room, and the operating room. The competition between specialties can lead to fights over turf and quality of care. While such issues can be "resolved" administratively, they are better resolved with data. The quality of care provided in each of these venues should be comparable, as mandated by the Joint Commission on Accreditation of Health Care Organizations (JCAHO) (1). Second, the field of endovascular interventions evolves as fast as new technology and techniques are developed. Changes are daily. Such rapid evolution may produce better outcomes but perhaps at the cost of a learning curve with increased complications. Only an unbiased outcome analysis can provide the information to see if overall quality of care is improved with new approaches. Third, there is a nationwide concern with patient harm due to medical errors. QI can help detect and address problems to reduce patient harm and increase benefit.

It should be noted that QI is not synonymous with presenting credentials or granting of privileges. Institutions require that physicians have appropriate credentials (i.e., training) before granting privileges. In this manner, quality of care is protected in an "up front" manner by having procedures performed only by trained personnel. A QI program maintains quality on an ongoing basis by examining whether procedures have been performed for appropriate indications, whether procedures have technically successful outcomes without complications with rates comparable to local and national standards, and whether patients are clinically better from these procedures. At the end of this chapter, a sample QI program for extremity and renal procedures is provided.

SCOPE OF CARE

A specific delineation of privileges is required for each member of the medical staff to perform endovascular procedures. Since there are now multiple specialties with different training guidelines for performing procedures (2–6), it seems that the American Heart Association (AHA) training criteria, which represents the only current interdisciplinary consensus-credentialing document, should be utilized (7). In addition to specifying specific case volumes and types needed for training, this document states that the outcomes of the training cases must be acceptable. It is likely that physicians and hospitals with a greater volume of cases would have better results (8,9), as has been shown for percutaneous coronary interventions. To achieve and maintain credentials for a specific procedure, an individual must show initial and continuing competence by adhering to quality improvement thresolds for indications, efficacy and safety. We believe that a trans-specialty QI program specific for vascular interventions should be in place with required participation for all individuals performing these interventions. In addition to procedure-specific credentialing, hospital accrediting organizations generally require an explicit statement of the patient population served, such as inpatients, outpatients, and most importantly, times during which those procedures are available. For example, routine scheduled cases are available five days a week, with emergency services available at any time as needed.

Delineation of privileges for a specific practitioner is usually granted by the chairman of the department or by a hospital-wide credentialing committee. The intent of the JCAHO is to provide similar levels of care throughout an institution, regardless of the department. Thus, when multiple services provide care, hospital-wide credentials guidelines should be in place. While multiple organizations have issued training standards for their membership for peripheral angioplasty, the AHA credentials statement is probably the most widely accepted and sole interdisciplinary credential document in widespread use (7).

SETTING UP A QI PROGRAM

The program should be based on objective criteria (10). In designing a QI program, the institution must:

1. assign specific responsibility for the clinical monitoring and evaluation program,
2. delineate the scope of care provided,
3. identify important aspects of care and indicators relating to them,
4. establish thresholds for evaluating the indicators,
5. collect and organize the data,

6. evaluate both the care and the procedure involving the care when specific thresholds are reached,
7. take specific actions to resolve identified problems,
8. perform follow-up evaluation to determine whether quality has improved and document this improvement, and
9. communicate relevant information to facility-wide QI programs.

The department chair is responsible for the QI program in his or her department. It is also the responsibility of the individual practitioner performing the procedure to appropriately document and record the procedure as well as any complications.

Endovascular procedures are monitored to determine the quality of their most important aspects of care (number 3 in the above list). These include appropriateness (indications), efficacy (effectiveness), and safety (complications). These quality indicators are procedure-specific. Some indications may be controversial. For example, some practitioners believe that percutaneous renal revascularization is justified to treat an asymptomatic renal artery stenosis in order to prevent later problems such as renal failure and hypertension. Others believe that appropriate candidates for such treatment should have hypertension resistant to at least three antihypertensive medications or developing azotemia or renal parenchymal loss. For this reason quality indicators are generally derived from published articles and consensus documents. For example, for peripheral vascular disease, the most widely accepted consensus document is the TransAtlantic Intersociety Consensus (TASC) document (11). The TASC group included members of interventional radiology, vascular surgery, and interventional cardiology societies from the United States and Europe. For renal disease, there is currently a consensus AHA document that includes reporting standards (12) and a single society QI document from the Society of Interventional Radiology (SIR) that includes indications and outcomes (13). For endovascular treatment of extracranial carotid artery stenosis, there is a single specialty QI document, but this field is changing so rapidly that any document may be rendered obsolete by new technology (14). There is a new multispecialty AHA document under creation to update the TASC document and include indications and outcomes for extremity, renal, and aortic aneurysmal disease. When available, this document should also provide useful benchmarks for QI programs. It is through the use of documents such as those mentioned that thresholds are set for the chosen indicators of care.

Data Collection

Data collection needs to be complete, unbiased, and accessible. Relying on practitioner generated procedure reports is easy but has limited value. Physicians are human beings and are subject to the bias of wanting to look good. The operator may consider some complications to be the expected outcome from a difficult case. Failures may be hidden by conversion to another procedure at the same sitting. Therefore, at least some cases must be reviewed from primary sources—patient records and procedure images. Someone independent of the operator should perform the review. Institutions may need to hire people and provide computer resources to obtain, record, and analyze QI data. Data sources generally consist of logs of vascular and interventional procedures done in the department, to include all specialties. A case log should include the patient's name, medical record number, operating physicians, indication, and specify the procedures performed. A complication log should also be maintained. These records and case logs are generally included in the department's confidential peer review file. Electronic logs are common; for example, the Hi-IQ® Electronic Database.

Evaluation

Review of indicators should be presented at a regular (monthly, quarterly) QI meeting. Cumulative data is ideally presented at the department meeting twice yearly. If thresholds are crossed, a review of policies and procedures should be undertaken. All physicians performing endovascular procedures in an institution should be monitored in the same fashion.

It is the responsibility of the individual physician to choose and perform those procedures best suited to the needs of his or her patient; the choice is based on the combination of published results and on the results achievable locally (15).

Actions to Improve Quality of Care

QI meetings should be viewed as educational, not punitive. Generally, adverse outcomes should be classified as avoidable or unavoidable, and means for preventing repeat events should be discussed; consensus should be attempted. If specific incidence thresholds are crossed, a specific plan should be formulated to rectify the problem. This might involve alteration of thresholds because the local service conditions or patient population is objectively different than the population from which thresholds were initially generated, or further training for some practitioners. Voluntary limitation of privileges should also be considered. Involuntary limitation of privileges may be considered if sufficient improvement has not occurred and should follow the hospital's medical staff by-laws and procedures.

Follow-Up

Follow up of actions taken is a critical component of QI to check if intended improvements have been achieved. The department report should include specific actions as well as follow up of previous actions. As defined in the institutional QI plan, the results of departmental meetings are reported to the hospital QI committee.

DEFINING OUTCOMES

Success and failure rates as well as complication rates are outcomes of interest, which are used in assessing the quality of endovascular procedures. Published outcomes may not reflect real community practice because published series often originate in institutions with high volumes and copious amounts of experience. Furthermore, there is probably a tendency to self-selection, so that only series with good results are submitted for publication. Thus, published results should be weighed against the experience of practicing physicians when generating outcome indicators during the guideline process (16). Outcome-based clinical practice guidelines from the SIR, for example, utilize a consensus process to evaluate the literature and inject a "reality check" for specific thresholds. Complication and technical success rates are also highly dependent on patient selection and factors. Thus, tailoring thresholds to an individual institution is reasonable and expected.

A procedure is initiated at the time of intention to treat; this may include attempts at passing a wire or catheter across a stenotic or occlusive lesion (17). Definitions of success and failure must be clear and uniformly applied.

Success

For diagnostic angiography, a successful study should provide a complete and adequate evaluation of the clinical problem. The study should be completed at a single session (18), and it should include inflow as well as a complete depiction of outflow (19). For diagnostic neuroangiography, for example, successful examination evaluates the intra- and extracranial circulation (20) and usually requires a selective study. Evaluating the carotid bifurcation alone is not sufficient for a complete diagnostic neuroangiogram (21).

Defining technical success for peripheral interventions such as angioplasty, lysis, and stenting is more complex than defining technical success for diagnostic procedures. While many definitions have been borrowed from conventional surgical revascularization operations (22), other definitions of success have been tailored for endovascular therapy. Reporting standards for unifying and standardizing endovascular procedures have been published (23) and include utilizing a combination of anatomical, hemodynamic, and clinical success. In the future, it is more likely that extended outcome assessments, including long-term clinical results, cost benefit analysis, functional status, and patient satisfaction indices will become more important (24). These long-term outcomes data are currently beyond the scope of most QI programs. However, since the principle aim of an interventionist is to relieve specific symptoms, it is reasonable to expect that these long-term quality measures will be mandated as part of future QI programs. Short- and medium-range technical and clinical success measures are proxies for these outcomes. The use of long-term and functional outcome data, such as freedom from stroke and ability to function independently, will become increasingly important to measure the effect of interventions in asymptomatic patients who undergo interventions aimed at averting catastrophic events, such as stroke related to carotid disease or aneurysm rupture. Some possible long-term and functional measures for extremity and renal procedures are included in the sample QI program at the end of this chapter.

Complications (Adverse Events)

Complications or adverse events are indicators of the safety of percutaneous procedures. If specific incidence thresholds are exceeded, a quality review should occur. Complications are most often categorized by outcomes (Table 1).

Major complications require detailed procedural review and are utilized to calculate complication rates for QI purposes (16). Minor complications are tracked, but are not used in the numerator data for complication rates. In clinical practice, the assignment of a specific adverse event to a complication category is often subjective. This inconsistent, variable description of complications has negative implications for the QI process, for patient care, and even for the validity and comparability of the scientific literature.

Consider the following similar clinical vignettes (25):

Vignette 1: Primary stenting of a common iliac artery stenosis results in a long flow limiting dissection, which extends from the focal target lesion down through the

Table 1 Classification of Complications by Outcome (Society of Interventional Radiology)

Minor complications
  No therapy, no consequence
  Nominal therapy, no consequence; includes overnight admission for observation only
Major complications
  Require therapy, minor hospitalization (<48 hours)
  Require major therapy, unplanned increase in level of care, prolonged hospitalization
    (>48 hours)
  Have permanent adverse sequelae
  Result in death

Source: From Ref. 22.

external iliac artery. This extended dissection is treated with two additional stents down to the mid common femoral artery.

Vignette 2: A patient with a proximal external iliac artery stenosis and superficial femoral artery occlusion is planned for staged procedures: iliac percutaneous translumenal angioplasty (PTA) with a subsequent femoral-popliteal bypass. During the iliac PTA, a large dissection extends down to the inguinal ligament necessitating stent placement into the proximal common femoral artery. The bypass is therefore taken from the proximal SFA rather than CFA as planned.

During a structured SIR Standards Committee survey, a group of experienced Interventional Radiologists categorized Vignette 1 as follows: 50% minor complication, 50% major complication. Vignette 2 was categorized as: 40% minor complication, 37% major complication, 14% not a complication (25). In fact in over 40% of 195 clinical vignettes surveyed, a consensus level of 80% agreement could not be achieved.

Similar exercises conducted with Interventional Cardiologists as well as an interdisciplinary group of Interventional Radiologists, Cardiologists, and Vascular Surgeons revealed similar inconsistencies in scoring complications vignettes (26,27). By developing a group of principles to guide categorization of complications and an iterative Delphi process, consensus could be reached in almost 90% (25). Using this process, the SIR hopes to create a reference list of adverse events that will allow more uniform categorization (16).

Radiation Injury

Although radiation injury is unlikely to occur during routine diagnostic arteriography, it can occur during prolonged procedures and complex interventions (28). After exposure to 200 rads two Gy, skin burns can develop; this exposure can be reached after about one hour of fluoroscopy over a single site in a single projection (29). Radiation exposure from filming is additive to fluoroscopy dose, especially if rapid frame cine is used (30). Fluoroscopy time is commonly recorded as a quality monitor, but it only roughly correlates with actual skin dose (31). Recently, the Food and Drug Administration has become concerned about radiation dose to patients during complex interventional procedures, and it is recommended that fluoroscopic exposure protocols be devised by institutions to assess potential for radiation injury (32). Some percutaneous endovascular reconstructions, vascular embolizations (especially complex intracerebral AVM treatments) and transjugular intrahepatic porto-system shunt placements (TIPS) are particularly problematic.

One society has recommended that radiation exposure be recorded for all patients, with exposure estimated as either fluoroscopy time plus number of radiographic exposures, dose area product, cumulative dose, or peak skin dose (33). The latter three measures require use of a radiation dosimeter, which is increasingly available on new angiographic equipment. Training in radiation safety should be a specific requirement for fluoroscopy privileges (34).

LEGAL IMPLICATIONS

Clinical practice guidelines can be used by both defense and plaintiff attorneys in malpractice litigations. While the plaintiff rather than the defense in court has used guidelines more frequently, data may be biased by cases being dropped if guidelines appear to support the defense (35). There is a general agreement that guidelines can reduce malpractice claims but non-compliance with accepted guidelines may actually place physicians at further risk.

Under the well-established legal theory of corporate liability, institutions are held responsible for the actions of independent physicians for care provided within its walls (36). An institution may be liable if it had knowledge or should have known that a particular physician was likely to provide substandard care and cause injury to a patient (37). For example, the institution may know that a physician has a complication rate significantly and persistently higher or a technical success rate lower than national QI standards. This evidence may be fortified if the physician has not met national accepted minimum training standards while others in the institution have.

ARCHIVING AND REPORTING

Appropriate reporting of interventional procedures and archiving of images is necessary for provision of high-quality care.

Evaluation of the completeness and accuracy of the written medical record and of acquired images should be part of the QI process. There is little federal regulatory guidance on the reporting and archiving of interventional procedures, although some do specify the minimum documentation needed to meet appropriateness and payment needs. There is a small body of state regulations covering archiving and reporting, which varies considerably between jurisdictions, and a recent guideline published by the SIR outlines appropriate film and written documentation (38). When state requirements exceed societal guidelines, physicians are advised to follow the more rigorous state regulations.

The written report and archived images serve four related purposes: (i) to document medical care, (ii) to guide any future diagnostic work up or therapy, (iii) to document procedures for appropriate coding, and (iv) to serve as an element of the QI and credentialing processes (38).

The medical record refers to all recorded medical information, including written and electronic data. Contrast agent dose, medications administered, and measures of radiation exposure must be part of the permanent medical record; if medical devices (e.g., stents) are inserted, appropriate identifying information such as product name, vendor, and lot numbers must be recorded.

Preprocedural documentation provides a baseline record and must clearly document the indication for any procedure; the preprocedural documentation must be written in the chart before initiation of the procedure or conscious sedation. In addition, pertinent physical examination, laboratory findings, American Society of Anesthesiology risk class, consent, and anticipated treatment plan must be documented.

A written (preliminary) post-procedure note is essential for communication to other personnel and should include at least a brief description of the percutaneous approach (puncture site), the procedure(s), operators, complications, and post-procedure monitoring and treatment plan. Administered medications and contrast load should also be recorded here, as they may guide post-procedure plans for hydration and sedation recovery (38).

The final procedural report should include the information provided in the preliminary report, but should also provide an extensive description of the technical aspects of the procedure as well as all diagnostic information: all access sites (including attempted accesses), guidance modalities, all catheters, wires, implanted devices, and other disposables used; hemostases methodology, consent, and each vessel catheterized.

Archived images are an important part of the medical record and should be saved in a permanently retrievable digital format or hard copy (38). Relevant anatomy and transient adverse events (e.g., emboli, even if successfully managed during the procedure) must be documented.

All pertinent imaging data must be saved as hard copy or in a permanent retrievable digital format. This includes documenting all anatomy that affects diagnosis and management, device position, complications, and any transient adverse event (e.g., emboli) successfully treated during the procedure. For digital angiography, a non-subtracted image is useful for orientation. The final position of all devices or implants (e.g., stents, caval filters, central venous catheters) placed with imaging guidance should be documented with imaging in addition to the pre-deployment images. After angioplasty, stenting, or lysis, images of the relevant runoff distal to the intervention should be archived. The image should also enable assessment of the effect of the device on target or non-target vessels.

SAMPLE QI PROGRAM

The appendix of this chpater is a possible QI program for extremity and renal angiography and interventions (39). This program may be helpful to readers as a guide for creating their own program tailored for their needs. For those who may wish to use this program as a model, the references have been numbered separately from the rest of this chapter. This QI program is designed to measure not only the usual variables of technical success and complications, but also indications and clinical outcomes.

To avoid bias, the indications for extremity angiography and interventions come from the TASC report. The indications for renal interventions come from the AHA and SIR. Outcomes are measured using questionnaires that assess walking (the Walking Impairment Questionnaire) and functional status (SF-36) (40,41). Other questionnaires are available. It is important that these be measured before and after intervention to determine improvement. If early revascularization is indeed beneficial, there should be a significant and sustained improvement in walking and functional status. If minimally stenotic lesions are being dilated, there should be little or no clinical improvement, even though minimally stenotic lesions can be treated with high success and low complication rates.

REFERENCES

1. JCAHO. Medical Staff Standard. The Comprehensive Accreditation Manual for Hospitals 1998; Medical Staff Standard 6.8:MS-79.
2. Levin DC, Becker GJ, Dorros G, Goldstone J, King SBd, Seeger JM, Spies JB, Spittell JA, Jr, Wexler L. Training standards for physicians performing peripheral angioplasty and other percutaneous peripheral vascular interventions. A statement for health professionals from the Special Writing Group of the Councils on Cardiovascular Radiology, Cardio-Thoracic and Vascular Surgery, and Clinical Cardiology, the American Heart Association. Circulation 1992; 86:1348–1350.
3. SCVIR. Society of Cardiovascular and Interventional Radiology: credentials criteria for peripheral, renal, and visceral percutaneous transluminal angioplasty. Radiology 1988; 167:452.
4. Spittell JA Jr, Nanda NC, Creager MA, Ochsner JL, Dorros G, Wexler L, Isner JM, Young JR. Recommendations for peripheral transluminal angioplasty: training and facilities. American College of Cardiology Peripheral Vascular Disease Committee. J Am Coll Cardiol 1993; 21:546–548.
5. Wexler L, Dorros G, Levin D, King S. Guidelines for performance of peripheral percutaneous transluminal angioplasty. The Society for Cardiac Angiography and Interventions, Interventional Cardiology Committee, Subcommittee on Peripheral Interventions. Cathet Cardiovasc Diagn 1990; 21:128–129.
6. White RA, Fogarty TJ, Baker WH, et al. Endovascular surgery credentialing and training for vascular surgeons. J Vasc Surg 1993; 17:1095–1102.
7. Levin DC, Becker GJ, Dorros G, Goldstone J, King SB 3rd, Seeger JM, Spies JB, Spittell JA Jr, Wexler L. Training standards for physicians performing peripheral angioplasty and other percutaneous peripheral vascular interventions. A statement for health professionals from the Special Writing Group of the Councils on Cardiovascular Radiology, Cardio-Thoracic and Vascular Surgery, and Clinical Cardiology, the American Heart Association. Circulation 1992; 86(4):1348–1350.
8. Hannan EL, Racz M, Ryan TJ, McCallister BD, Johnson LW, Arani DT, Guerci AD, Sosa J, Topol EJ. Coronary angioplasty volume-outcome relationships for hospitals and cardiologists. J Am Med Assoc 1997; 277:892–898.
9. Kimmel SE, Berlin JA, Laskey WK. The relationship between coronary angioplasty procedure volume and major complications. J Am Med Assoc 1995; 274:1137–1142.
10. SIR Standards of Practice Committee, July 1989. Guidelines for establishing a Quality Assurance Program in vascular and interventional radiology. J Vasc Interv Radiol 2003; 14:S203–S207.
11. Dormandy JA, Rutherford RB. TASC Working Group. Management of Peripheral Arterial Disease (PAD). Trans Atlantic Inter-Society Concensus (TASC). J Vasc Surg 2000; 31(1 Pt 2):S1–S296.
12. Rundback J, Sacks D, Kent K, Christopher Cooper, Daniel Jonse, Timothy Murphy, kenneth Rosenfield, Christopher White, Michael Bettmann, Stanley Cortell, Jules Puschett, Daniel G. Clair, Patricia Cole. Guidelines for the reporting of renal artery revascularization in clinical trials. Circulation 2002; 106:1572–1585.
13. Martin LG, Rundback JH, Sacks D, John FC, Chet RR, Alan HM, Steven GM, Marc SS, Mark IS, Curtis AL. Quality improvement guidelines for angiography, angioplasty, and stent placement in the diagnosis and treatment of renal artery stenosis in adults. J Vasc Interv Radiol 2002; 13:1069–1083.
14. Connors JJ, Sacks D, Becker GJ, Barr JD. Carotid artery angioplasty and stent placement: quality improvement guidelines to ensure stroke risk reduction. J Vasc Interv Radiol 2003; 14:S317–S319.
15. Hertzer NR. Outcome assessment in vascular surgery—results mean everything. J Vasc Surg 1995; 21:6–15.

16. Sacks D, McClenny TE, Cardella JF, Lewis CA. Society of Interventional Radiology Clinical Practice Guidelines. J Vasc Interv Radiol 2003; 14:S199–S202.

17. Sacks D. Angiography and percutaneous vascular interventions: complications and quality improvement. In: Rutherford RB, ed. Vascular Surgery. 5th ed. Philadelphia: WB Saunders, 1999:796–812.

18. Singh H, Cardella JF, Cole PE, Clement JG, McCowan TC, Timothy LS David S, Curtis AL. Quality improvement guidelines for diagnostic arteriography. J Vasc Interv Radiol 2002; 13:1–6.

19. Pentecost MJ, Criqui MH, Dorros G, Goldstone J, Johnston KW, Martin EC, Ring EJ, Spies JB. Guidelines for peripheral percutaneous transluminal angioplasty of the abdominal aorta and lower extremity vessels. A statement for health professionals from a special writing group of the Councils on Cardiovascular Radiology, Arteriosclerosis, Cardio-Thoracic and Vascular Surgery, Clinical Cardiology, and Epidemiology and Prevention, the American Heart Association. Circulation 1994; 89:511–531.

20. Citron S, Wallace R. Standards of Practice Committee of the SCVIR. Quality improvement guidelines for adult diagnostic neuroangiography. Cooperative study between ASITN, ASNR, and SIR. J Vasc Interv Radiol 2000; 11:129–134.

21. Ullrich C, Moore A, Parsons R. The arteriographic diagnosis of extracranial cerebrovascular disease. In: Robicsek F, ed. Extracranial Cerebrovascular Disease: Diagnosis and Management. New York: Macmillan, 1986:108–140.

22. Rutherford RB, Baker JD, Ernst C, Johnston KW, Porter JM, Ahn S, Jonse DN. Recommended standards for reports dealing with lower extremity ischemia: revised version. J Vasc Surg 1997; 26:517–538.

23. Sacks D, Marinelli DL, Martin LG, Spies JB. Reporting standards for clinical evaluation of new peripheral arterial revascularization devices. Technology Assessment Committee [published errata appear in J Vasc Interv Radiol 1997 May–June; 8(3):492 and 1997 July–August; 8(4):658]. J Vasc Interv Radiol 1997; 8:137–149.

24. McDaniel MD, Nehler MR, Santilli SM, William RH, Judith GR, Jerry Goldstone, Walter JM, John VW. Extended outcome assessment in the care of vascular diseases: revising the paradigm for the 21st century. J Vasc Surg 2000; 32(6):1239–1250.

25. Bakal C. Categorization of procedure related complications: results of the SIR Task Force. SIR Annual Scientific Meeting, Salt Lake City, March 28, 2003.

26. Bakal C. Categorization of medical errors and complications. ACC Heart House, June 18, 2002, Bethesda.

27. Bakal C. Categorization of complications: can there be consensus? Vascular Centers Third Annual Meeting, Atlanta, April 29, 2001.

28. Mettler FA Jr, Koenig TR, Wagner LK, Kelsey CA. Radiation injuries after fluoroscopic procedures. Semin Ultrasound CT MR 2002; 23(5):428–442.

29. Wagner LK, Eifel PJ, Geise RA. Potential biological effects following high X-ray dose interventional procedures. J Vasc Interv Radiol 1994; 5:71–84.

30. Norbash AM, Busick D, Marks MP. Techniques for reducing interventional neuroradiologic skin dose: tube position rotation and supplemental beam filtration. AJNR Am J Neuroradiol 1996; 17:41–49.

31. Miller DL, Balter S, Cole PE, Lu HL, Beth AS. Radiation doses in interventional radiology procedures. The RAD-IR Study. Part I: overall measures of dose. J Vasc Interv Radiol 2003; 14:711–727.

32. FDA. Important information for physicians and other healthcare professionals: recording information in the patient's medical record that identifies the potential for serious X-ray-induced skin injuries following fluoroscopically guided procedures. Rockville, MD: Center for Devices and Radiological Health, Food and Drug Administration, September 15, 1995.

33. Miller DL. Quality improvement guidelines for reporting patient radiation dose. J Vasc Interv Radiol. In press.

34. Cardella JF, Miller DL, Cole, Patricia E, Lewis CA. Society of Interventional Radiology Position Statement on Radiation Safety. J Vasc Interv Radiol 2003; 14:S387.

35. Hyams AL, Brandenburg JA, Lipsitz SR, Shapiro DW, Brennan TA. Practice guidelines and malpractice litigation: a two-way street. Ann Intern Med 1995; 122:450–455.

36. McLean D. Credentialing & Privileging: One Size Doesn't Fit All. http://www.amda.com (10/6/2003).

37. Feegel JR. Liability of health care entities for negligent care. In: American College of Legal Medicine, ed. Legal Medicine. 3rd ed. St. Louis, MO: Mosby-Yearbook, 1995:156.

38. Omary RA, Bettmann MA, Cardella JF, Bakal CW, Schwartzberg MS, Sacks D, Rholl KS, Meranze SG, Lewis CA. Quality improvement guidelines for the reporting and archiving of interventional radiology procedures. J Vasc Interv Radiol 2002; 13(9): 879–881.

39. Sacks D. Developing an institution-wide quality assurance program. Vascular Centers 2002 Annual Meeting, Atlanta, May 2002.

40. Hiatt WR, Hirsch AT, Regensteiner JG, Brass EP. Clinical trials for claudication. Assessment of exercise performance, functional status, and clinical end points. Vascular Clinical Trialists. Circulation 1995; 92:614–621.

41. Ware JE Jr, Sherbourne CD. The MOS 36-item short-form health survey (SF-36). I. Conceptual framework and item selection. Med Care 1992; 30:473–483.

APPENDIX: A QUALITY ASSURANCE PROGRAM FOR PERIPHERAL VASCULAR DIAGNOSTIC AND THERAPEUTIC PROCEDURES

General Issues

The QA program will need to include both diagnostic and therapeutic vascular procedures done by different vascular specialties, i.e., interventional radiology, cardiology, and vascular surgery. The following categories of information need to be acquired:

A. Indications for the procedure
B. Duration of symptoms (acute versus chronic ischemia)
C. Technical success/failure
D. Technical complications
E. Measurement of radiation exposure and contrast use
F. Measurement of frequency with which diagnostic and therapeutic procedures are performed on the same day for percutaneous procedures
G. Clinical categorization of disease severity prior to the procedure
H. Improvement following intervention. Because the QA process will focus on clinical outcomes, data collection will primarily be focussed on clinical outcomes rather than anatomic measures of patency of treated vessels
I. Durability of improvement (including the number of reinterventions in the target organ to maintain improvement)

Quality thresholds are listed when possible. For some categories, such as radiation exposure, contrast use, improvement, and durability of improvement quality thresholds are not defined, but outcomes still need to be followed.

References for the Appendix can be found on p. 26.

Diagnostic Extremity Arteriography

    A. Indications

        1. Claudication

            a. TransAtlantic Inter-Society Consensus (TASC) Recommendation #18 (1): Angiography in a patient with intermittent claudication is usually indicated only when a decision has been made to intervene should a suitable lesion be identified (i.e., the patient should meet the indications for intervention as listed immediately below).

            b. TASC Recommendation #21 (1): Intervention in a patient with intermittent claudication is indicated only if:

                i. There is a lack of response to exercise therapy and risk factor modification.

               ii. The patient has a severe disability, either unable to perform normal work or with very serious impairment of other activities.

             iii. Absence of other disease that would limit exercise even if the claudication were improved.

             iv. The patient has appropriate natural history and prognosis.

              v. Treatment of the lesion must have low risk and a high probability of initial and long-term success.

        2. Critical limb ischemia
Defined as chronic ischemic rest pain, ulcers, or gangrene attributable to objectively proven arterial disease (TASC Recommendation #73) (1). Usually the presence of critical limb ischemia is sufficient indication for diagnostic and interventional procedures.

            Threshold for appropriate indications = 95% (Table A-1)

    B. Duration of symptoms
Acute and chronic symptoms are due to different pathology and have different therapies. Duration of symptoms are categorized as follows (2):

        a. Hyperacute ($<$ 24 hours).

        b. Acute A (1–7 days).

        c. Acute B (8–14 days).

        d. Subacute (14 days–3 months).

        e. Chronic ($>$3 months).

    C. Technical success
The extremity arteries should be evaluated so that all disease potentially related to patient symptoms has been adequately evaluated. The extremity arteries should be adequately visualized from the distal aorta to the foot. The iliac artery bifurcation should be imaged free of overlap that may obscure lesions. The common femoral artery bifurcation should be imaged free of overlap that may obscure lesions.

            Threshold for technical success = 95% (Table A-1)

Table A–1 Diagnostic Angiography Quality Improvement Standards

Indicators	Threshold (%)
I. Indications	95
II. Success rates	95
III. Complications	
a. Puncture site	
1. Hematoma (requiring transfusion, surgery, or delayed discharge)	0.5
2. Occlusion	0.2
3. Pseudoaneurysm/arteriovenous fistula	0.2
b. Catheter induced, other than puncture site	
1. Distal emboli	0.5
2. Arterial dissection/subintimal passage	0.5
3. Subintimal injection of contrast	0.5
c. Contrast induced renal failure	0.2
(elevation in baseline serum creatinine or blood urea nitrogen requiring care that delays discharge, requires unexpected admission or readmission or that results in permanent impairment of renal function)	
IV. Overall procedure threshold for major complications	1
The overall procedure threshold for major complications is determined by the following formula: (No. of patients undergoing only diagnostic arteriography with complications)/(No. of patients undergoing only diagnostic arteriography) × 100.	

Source: From Ref. 19.

D. Technical complications

Complications are graded using the society of international radiology (SIR) categories of major and minor complications. It is expected that the current definitions will be modified in the near future to include adverse events that do not produce current symptoms but have the potential to produce measurable harm to the patient in the future. SIR will also be publishing guidelines to be used for assigning categories of complication to specific events. These revisions will be adopted by the QA process. The current categories are as follows (3):

Minor complications:

a. No therapy, no sequela.
b. Minor therapy or minor sequela, includes unplanned overnight hospital admission for observation only (<24 hours).

Major complications:

c. Requires major therapy or unplanned hospitalization (24–48 hours).
d. Requires major therapy, unplanned increase in the level of care, prolonged hospitalization (>48 hours).
e. Permanent adverse sequelae.
f. Death.

Classification of major complications are listed in Table A–2

Table A–2 Classification of Complications by Outcome (Society of Interventional Radiology)

Grade	Category	Clinical description	Objective criteria
0	0	Asymptomatic—no hemodynamically significant occlusive disease	Normal treadmill or reactive hyperemia test
I	1	Mild claudication	Completes treadmill exercise (five minutes at 2 mph on 12% incline) postexercise ankle pressure is >50 mmHg but at least 20 mmHg <resting value
	2	Moderate claudication	Between categories 1 and 3
	3	Severe claudication	Cannot complete standard treadmill exercise and postexercise ankle pressure <50 mmHg
II	4	Ischemic rest pain	Resting ankle pressure <40 mm Hg; flat or barely pulsatile ankle or metatarsal plethysmographic tracing (PVR); toe pressure <30 mmHg
III	5	Minor tissue loss-nonhealing ulcer, focal gangrene with diffuse pedal ischemia	Resting ankle pressure <60 mm Hg ankle or metatarsal PVR flat or barely pulsatile; toe pressure <40 mmHg
	6	Major tissue loss extending above transmetatarsal level, functional foot no longer salvageable	Same as category 5

Source: From Ref. 12.

E. Measurement of radiation exposure and contrast use

Radiation exposure can be measured in multiple ways. The ideal measurement is that of peak cumulative skin exposure, but this is not possible with the current imaging equipment. Measurement of fluoroscopy time is easy to acquire but crude, as it does not take into account the amount of radiation during fluoroscopy or imaging. The current imaging systems are capable of reporting dose area product and specifying which part of the dose comes from fluoroscopy versus digital imaging, but again do not specify where in the body the radiation exposure occurred. For these reasons, the recommendation is that radiation exposure be reported at a minimum using fluoroscopy time plus number of images obtained (4). Patients should be tracked according to FDA guidelines (5–7). These guidelines require reporting of radiation exposure for procedures that are likely to approach 2 Gy (200 R) for any body part. While radiation exposure is due to the combined exposure from fluoroscopy and image acquisition, with current digital imaging at 1–2 frames/sec, the majority of radiation exposure from most procedures comes from fluoroscopy. A fluoroscopy time of one hour during the procedure has been previously used as a quality threshold (8) and therefore all cases with a fluoroscopy time of 60 minutes or longer should be reported. In addition, due to the high radiation exposure from cineradiography at frame rates of 15–30 frames/sec (9), non-cardiac imaging using cineradiography should also be reported.

Contrast use depends on the volume and concentration of contrast used. This is best expressed as grams of iodine used. Only iodinated contrast used will be tracked. Alternative contrast agents such as carbon dioxide (toxicity is not related to total dose) and gadolinium (toxicity is rare and dose should be less than 50 cc) will not be tracked. For procedures done at one sitting the total iodinated contrast dose will be calculated in addition to the dose from the tracked procedure. This includes contrast from diagnostic peripheral arteriography that precedes interventions, and contrast from cardiac procedures performed at the same sitting as peripheral procedures.

 F. Measurement of frequency with which diagnostic and therapeutic procedures are performed on the same day. This is applicable to therapeutic procedures only.
 G. Clinical categorization of disease severity prior to the procedure
 For chronic ischemia:

   1. Ankle/brachial index or pulse-volume recording.
   2. Assessment of walking impairment with WIQ (10).
   3. Assessment of general quality of life with SF-36 (11).
   4. Use of Rutherford categories of chronic ischemia (Table A–4) (12).
   For acute ischemia:
   Use of Rutherford categories of acute ischemia (12) (Table A–3).

 H. Improvement following intervention: not applicable.
 I. Durability of improvement: not applicable.

Table A–3 Clinical Categories of Acute Limb Ischemia

Category	Description/ prognosis	Sensory loss	Muscle weakness	Doppler signals	
				Arterial	Venous
I. Viable	Not immediately threatened	None	None	Audible	Audible
II. Threatened					
a. Marginally	Salvageable if promptly treated	Minimal (toes) or none	None	Inaudible	Audible
b. Immediately	Salvageable with immediate revascularization	More than toes Associated with rest pain	Mild, moderate	Inaudible	Audible
III. Irreversible	Major tissue loss or permanent nerve damage inevitable	Profound anesthetic	Profound paralysis (rigor)	Inaudible	Inaudible

Source: From Ref. 12.

Table A–4 Recommended Scale for Gauging Changes in Clinical Status for Chronic Limb Ischemia

Grade	Description
+3	*Markedly improved*: no ischemic symptoms; any foot lesions completely healed; ABI > 0.9
+2	*Moderately improved*: no open foot lesions; still symptomatic but only with exercise and improved by at least one category; ABI not normalized but increased by > 0.10
+1	*Minimally improved*: > 0.10 increase in ABI but no categorical improvement or vice versa (i.e., upward categorical shift without an increase in ABI of > 0.10
0	*No change*: no categorical shift and < 0.10 change in ABI
−1	*Mildly worse*: no categorical shift but ABI decrease > 0.10, or downward categorical shift with ABI decrease < 0.10
−2	*Moderately worse*: one category worse or unexpected minor amputation
−3	*Markedly worse*: more than one category worse or unexpected major amputations

Note: Categories refer to chronic limb ischemia (Table A–3).
Abbreviations: ABI, ankle/brachial index.
Source: From Ref. 12.

Extremity Interventions

Interventions included in the QA process are percutaneous revascularizations (angioplasty, atherectomy stent, lysis, etc.).

A. Indications for revascularization

1. Claudication: TASC Recommendation 21 as listed in diagnostic extremitry angiography section A.1.b above (1).
2. Critical limb ischemia: Usually the presence of critical limb ischemia is sufficient clinical indication for diagnostic and interventional procedures.
3. Stenosis > 50% diameter. For stenoses < 70% diameter there should be a trans-stenotic pressure gradient > 10 mm systolic or > 10% (3).
4. Femoral popliteal stenting is indicated only in treatment of acute balloon angioplasty failure or complications (TASC Recommendation 36) (1).

Threshold for appropriate indications = 95%

B. Duration of symptoms
Acute and chronic symptoms are due to different pathology and have different therapies. Duration of symptoms are categorized as follows (2):

a. Hyperacute (< 24 hours)
b. Acute A (1–7 days)
c. Acute B (8–14 days)
d. Subacute (14 days–3 months)
e. Chronic (>3 months)

C. Technical success
A procedure may be technically successful and clinically unsuccessful, for example if there is severe untreated disease elsewhere in the leg or if the patient's symptoms were not due to ischemia.

   1. Technical success is judged on "intention to treat." For example, failure to cross a stenosis with a guide wire is a failure of the intended revascularization therapy (angioplasty, stent, lysis). The intention is stated in the chart prior to the procedure being attempted.
   2. Technical success for percutaneous revascularzation other than lysis is stratified by lesion morphology as listed in TASC Recommendations #31 for iliac lesions and #34 for femoropopliteal lesions (1).
   3. To be considered technically successful, in the immediate post-procedure period the intervention must meet the criteria for both anatomic and hemodynamic success as defined below (12,13).

      A. Anatomic: <30% final residual stenosis measured at the narrowest point of the vascular lumen.
      Continued anatomic: <50% recurrent stenosis.
      B. Hemodynamic: ankle-brachail index (ABI) or thigh-brachial index (TBI) improved by 0.1 or greater above baseline and not deteriorated by >0.15 from the maximum early post-procedure level, or pulse volume recording distal to the reconstruction maintained at 5 mm above the preoperative tracing (only for patients with incompressible vessels). If intravascular pressures are obtained, the gradient across the treated segment should be <10 mmHg or <10% either with or without vasodilation (3).

   4. Since stents are frequently reserved for PTA failures in the extremities, PTA and stents will be considered combination percutaneous therapy and the PTA will not be categorized as a technical failure if a stent is subsequently placed at the same encounter.
   5. Technical success for lytic cases is defined as restorations of antegrade flow and complete or near complete (95% by volume) removal of the thrombus. This definition allows evaluation of lysis separately from the adjunctive procedure(s), if needed (2).

      Thresholds for technical success for extremity PTA and iliac stenting are listed in Tables A–5 and A–6. Thresholds for technical success for lysis are not defined

D. Complications
Complications are graded using the SIR categories of major and minor complications.

   Thresholds for complications for extremity PTA and iliac stenting are listed in Tables A–5 and A–6. Thresholds for complications for lysis are not defined

E. Measurement of radiation exposure and contrast use.
Radiation exposure is tracked as fluoroscopy time plus number of images, or using radiation dosimetrics (dose area product, etc.). Patients with

Table A–5 Peripheral Angioplasty Quality Improvement Standards

Indicator	Threshold (%)
I. Indications	95
II. Success	
a. Iliac	95
b. Superficial femoral and popliteal	90
c. Tibial and peroneal	80
III. Complications	
a. Emergency surgery	3
b. Severe bleeding or hematoma	4
c. Puncture site occlusion	0.5
d. Angioplasty site occlusion	3
e. Distal embolization causing tissue damage	1
f. Vessel perforation requiring surgery	0.5

Source: From Ref. 20.

expected exposures of two Gy are tracked for skin injury. Contrast dose is reported.

F. Measurement of frequency with which diagnostic and therapeutic procedures are performed on the same day.

Diagnostic and interventional procedures should be performed on the same day. Given the ability to use 1/2-strength contrast with digital subtraction angiography, contrast loads are not a problem in patients with normal renal function.

The threshold for same day diagnosis and interventions for extremity procedures is 95%

G. Clinical categorization of disease severity prior to the procedure (same as for diagnostic procedures)
For chronic ischemia:

1. Ankle/brachial index or pulse-volume recording.
2. Assessment of walking impairment with WIQ (10).
3. Assessment of general quality of life with SF-36 (11).
4. Use of Rutherford categories of chronic ischemia (12) (Table A–3).
For acute ischemia:
Use of Rutherford categories of acute ischemia (12) (Table A–4) as per TASC Recommendation #44 (1).

H. Improvement following interventions

1. Hemodynamic: ABI or TBI improved by 0.1 or greater above baseline and not deteriorated by >0.15 from the maximum early post-procedure level, or pulse volume recording distal to the

Table A–6 Aortoiliac Stent Quality Improvement Standards

Indicator	Threshold (%)
I. Indications	95
II. Success	
a. Crossing the stenosis	
1. Short stenosis <3 cm	98
2. Long stenosis >3 cm	95
b. Crossing the occlusion	
1. Short occlusion < 6 cm	85
2. Long occlusion >6 cm	Insufficient data
c. Attempted percutaneous stent placement	98
d. Successful percutaneous vascular access for stent placement	99
e. Successful stent deployment	98 if lesion is crossed
f. Patency	
1. Short stenosis	90 @ 1 year
2. Long stenosis	85 @ 1 year
3. Chronic occlusion	70 @ 1 year

III. Complications	Reported rate	Threshold (%)
a. Stent related	2%	3
1. Thrombosis (periprocedural <30 days)		
2. Dislodgment/malposition		
3. Pseudoaneurysm at stent site		
b. Arterial injury prior to stent deployment	2%	3
1. Pseudoaneurysm, rupture, perforation after angioplasty at the treated segment		
c. Puncture site (major)	4%	4
1. Large hematoma, bleeding, thrombosis, pseudoaneurysm, arteriovenous fistula		
d. Distal embolization associated with:		
1. Stenosis	1%	2
2. Occlusion	3–6%	7
e. Post-procedure myocardial infarction	1%	2
f. Mortality within 30 days	1%	2

III. Complications	Reported rate	Threshold (%)
IV. Overall Major Complications		
a. Stenosis	4%	6
b. Occlusion	9%	10

(Continued)

Table A–6   Aortoiliac Stent Quality Improvement Standards (*Continued*)
Note:
It is considered a technical failure of percutaneous therapy when an endovascular procedure (arteriogram, angioplasty, atherectomy, vascular stent or stent/graft) initially intended to be performed percutaneously is converted to an open surgical procedure because of a failure to obtain vascular access. Similarly, the conversion of a percutaneous procedure to an open procedure due to a failure to cross lesion is considered a failure of the percutaneous procedure. These technical failures require a major unplanned increase in the level of care even if the procedure is subsequently completed through an open access. If the patient has also been injured during the failed attempt to enter the vessel percutaneously or cross the lesion, the procedure is a failure with a complication.

Rarely, endovascular procedures will be performed open without an attempt at a percutaneous approach. These are procedures which are intended to be combined with an open bypass operation at the same access site, which involve decides too large to be inserted percutaneously, or involve access sites that are so severely diseased or occluded that percutaneous access is not possible. Routine angioplasty, atherectomy, and stent placement is a percutaneous procedure. For this reason a threshold of 98% has been set for attempted percutaneous stent placement. It is expected that 99% of percutaneous vascular access attempts will be successful. Therefore, including failures of percutaneous vascular access, fewer than 3% of stents should be placed during an open surgical procedure.
Source: From Ref. 20.

reconstruction maintained at 5 mm above the preoperative tracing (only for patients with incompressible vessels) (3,12).

2. Clinical:

   a. Rutherford criteria for improvement of chronic limb ischemia (12) (Table A–4).
   b. Patel classification for improvement of acute limb ischemia treated with thrombolysis (Table A–7) (2).
   c. WIQ (10) for chronic limb ischemia.
   d. SF-36 (11) for chronic limb ischemia.

I. Durability of improvement

   1. Follow-up intervals should be roughly 1, 3, 6, 12 months and then yearly.
   2. Results are reported in lifetable format (14) for binary data (patency, hemodynamic improvement, clinical improvement by Rutherford criteria (12), improvement in WIQ or SF-36 above a significant threshold).
   3. Surgical bypass of a vessel previously treated with percutaneous revascularization is considered a failure of the percutaneous therapy.
   4. Results for continuous data (WIQ, SF-36) are reported as average improvement per patient, and average improvement in all patients treated.
   5. The number and type of revascularization re-interventions over time for the same limb is recorded per patient and per group.

Diagnostic Renal Arteriography for Evaluation of Renal Artery Stenosis

   A. Indications
   Clinical signs of renovascular hypertension or ischemic nephropathy or a cardiac disturbance syndrome are present (Table A–8) and there is one of the following conditions (15):

Table A–7 Recommended Scale for Gauging Changes in Clinical Status in Acute Limb Ischemia After Thrombolysis

−1	Ischemia is worse (by at least one major or minor category from SVS/ISCVS Clinical Categories of Acute Limb Ische)
0	No change (failure)
+1	Ischemia improved

  a. Revascularization with thrombolytic methods alone
   i. amputation necessary but at a lesser level[a]
  b. Adjunctive surgical revascularization necessary but at a lesser level[b]
   i. amputation necessary but at a lesser level[a]
  c. Adjunctive endovascular revascularization necessary (angioplasty, stent, atherectomy, etc.)
   i. amputation necessary but at a lesser level[‡]

Note: The categories a, b and c do not imply greater or lesser degrees of success
[a]Levels of amputation
  1. Above the knee
  2. Below the knee
  3. Transmetatarsal
  4. Toe
[b]Levels of surgical revascularization
  1. Major:
  Insertion of new bypass graft
  Replacement of an existing bypass graft
  Excision or repair of an aneurysm
  2. Moderate:
  Graft revision, patch angioplasty
  Endarterectomy
  Profundaplasty
  3. Minor
  Thrombectomy/embolectomy
  Fasciotomy
Source: From Ref. 2.

1. Noninvasive vascular imaging is suggestive that a renal artery stenosis of more than 50% is present.
2. Progression of a hemodynamically significant renal artery stenosis is indicated by noninvasive vascular imaging.
3. Noninvasive vascular imaging is technically inadequate, equivocal, or cannot be performed.
4. Onset of hypertension occurs in a patient less than 30 years of age.
5. Renal artery fibromuscular dysplasia is suspected as the etiology of the hypertension.
6. There is recent onset of hypertension in a patient 60 years of age or older.
7. There is loss of renal mass or deterioration of renal function while hypertension is being controlled medically, especially when being treated with angiotensin converting enzyme inhibitors or angiotensin II receptor blockers.

Threshold for appropriate indications = 95%

B. Duration of symptoms
Generally not relevant for renal artery stenosis.

Table A–8   Clinical Features Suggestive of Renovascular Hypertension

Onset of hypertension before 30 years of age, especially without a family history, or recent
  onset of signifcant hypertension after 55 years of age
An abdominal bruit, particularly if it continues into diastole and is lateralized
Accelerated or resistant hypertension
Recurrent (flash) pulmonary edema
Renal failure of uncertain cause, especially with a normal urinary sediment
Coexisting diffuse atherosclerotic vascular disease, especially in heavy smokers
Acute renal failure preecipitated by antihypertensive therapy, particularly ACE inhibitors or
  angiotensin II blockers

Source: From Ref. 21.

C.   Technical success/failure
     A technically successful study images the renal vasculature from the
     aorta to the renal parenchyma. The renal artery ostium is seen in profile.
     Aortography (catheter based or noninvasive) is performed prior to selec-
     tive renal arteriography **(threshold of 95%)**. Patients with azotemia can be
     imaged using alternative contrast agents such as CO_2 or gadolinium to
     reduce the risk of contrast nephrotoxicity.

     Threshold for technical success = 95%

D.   Technical complications
     Complications are graded using the SIR categories of major and minor
     complications.

     Thresholds for technical complications are listed in Table A–1 .

E.   Radiation exposure and contrast use
     Radiation exposure is tracked as fluoroscopy time plus number of images,
     or using radiation dosimetrics (dose area product, etc.). Patients with
     expected exposures of two Gray are tracked for skin injury.
     Contrast dose is reported.
F.   Measurement of frequency with which diagnostic and therapeutic proce-
     dures are performed on the same day. This is applicable to therapeutic
     procedures only.
G.   Clinical categorization of disease severity prior to the procedure

     1.   Blood pressure.
     2.   Creatinine (creatinine clearance only if available).
     3.   Number of antihypertensive drugs.
     4.   Number of defined daily doses (16) if possible.

H.   Improvement following intervention: not applicable.
I.   Durability of improvement: not applicable.

Renal Artery Interventions

A.   Indications for the procedure (15,17)
     Presence of a hemodynamically significant renal artery stenosis (greater

than 50% luminal stenosis and greater than a 20 mmHg systolic pressure gradient and there is one of the following conditions:

1. Hypertensive control

    a. A reasonable likelihood of cure of renovascular hypertension.

        i. Onset of hypertension before age 30.
        ii. Recent onset of hypertension after age 60.
        iii. Stenosis is caused by fibromuscular hyperplasia.

    b. Hypertension is "refractory" to medical control with at least three medications of different classes including a diuretic.
    c. Hypertension is "accelerated," i.e., there is sudden worsening of previously controlled hypertension.
    d. Hypertension is "malignant," i.e., is associated with end-organ damage such as left ventricular hypertrophy, congestive heart failure, visual or neurological disturbance, grade III–IV retinopathy.
    e. Hypertension with a unilateral small kidney ipsilateral to the renal artery stenosis.
    f. The patient is intolerant or non-compliant with antihypertensive medical treatment.

2. Renal salvage

    a. Unexplained worsening of renal function.
    b. Loss of renal mass, especially while under surveillance during medical antihypertensive treatment.
    c. Impairment of renal function or acute renal failure secondary to antihypertensive medication, particularly with an angiotensin converting enzyme inhibitor.
    d. Progression of a hemodynamically significant renal artery stenosis while under surveillance.

3. Cardiac disturbance syndrome

    a. Recurrent "flash" pulmonary edema secondary to impaired left ventricular function.
    b. Unstable angina.

Threshold for appropriate indications = 95%

B. Duration of symptoms
   Generally not relevant for renal artery stenosis.
C. Technical success/failure

    1. Technical success is judged on "intention to treat." For example, failure to cross a stenosis with a guide wire is a failure of the intended revascularization therapy (angioplasty, stent, lysis). The intention is stated in the chart prior to the procedure being attempted.
    2. Since stents are frequently reserved for PTA failures in the renal arteries, PTA and stents will be considered combination percutaneous therapy and the PTA will not be categorized as a technical failure if a stent is subsequently placed at the same encounter.

3. To be considered technically successful the renal artery intervention must meet the criteria for both anatomic and hemodynamic success as defined below (17).

   a. Anatomic:

      i. $< 30\%$ final residual stenosis measured at the narrowest point of the vascular lumen.
      ii. A renal artery stent should project into the aorta $< 2\,mm$.

   b. Hemodynamic: The intravascular pressure gradient across the treated segment should be $< 20\,mmHg$ systolic or $< 10\,mm$ mean. If there is no residual stenosis, a post procedure pressure gradient is not needed.

Threshold for technical success is 90%

D. Technical complications
   Complications are graded using the SCVIR categories of major and minor complications.

Threshold for technical complications is listed in Table A–9

E. Measurement of radiation exposure and contrast use
   Radiation exposure is tracked as fluoroscopy time plus number of images, or using radiation dosimetrics (dose area product, etc.). Patients with expected exposures of two Gy are tracked for skin injury.
   Contrast dose is reported.

F. Measurement of frequency with which diagnostic and therapeutic procedures are performed on the same day.

Table A–9 Percutaneous Renal Revascularization Quality Improvement Standards

	Reported rate (%)	Threshold (%)
Indications		95
Technical success	80–99	90
Specific major complications		
30 day mortality	1	1
Secondary nephrectomy	<1	1
Surgical salvage operation	1	2
Symptomatic embolization	3	3
Main renal artery occlusion	2	2
Branch renal artery occlusion	2	2
Access site hematoma requiring surgery or prolonging hospital stay	5	5
Acute renal failure	2	2
Worsening of chronic renal Failure requiring an increase in the level of care	2	5

Note: Overall threshold for complications of percutaneous renal revascularization 10%.
Source: From Ref. 15.

Diagnostic and interventional procedures should be performed on the same day. Given the ability to use 1/2-strength contrast with digital subtraction angiography, contrast loads are not a problem in patients with normal renal function. In patients with azotemia, alternative contrast agents such as CO_2 and gadolinium should be used. Renal interventions may be delayed in the presence of unstable coronary artery disease requiring percutaneous or surgical intervention.

Unless there is unstable coronary artery disease, the threshold for same day diagnosis and interventions for renal procedures is 95%

G. Clinical categorization of disease severity prior to the procedure

1. Blood pressure.
2. Creatinine (creatinine clearance only if available).
3. Number of antihypertensive drugs.
4. Number of defined daily doses (16) if possible.

H. Improvement following intervention

1. For interventions to treat hypertension, improvement can be measured as follows (16,18):

   a. Cure—diastolic blood pressure < 90 mmHg and systolic blood pressure <140 mmHg off anti-hypertensive medications.
   b. Improvement—diastolic blood pressure < 90 mmHg and/or systolic blood pressure <140 mmHg on the same or reduced number of medications (or reduced number of defined daily doses) as described by the World Health Organization (16) or a reduction in diastolic blood pressure by at least 15 mmHg using the same or reduced number of medications.
   c. Failure—no change or inability to meet above criteria for cure or improvement.
   d. Benefit—cure or improvement.

2. For interventions to treat loss of renal function

   a. The simplest but least accurate method to assess improvement is to measure serum creatinine. This is required. Improvement is considered a drop in creatinine by $>20\%$ in patients with azotemia.
   b. Slightly better but more involved is measurement of creatinine clearance.
   c. Ideally, but probably not achievable outside of a research study, is reporting of improvement as changes in the rate of decline of creatinine clearance over time (17).

I. Durability of improvement

1. Follow-up intervals should be roughly 1, 3, 6, 12 months and then yearly.
2. Results are reported in lifetable format for binary data (cure or improvement of hypertension, or improvement in renal function).

Table A–10 Summary of Thresholds from Tables A–1, A–5, A–6, and A–9

	Extremity anglography (%)	Extremity PTA (%)	Iliac stent (%)	Renal angiography	Renal PTA/ stent (%)
Indications	95	95	95	95	95
Technical success	95	80–95	85–98	95	90
Overall major complications	1	NA	6–10	1	10
Same day Dx and Rx		95	95		95

Abbreviations: PTA, angioplasty; Dx, diagnostic procedure; Rx, therapeutic procedure.

3. Surgical bypass of a vessel previously treated with percutaneous revascularization is considered a failure of the percutaneous therapy.
4. Results for continuous data (creatinine) are reported as average improvement per patient, and average improvement in all patients treated)
5. The number and type of revascularization re-interventions over time for the same renal vessel is recorded per patient and per group.

The thresholds for extremitry angiography, extremitry PTA, iliac stent, renal angiography, and renal PTA/stent are summarized in Table A-10.

References

1. Dormandy J, Rutherford R. Group at TW Management of Peripheral Arterial Disease (PAD). TransAtlantic Inter-Society Consensus (TASC). J Vasc Surg 2000; 31(suppl): S1–S296.
2. Patel N, Sacks D, Patel RI, Moresco KP, Ouriel K, Gray R, Ambrosius WT, Lewis CA. SCVIR reporting standards for the treatment of acute limb ischemia with use of transluminal removal of arterial thrombus. J Vasc Interv Radiol 2001; 12:559–570.
3. Sacks D. Angiography and percutaneous vascular interventions: complications and quality improvement. In: Rutherford RB, ed. Vascular Surgery. Philadelphia: WB Saunders, 1999:796–812.
4. Miller DL. Balter S, Wagner LK, Cardella J, Clark T, Neithamer CD Jr, Schwartzberg MS, Swan TL, Towbin RB, Rholl KS, Sacks D. Quality improvement guidelines for recording patient radiation dose in the medical record. J Vasc Interv Radiol. 2004; 15:423–429.
5. FDA. Important information for physicians and other healthcare professionals: recording information in the patient's medical record that identifies the potential for serious x-ray-induced skin injuries following fluoroscopically guided procedures. Rockville, MD:Center for Devices and Radiological Health, Food and Drug Administration, September 15, 1995.
6. FDA. Public health advisory: avoidance of serious x-ray-induced skin injuries following fluoroscopically guided procedures. Rockville, MD: Center for Devices and Radiological Health, Food and Drug Administration, September 30, 1994.
7. FDA. Important information for physicians and other health care professionals. Avoidance of serious x-ray-induced skin injuries to patients during fluoroscopically-guided procedures. Rockville, MD: Center for Devices and Radiologic Health, Food and Drug Administration, September 9, 1994.

8. Ayoub DM, Muehle CM. Differences in outcomes of percutaneous endovascular lower extremity interventions: Interventional radiology versus surgery. J Vasc Interv Radiol (supp) 1997; 8:214.

9. Cardella JF, Casarella WJ, DeWeese JA, et al. Optimal resources for the examination and endovascular treatment of the peripheral and visceral vascular systems. AHA Intercouncil report on peripheral and visceral angiographic and interventional laboratories. Circulation 1994; 89:1481–1493.

10. Hiatt WR, Hirsch AT, Regensteiner JG, Brass EP. Clinical trials for claudication. Assessment of exercise performance, functional status, and clinical end points. Vascular Clinical Trialists. Circulation 1995; 92:614–621.

11. Ware JE, Jr, Sherbourne CD. The MOS 36-item short-form health survey (SF-36). I. Conceptual framework and item selection. Med Care 1992; 30:473–483.

12. Rutherford RB, Baker JD, Ernst C, et al. Recommended standards for reports dealing with lower extremity ischemia: revised version. J Vasc Surg 1997; 26:517–538.

13. Sacks D, Marinelli DL, Martin LG, Spies JB. Reporting standards for clinical evaluation of new peripheral arterial revascularization devices. Technology Assessment Committee [published errata appear in J Vasc Interv Radiol 1997 8(3):492 and 1997; 8(4):658]. J Vasc Interv Radiol 1997; 8:137–149.

14. Peto R, Pike MC, Armitage P, et al. Design and analysis of randomized clincl trials requiring prolonged observation of each patient. I. Introduction and design. Br J Cancer 1976; 34:585–612.

15. Martin LG, Rundback JH, Sacks D, et al. Quality improvement guidelines for angiography, angioplasty, and stent placement in the diagnosis and treatment of renal artery stenosis in adults. J Vasc Interv Radiol 2002; 13:1069–1083.

16. WHO. Main principles for the establishment of defined daily doses. Guidelines for ATC classification and DDD assignment. Oslo, Norway: WHO collaborating Centre for Drug Statistics Methodology, 1995:22–31.

17. Rundback J, Sacks D, Kent K, et al. Guidelines for the Reporting of Renal Artery Revascularization in Clinical Trials. Circulation 2002; 106:1572–1585.

18. Working Group on Renovascular Hypertension. Detection, evaluation, and treatment of renovascular hypertension. Final report. Working Group on Renovascular Hypertension. Arch Intern Med 1987; 147:820–829.

19. Singh H, Cardella J, Cole P, et al. Quality improvement guidelines for diagnostic arteriography. J Vasc Interv Radiol 2002; 13:1–6.

20. SCVIR. Guidelines for establishing a quality assurance program in vascular and interventional radiology. J Vasc Interv Radiol 2003; 14:S203–S207.

21. The sixth report of the Joint National Committee on prevention, detection, evaluation, and treatment of high blood pressure. Arch Intern Med 1997; 157:2413–2446.

2

Complications of Endovascular Procedures at the Target Site

Alan B. Lumsden, Eric K. Peden, Ruth L. Bush, and Peter H. Lin
Division of Vascular Surgery and Endovascular Therapy, Michael E. DeBakey Department of Surgery, Baylor College of Medicine, and The Methodist Hospital, Houston, Texas, U.S.A.

As endovascular techniques are performed more frequently, the number of interventionalists increases, and the array of endovascular techniques continues to expand, we will increasingly encounter complications from these procedures. Some of these complications are simply a function of the access: arteriovenous fistula (AVF), bleeding, and pseudoaneurysm. Others are specific to the type of procedure being performed on the target vessel: renal artery dissection and stent migration from iliac veins. Furthermore, with each new device so unexpected and occasionally unique, complications are identified and treatment strategies gradually refined: aortic stent graft migration, failure in inferior vena cava (IVC) filter retrieval, embolization protection device occlusion, and femoral artery infection with closure devices. Consequently, the interventionalist must be aware of these complications and salvage options. In this chapter we describe some of the more commonly encountered complications and discuss their management.

ACCESS SITE COMPLICATIONS

The frequency of groin complications following an endovascular procedure varies dependent on the type of procedure being performed. Because of the very large number of coronary interventions performed compared with peripheral procedures, reports of groin complications tend to be predominantly following those interventions. Following cardiac catheterization the incidence of groin complications is 0.05–0.7%, whereas following percutaneous transluminal angioplasty the incidence is much higher 0.7–9.0% (1–3).

Peripheral vascular complications include hematoma, pseudoaneurysms, AVF, acute arterial occlusions, cholesterol emboli, and infections that occur with an overall incidence of 1.5–9% (1). In descending order of frequency they are: pseudoaneurysm, groin hematoma, re-bleeding, AVF, arterial occlusion, and distal embolization (Fig. 1). The anatomical distribution of access site complications, showing the predominance

• Pseudoaneurysm	61.2%
• Hematoma	11.2%
• AVF	10.2%
• External Bleeding	6.1%
• Retroperitoneal Hematoma	5.1%
• Arterial thrombosis	3.1%
• Groin Abscess	2.0%
• Mycotic Aneurysm	1.0%

Figure 1 Type of complications requiring surgical intervention.

within the common femoral, superficial, and profunda femoris is shown in Figure 2. As a result of the increasing use of groin closure devices, the unusual complication of arterial infection has been increasingly reported recently (4,5). Acceptable threshold incidences for these complications have been described by the Society for Interventional Radiology (Fig. 3) (6).

Groin Hematoma

This varies from being trivial to potentially life threatening (Figs. 4 and 5). Sudden onset of massive bleeding can occur (Fig. 6). Symptoms vary from mild groin discomfort to

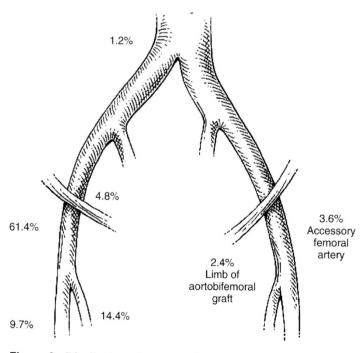

Figure 2 Distribution of puncture sites associated with groin complications.

Complication	Threshold
Hematoma	3%
Occlusion	0.5%
Pseudoaneurysm	0.5%
Arterial venous fistula	0.1%
Catheter-induced complications	
Arterial dissection	2%
Subintimal injection	1%
Cerebral arteriography	
All neurologic complications	4%
Permanent neurologic complications	1%
Contrast reactions	
All reactions	3%
Major reactions	0.5%
Contrast-induced renal failure	10%

Figure 3 Society for Interventional Radiology (SIR) threshold complication rate for quality assurance following groin puncture and angiography.

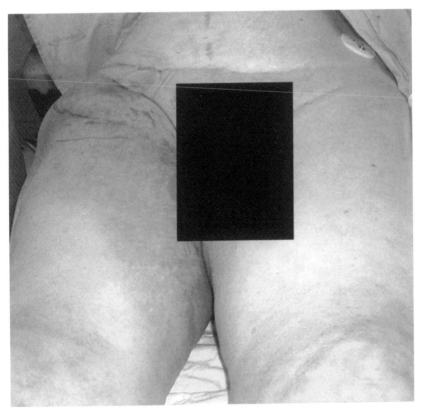

Figure 4 Thigh enlargement from a large groin hematoma. Note the minimal amount of ecchymosis at this stage.

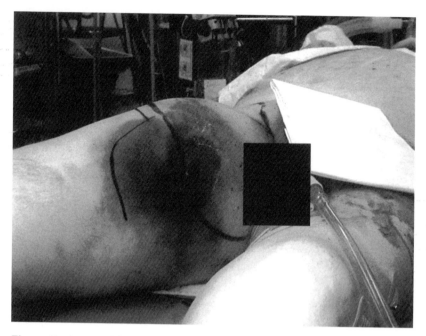

Figure 5 A tense thigh hematoma which has been observed. There is extensive ecchymosis and early skin compromise.

severe pain, huge swelling and potential necrosis of the overlying skin from pressure of the hematoma. Initially there is minimal ecchymosis, but this develops later. As the patient ambulates, the ecchymosis extends down the thigh, changing colors to a more yellowish appearance. The patient with a hematoma under observation should be

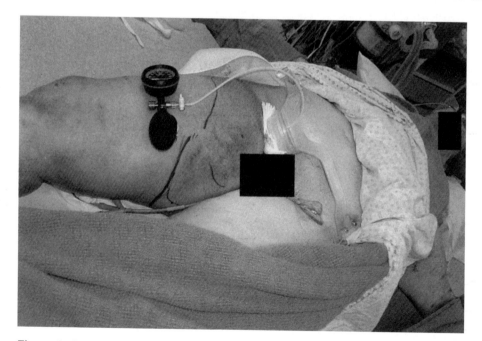

Figure 6 Massive thigh hematoma developing despite an external compression device.

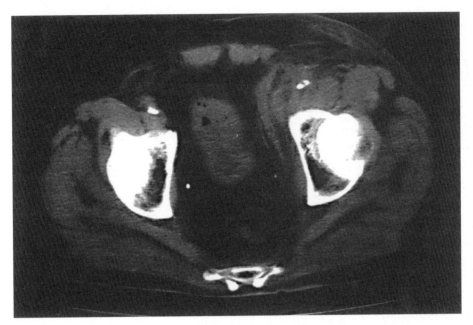

Figure 7 CT scan showing left groin hematoma around the femoral vessels and in the subcutaneous tissues.

cautioned about these developments. Eventually the discoloration will extend into the leg below the knee and does not represent new bleeding. Extent of a hematoma and presence or absence of retroperitoneal extension is best determined by CT scanning (Fig. 7). Rarely can active bleeding be seen by angiography. This degree of bleeding will be associated with hemodynamic instability (Fig. 8).

Indications for groin exploration and hematoma evacuation are severe pain, progressive enlargement, skin compromise or evidence of femoral nerve compression (See below under retroperitoneal hematoma). There is a high incidence of wound infection following hematoma evacuation.

Wounds should be irrigated with antibiotic solution and drained. It is not often possible to close the underlying adipose tissue following evacuation of large hematomas.

Arteriovenous Fistula (AVF)

The most common cause of AVF is inadvertent puncture of the profunda femoris artery and the vein, which crosses between it and the superficial femoral artery. Fistulae are usually asymptomatic and detected clinically by the presence of a palpable thrill in the groin or by auscultating a continuous bruit. The overwhelming majority does not give rise to signs of cardiac failure. Duplex ultrasound confirms the presence of a fistula showing the characteristic systolic–diastolic flow pattern with arterialization of the venous signal (Fig. 9A and B). Kresowik et al. (7) in a prospective duplex examination of 144 patients undergoing coronary angioplasty noted a 2.8% incidence of AVF. Kent et al. (8) in contrast, using the detection of an audible bruit as a trigger for duplex scanning reported a 0.3% incidence, although this clearly will underestimate the true incidence. Fistulae usually do not close spontaneously,

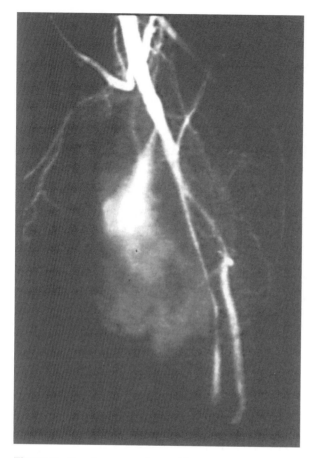

Figure 8 Rarely seen angiographic appearance of active bleeding from a puncture site in the femoral artery.

therefore operative repair is indicated when they are detected. Fistulae progressively enlarge with time, therefore expeditious intervention is warranted.

Risk factors for development of an AVF include: female gender, hypertension, left femoral puncture, and periprocedural anticoagulation. The increased incidence associated with left groin puncture may be a function of the physician standing on the patients right side and the wrong angle of approach resulting in arterial and venous puncture (9).

Surgical repair is performed by dissection of the artery until brisk arterial bleeding identifies the defect. The artery is then controlled either by clamping or digital pressure. The venous bleeding is usually easily controlled with direct pressure, until repair can be effective. The defect in the artery is first repaired with interrupted prolene followed by repair of the vein. Usually only one or two horizontal mattress sutures are required in each vessel (10).

In our opinion, there is no current role for use of covered stents in management of AVF or pseudoaneurysms.

Recently there have been reports using stent grafts to treat femoral AVF. Only those fistulae that are remote and form the origin of the profunda femoris artery should be considered, so that the profunda orifice is not covered during

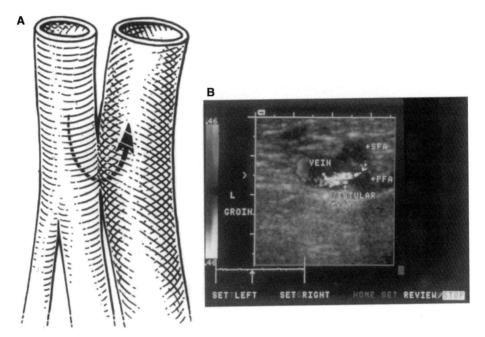

Figure 9 (**A**) Diagram of an arteriovenous fistula (AVF). (**B**) Typical duplex appearance of fistula.

deployment. Only very short-term data currently exist for this approach. Consequently, it should remain a secondary option in patients for whom surgery would be challenging (11).

Pseudoaneurysm

Pseudoaneurysm following arterial puncture results from failure in closure of the arteriotomy site, with contained bleeding into the soft tissue around the artery (Fig. 10). Blood flows in and out of the artery. Pseudoaneurysm can occur in any vessel that is punctured, although it most frequently develops in the femoral artery. Pseudoaneurysms can be difficult to detect if accompanied by a hematoma. However, the presence of expansile pulsation and tenderness should raise suspicion and lead to diagnosis by duplex scanning (Fig. 11). The duplex examination should note the size and the likely source of the pseudoaneurysm. Some are complex and appear to have multiple lobes; others are a single, simple cavity. The neck of the pseudoaneurysm should be defined, whether it is a single wide neck or whether it is a long, tortuous, narrow neck (the latter are easier to compress). Femoral pseudoaneurysms occur in approximately 1% femoral artery punctures. Knight et al. (12) noted three independent risk factors for pseudoaneurysm: female gender, interventional procedures (versus diagnostic studies), and no closure device. Women have smaller arteries which may be more difficult to access and more difficult to compress. Interventions require a larger diameter sheath size. Although closure devices may reduce the risk of bleeding complications and pseudoaneurysms, they may be associated with a slight increase in the number of thrombotic and infective complications.

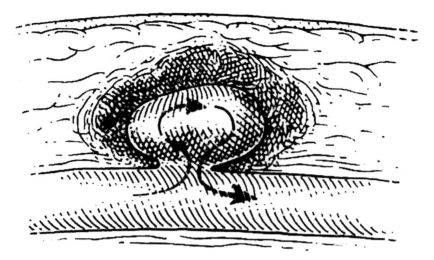

Figure 10   Diagram of typical femoral pseudoaneurysm.

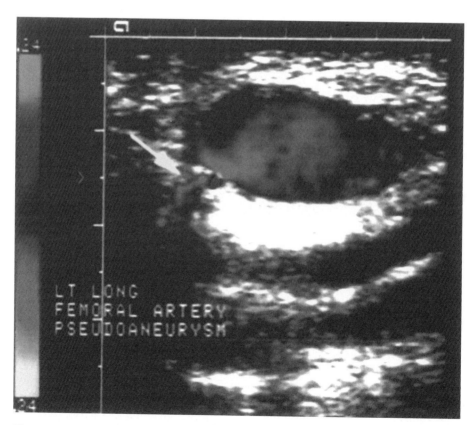

Figure 11   Duplex examination of pseudoaneurysm showing tract from the femoral artery into the pseudoaneurysm cavity.

Complications following arterial repair.

Aspiration pneumonia	1.05%
Neuralgia	5.25%
Wound bleeding	7.35%
Retroperitoneal bleeding	2.1%
Lymph leak	1.05%
Limb swelling	1.05%
Myocardial infarction	1.05%
Septicemia	2.1 %
Death	3.1%

Figure 12 Postoperative complications following open repair of the femoral artery following arterial puncture.

There are now a variety of approaches for treatment of pseudoaneurysm.

Surgical Repair: Surgical repair has been the main therapy (10,13). Rationale for prompt surgical intervention has been the belief that there was a low spontaneous incidence of resolution. This clearly is a concept that has been challenged and complications following groin exploration are not uncommon (Fig. 12). It was believed that an aggressive approach would result in relief of groin pain, prevention of progressive enlargement and rupture, skin necrosis, and compression neuropathy. The femoral artery is exposed through a groin incision. Techniques vary, some surgeons opting to gain full control of the artery prior to exposing the puncture site. Sliding down the external oblique and identifying the femoral artery as it enters the thigh can obtain proximal control. Rolling the inguinal ligament superiorly or dividing the external oblique fibers permits exposure of the external iliac artery. Gaining proximal control is particularly important with a large hematoma or large pseudoaneurysm. An alternate approach: Knowing that the arterial defect is usually only a 2–3 mm puncture site, enter the pseudoaneurysm directly, controlling the bleeding digitally and over-sewing the puncture site with Prolene. It is extremely important to ensure that the arterial wall is exposed prior to repair. A common error is to mis-identify a hole in the fascia as the arterial defect and therefore place sutures within the fascia. This can lead to recurrent pseudoaneurysm formation or persistent bleeding. We do not routinely explore the posterior wall of the artery.

Observation: Observation is very reasonable for small pseudoaneurysms are not associated with a lot of discomfort. Most small pseudoaneurysms will thrombose spontaneously within two to four weeks. It is likely that concurrent anticoagulation decreases the likelihood that spontaneous thrombosis will occur.

Ultrasound-guided compression: The neck of the pseudoaneurysm, identified as a high velocity jet, is localized with ultrasound and direct compression applied with the transducer. Pressure is increased until the jet is obliterated and continued for 20-minute intervals. Mean time to thrombosis is 22 minutes, but some require up to 120 minutes This, however, may be associated with significant discomfort; consequently, sedation and analgesia is always required. This is also very labor intensive because it requires a dedicated technician to apply pressure.

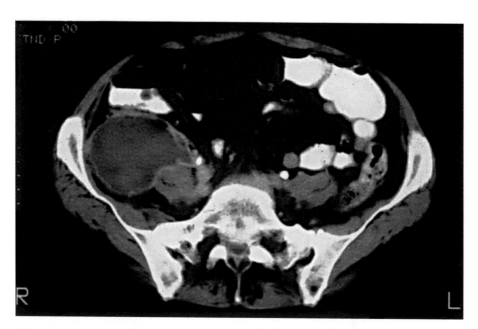

Figure 13   Hematoma lateral to the psoas major muscle within the retroperitoneal space.

Ultrasound-guided thrombin injection: This is an off-label use for thrombin, but it is very successful in inducing thrombosis of pseudoaneurysm and thereby avoiding surgery (14,15).

Retroperitoneal Hematoma (RPH)

Retroperitoneal hematoma (RPH) following groin puncture is an infrequent (0.15% incidence) but morbid complication (16). It is perhaps the most feared complication of groin puncture. The term refers to blood contained within the retroperitoneum, but several patterns occur. An iliopsoas hematoma occurs when blood enters and is confined within the fascia of the iliopsoas muscle. The psoas muscle contains the lumbar plexus; this pattern of hematoma may more likely be associated with compression neuropathy (Fig. 13). In contrast the space between the peritoneum and retroperitoneal structures is potentially vast and can contain huge quantities of blood, which may be very difficult to detect clinically (Fig. 14). These hematomas can lead to dramatic elevation and compression of the ipsilateral kidney.

Any patient who has had groin puncture and who develops lower abdominal pain should be suspected of having an RPH. Abdominal examination usually shows tenderness only. Occasionally palpable fullness may be detected. Thigh pain, numbness, or quadriceps weakness should lead to suspicion of RPH and femoral nerve compression, and mandates urgent CT scanning and possible decompression. Post-catheterization anticoagulation and high arterial puncture are the principal risk factors ($p < 0.001$). Early recognition is essential and should be prompted by a falling hematocrit, lower abdominal pain, or neurological changes in the lower extremity.

There should be a low threshold for performing abdomino-pelvic CT scans in such patients, which is diagnostic. Management of RPH must be individualized: (1) Patients with neurological deficits in the ipsilateral extremity require urgent

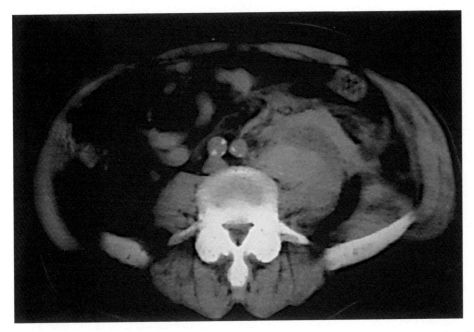

Figure 14 Hematoma within the psoas fascia, which invests the muscle and contains the lumbar plexus.

decompression of the hematoma; (2) Anticoagulation should be stopped or minimized; and (3) Hematoma progression by serial CT necessitates surgical evacuation and repair of the arterial puncture site.

MISCELLANEOUS COMPLICATIONS OF FEMORAL PUNCTURE

Acute thrombosis of the femoral artery occurs infrequently and manifests as typical lower extremity ischemia. It has been associated with insertion of devices, but more recently several series report its occurrence with groin closure devices (17,18). Exploration of the femoral artery usually reveals a large posterior plaque, which has been elevated with thrombosis of the residual lumen. Femoral endarterectomy patch angioplasty and balloon catheter embolectomy of the external iliac and superficial femoral artery is the most commonly required procedure. Distal embolization is more commonly due to passage of catheters and the intervention performed from groin puncture alone but can result in trash foot (Fig. 15). Rarely catheter/wire passage can result in arterial perforation and, more rarely, mycotic pseudoaneurysm (Fig. 16). Femoral endarteritis and mycotic femoral artery aneurysm have also been reported as a result of the use of percutaneous closure devices. Fortunately, the incidence of this complication is low (0.7%). Obesity and diabetes mellitus increase the risk of this complication. Gram-positive cocci are the most common pathogen (19–22).

Axillary and Brachial Artery Puncture

All of the complications described above for femoral puncture have been described as also complicating axillary artery and brachial arterial puncture. However, there is

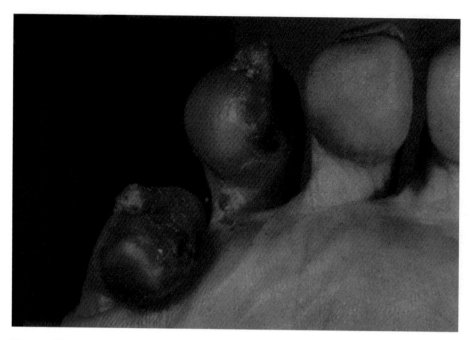

Figure 15 Toe ischemia (trash foot) as a result of distal embolization.

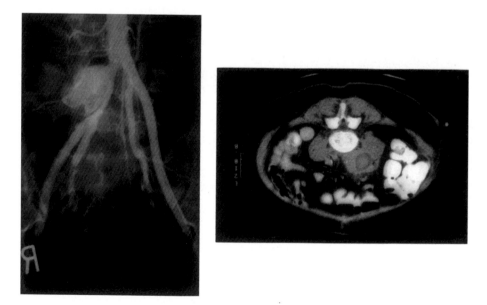

Figure 16 Mycotic pseudoaneurysm as a result of common iliac perforation and retroperitoneal hematoma.

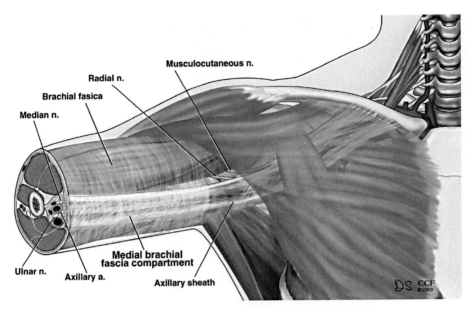

Figure 17 Anatomy of the brachial and axillary neurovascular bundles.

a higher incidence of neuropraxia, involving the median nerve or other branches of the brachial plexus.

In a recent prospective study of cardiac catheterization via the femoral artery, damage to the adjacent femoral nerve occurred in 20 out of 9585 cases (0.2%) and, although initially disabling, was reported to be almost completely reversible (20,21). Frequency of nerve injury to nerves of the brachial plexus is between 0.4% and 12.7% (23), and there are three potential mechanisms. Hematoma formation is likely the most common. The hematoma forms within a fascial compartment containing the neurovascular bundle resulting in nerve compression (Fig. 17). Second, direct nerve damage caused by the needle, catheter or introducer sheath may occasionally be the etiology. Lastly, nerve damage may be due to nerve ischemia caused by varying degrees of arterial thrombosis, which may be contributory in a minority of patients.

Time to symptom onset varies from immediately to three days (mean 12 hours) (22). Pain at the puncture site is the most common symptom. The pain may radiate down the arm. Muscle weakness accompanied by numbness indicates more severe symptoms and mandates immediate intervention. Swelling from a hematoma is inconsistent; even a small strategically placed hematoma can result in nerve compression (Fig. 18). The size of a hematoma or presence of ecchymosis does not correlate with either the severity of symptoms or degree of nerve damage.

SURGICAL THERAPY

The treatment principles consist of: (1) awareness of the possibility of nerve compression following axillary or brachial artery puncture, (2) evaluation of the hand post-procedure for pain or sensory or motor dysfunction, and (3) early surgical

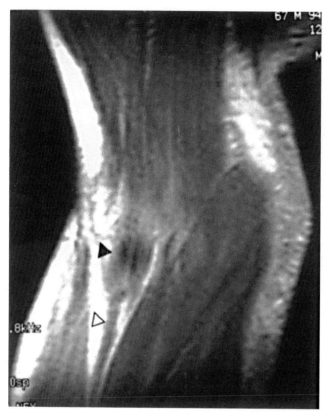

Figure 18 T1 weighed MRI of the forearm. The black arrow indicates a small hematoma at the antecubital fossa; the white arrow indicates the radial artery as it crossed the antecubital fossa.

decompression for any pain in excess of that anticipated from arterial puncture or the presence of a motor sensory deficit.

The artery should be surgically exposed, any hematoma evacuated, and the puncture site repaired with Prolene. The fascia of the neurovascular bundle is widely opened and any perineural hematoma evacuated. The deep fascia of the forearm is not closed; only the subcutaneous fat and skin should be approximated.

The functional outcome from a missed nerve injury is poor and most patients, although having some improvement, report persistent sensory or motor impairment (Fig. 19). A few patients develop disabling pain syndromes (22).

COMPLICATIONS RELATED TO PASSAGE OF CATHETERS AND DEVICES

As a wire, catheter, or device is passed through a blood vessel, it can injure the vessel wall directly. For example, glide wires are notorious for entering the vessel wall and continuing to track in an intramural position. Lack of blood return through a catheter should raise suspicion of dissection. Hand injection of 3–5 cc of dye will confirm catheter position by the appearance of a spot of dye, which fails to wash out. The catheter should be pulled back until blood return is obtained and a wire used to

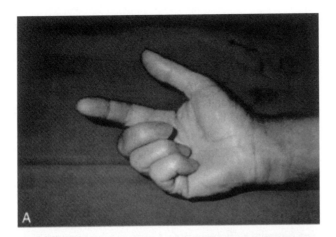

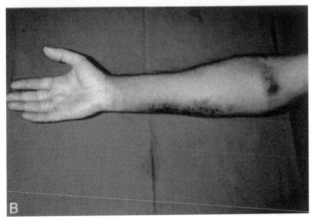

Figure 19 (**A**) Orator's hand posture: The patient has been asked to make a fist. The hand is held in an "orator's hand" posture. This is typical of a high median nerve palsy, in which there is paralysis of the flexor pollicis longus, and the flexor digitorum profundus of the second digit. This leads to an inability to pinch together the thumb and index finger. (**B**) The extensive bruising of the right forearm was noted two days after the angiogram in patient A.

navigate the true lumen. These types of dissections, when identified, are usually of no clinical consequence.

Microembolization can occur following passage of any endovascular device. It is particularly likely to happen in patients with severe atheromatous disease. Stroke from catheter manipulation in an atheromatous aortic arch is well recognized. Catheters and wires should be kept out of the arch unless access is necessary for the procedure, and manipulation should be minimized.

When wires are passed blindly, they can enter side branches or even the supra-aortic trunks. Even at the femoral access site, wires may deflect inferiorly down the SFA profunda, or may deflect superiorly up the circumflex iliac artery. Femoral arterial injury will result from attempts at sheath introduction when the wire is misplaced in these positions. Good technique: Imaging of the wire and control of the wire tip are fundamental. It is possible for inadvertent perforation of organs to occur, e.g., renal perforation if the wire enters a renal artery and is not visualized. Wires entering the supra-aortic trunks can lead to cerebrovascular ccident.

INTERVENTION-SPECIFIC COMPLICATIONS

These can broadly be classified in the following way: infection, bleeding, rupture, dissection, embolization, occlusion, restenosis. These complications can occur essentially with any intervention, however, the frequency and significance of each varies depending on the type of intervention being performed.

Device Infection

Infection of endovascular devices has generally been rare. Given the huge number of coronary procedures performed including stent implantation, reports on infection of these devices are remarkably uncommon. Antibiotic prophylaxis has been sporadic and its necessity questioned. However, the advent of stent grafting has clearly been associated with increasing reports of device infection. Two mechanisms exist: infection at the time of implantation, and seeding of an implanted graft via bacteremia. Unlike aortic graft infections, which are indolent, slowly progressive, and present years after implantation, infections of endografts are rapidly progressive, resulting in rapid conformational changes and rupture of the aneurysm. The patient shows all of the classic signs of sepsis and the device must be removed with aortic reconstruction performed using the standard techniques for aortic graft infection. Fiorani et al. (24) recently reported on endovascular graft infection in an international study. The authors' conclusions: Endograft infection occurs in 0.45% of cases, 65% of which presented with abdominal infection, groin abscess, and septic embolization. The remaining 35% had vague symptoms only. Overall mortality rate was 27.4%. *Staphylococcus aureus* was the offending organism in 54.5% of cases.

There have also been increasing reports of infection in bare stents. This is particularly likely to occur if stents are placed in patients with long periods of catheterization (such as for lysis) (23). Stent infection results in septic arteritis within the wall of the host artery, pseudoaneurysm formation, and rupture (Fig. 20). Seeding of stents also appears to occur. Usually arterial resection and reconstruction with autogenous tissue is necessary (25).

Fibrinolysis

Lytic agents activate plasminogen to form plasmin, which breaks fibrin into fibrin degradation products resulting in clot lysis. In appropriately selected patient groups, complications are minor and most commonly related to local bleeding at the site of catheter entry: hematoma, retroperitoneal bleeding, and pseudoaneurysm. In the majority of cases, these may be controlled by local application of pressure. There should be a high index of suspicion of retroperitoneal hematoma in any patient receiving lytic therapy who demonstrates a fall in hematocrit and no obvious source of blood loss. This can be easily confirmed with an abdominal CT scan. Development of a retroperitoneal hematoma usually requires discontinuation of therapy. Bleeding from an anastomosis is usually a problem only in recently implanted or infected grafts. Distal embolization is, in theory, more likely during graft lysis than

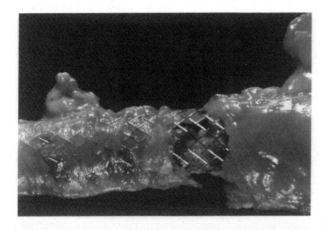

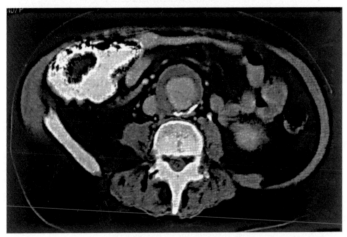

Figure 20 Mycotic aortic aneurysm complicating infection of an iliac Wallstent®. This occurred following prolonged lysis followed by stent placement. Infection in the artery has resulted in destruction of the iliac artery wall and extension into the aorta. *Source*: From Ref. 23.

lysis of native vessels due to the more extensive thrombus formation. Transgraft bleeding is a concern only in recently placed Dacron grafts. Cerebrovascular accident is an uncommon, but dreaded, complication of lytic therapy. There are no specific factors that increase this risk other than a history of cerebrovascular accident. History of a cerebrovascular accident within the prior two months is an absolute contraindication to lytic therapy. The National Institutes of Health Consensus Panel also recommend against the use of fibrinolytic therapy in patients with sustained systolic pressures greater than 200 mmHg, or diastolic pressures greater than 110 mmHg.

Aortic Stent Grafts

Numerous complications have now been described which are relatively specific for aortic stent grafting. Iliac artery dissection and rupture can occur with device insertion. This is particularly likely in patients with small, calcified iliac arteries, especially those with intercurrent occlusive disease. Increasing awareness of this problem has led to the development of alternate approaches such as insertion of an iliac conduit using a retroperitoneal approach to avoid such difficult iliac arteries. Misplacement can result in coverage of the renal arteries and lead to development of renal failure. Occlusion of the inferior mesenteric artery or hypogastric arteries can lead to colon ischemia.

Embolization or coverage of the internal iliac arteries results in buttock claudication in 30% of cases. Pelvic ischemia syndromes, cauda equina ischemia and colon ischemia, can also occur.

There have recently been increasing numbers of reports of infection occurring in aortic stent grafts. This is most commonly due to hematogenous seeding and leads to rapidly progressive infection, presumably because of the favorable environment of a stent graft surrounded by thrombus. Pain, rapid aneurysm expansion, and rupture are the usual clinical sequence.

Consequences and complications of endoleaks are beyond the scope of this chapter.

Renal Angioplasty and Stenting

Renal angioplasty is one of the most difficult endovascular procedures. Gaining atraumatic access to the renal artery and establishing a stable platform for intervention are the keys to avoiding complications. Traumatic crossing of a renal stenosis can result in dissection of the renal artery, a condition that must be recognized and is usually successfully treated by renal stenting (Fig. 21). Failure to recognize this

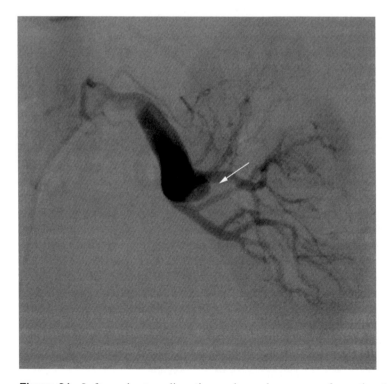

Figure 21 Left renal artery dissection and pseudoaneurysm formation (*white arrow*).

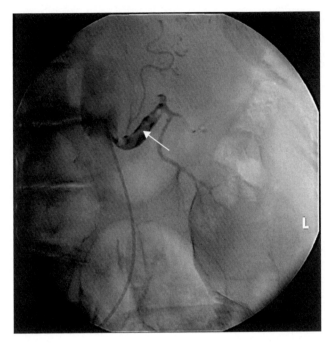

Figure 22 Thrombosis of left renal artery following percutaneous transluminal angiography (PTA). The thrombus is seen extending into the distal main renal artery.

complication can result in renal artery thrombosis (Fig. 22). Renal artery occlusion threatens the viability of the kidney and mandates immediate intervention. This includes thrombolysis, stenting, and occasionally surgical bypass grafting.

Renal angioplasty is set up with the tip of the guidewire always visible in the peripheral image field. Inadvertent advancement of the wire can result in perforation of the renal parenchyma and perinephric or subcapsular hematoma (Fig. 23). Most

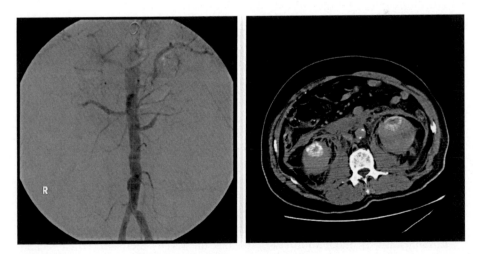

Figure 23 Marked angiographic pruning of the renal arteries due to bilateral subcapsular hematoma as a result of guidewire trauma.

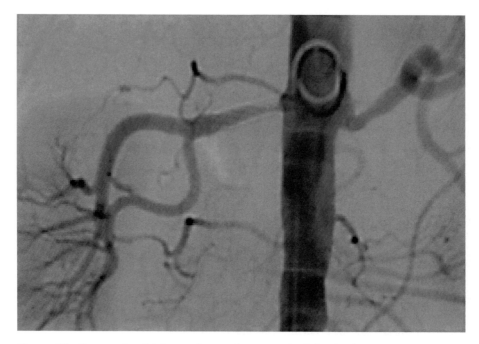

Figure 24 Restenosis of right renal stent three months following implantation.

of these hematomas can be managed by anticoagulation reversal and observation, however, branch renal vessel embolization may be required.

Microembolization may account for the deterioration in renal function, which occurs in some patients following renal stenting. This is usually implied rather than documented, although cholesterol embolization has been documented on renal biopsy.

Restenosis (Fig. 24) remains the Achilles heel of renal stenting with rates reported as high as 20%. This can result in return of hypertension or deterioration in renal function. Repeat angioplasty is required; surgical bypass can be significantly more complicated if stents extend well beyond the ostia of the renal arteries.

Iliac Angioplasty and Stenting

The most common problem encountered with iliac angioplasty is subintimal passage of the guidewire, which tracks on up into the aortic wall. This is prevented by observing the movement of the wire as it crosses the lesion. Suspicion of subintimal passage is raised by failure to aspirate blood from the catheter and hand injection of 2–3 cc of dye, which forms a spot in the aortic wall and fails to wash out. The catheter and wire are retrieved and the lesions re-crossed. Failure to recognize a subintimal location can lead to catastrophic problems if devices are then advanced over the subintimal wire.

Restenosis occurs in 10–20% of cases and can lead to complete stent occlusion (Fig. 25).

Embolization is uncommon (Fig. 26), but the risk is increased when recanalizing total occlusions. It can also occur as a result of thrombus formation on the implanted stent (Fig. 27 A–C).

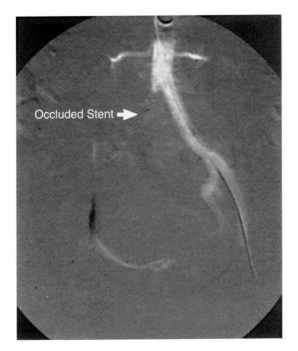

Figure 25 Occluded right common iliac stent.

Iliac rupture is remarkably uncommon, but is a particular risk in small calcified iliac arteries, especially the external iliac artery (Fig. 28). In these high-risk patients, a stent graft (Viabahn®, Wallgraft®) should be immediately available to seal a rupture.

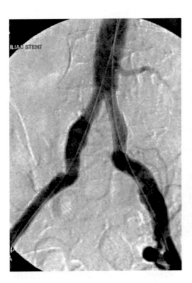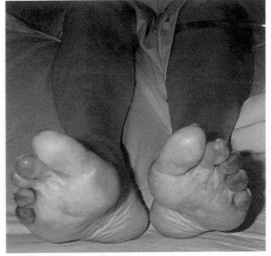

Figure 26 Distal embolization following kissing iliac stents.

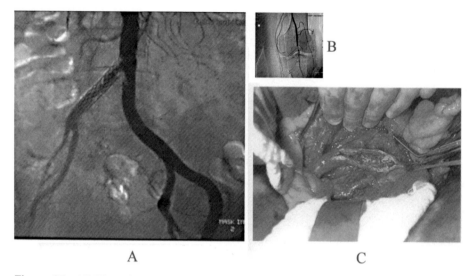

Figure 27 (**A**) Thrombus has formed inside the right common iliac stent. (**B**) Embolization occurred distal to the popliteal artery. (**C**) The stent was removed and a Dacron patch applied to the iliac artery .

Venous Interventions

Venous angioplasty and stenting are performed for central venous stenoses such as that occur with dialysis access or in the left common iliac vein in May-Thurner syndrome. Venous lesions, especially those associated with dialysis access, are

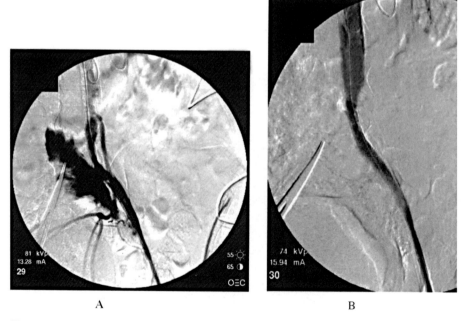

Figure 28 (**A**) Iliac rupture following percutaneous transluminal angiography (PTA) resulting in dye extravasation. (**B**) Successfully treated by Wallgraft deployment.

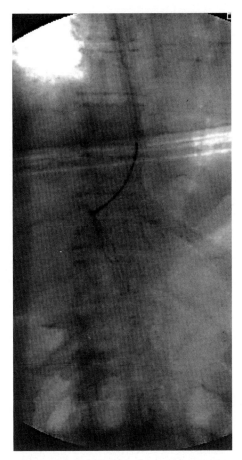

Figure 29 Maldeployed Greenfield (legs bound by thrombus formation) filter undergoing retrieval with gooseneck snare.

notoriously difficult to dilate, often require very high balloon pressures (up to 30 atmospheres), and can result in venous rupture. Most of these venous ruptures are self limiting and seal either spontaneously or within a few minutes of balloon tamponade.

IVC Filter Complication Rates

Complications	Reported Rates (%)	Threshold %
Death	0.12	<1
Recurrent pulmonary embolism	0.5-6	5
IVC occlusion	2.0-30	10
Filter embolization	2.0-5.0	2

Figure 30 Society for Interventional Radiology (SIR) threshold complication rates for inferior vene cava (IVC) filter placement.

IVC penetration	0–41%
Migration	0–18%
Fracture	2–10%
Access site thrombosis	
– all	0–25%
– occlusive	3–10%
Insertion problems	5–50%

Figure 31 Reported complications and their frequency following IVC filter placement.

Stent deployment in central veins is associated with the highest incidence of device migration. Because of the highly compliant nature of the veins and their ability to change dramatically in diameter, stent migration can occur. Careful measurement, over sizing, and ensuring a secure proximal anchor for the stent is important. Migrated Wallstents can usually be retrieved using a snare (Gooseneck® or EN-snare®); since they will compress when pulled into a sheath, they usually can be removed percutaneously (26). Retrieved nitinol of balloon-expanded stents usually require a surgical cut down for retrieval (27).

IVC filters are widely used. Specific filter complications include: IVC occlusion, caval penetration, filters migration, and maldeployment (Figs. 29–31). Wire prolapse is unique to the birds nest filter and is usually asymptomatic. Guidewire entrapment, usually with J-wires is another complication unique to IVC filters. Care must be taken in advancing and retrieving guidewires in the venous system when IVC filters are present (28).

REFERENCES

1. Nasser TK, Mohler ER 3rd, Wilensky RL, Hathaway DR. Peripheral vascular complications following coronary interventional procedures. Clin Cardiol 1995; 18(11):609–614.
2. Zahn R, Thoma S, Fromm E, Lotter R, Zander M, Seidl K, Senges J. Pseudoaneurysm after cardiac catheterization: therapeutic interventions and their sequelae: experience in 86 patients. Cathet Cardiovasc Diagn 1997; 40(1):9–15.
3. Fransson SG, Nylander E. Vascular injury following cardiac catheterization, coronary angiography, and coronary angioplasty. Eur Heart J 1994; 15(2):232–235.
4. Dangas G, Mehran R, Kokolis S, Feldman D, Salter LF, Pichard AD, Kent KM, Lansky AJ, Stone GW, Leon MB. Vascular complications after percutaneous coronary interventions following hemostasis with manual compression versus arteriotomy closure devices. J Am Coll Cardiol 2001; 38(3):638–641.
5. Toursarkissian B, Mejia A, Smilanich RP, Shireman PK, Sykes MT. Changing patterns of access site complications with the use of percutaneous closure devices. Vasc Surg 2001; 35(3):203–206.
6. Singh H, Cardella JF, Cole PE, Grassi CJ, McCowan TC, Swan TL, Sacks D, Lewis CA. SCVIR Standards of Practice Committee. Society of Cardiovascular & Interventional Radiology. Quality improvement guidelines for diagnostic arteriography. J Vasc Interv Radiol 2002; 13(1):1–6.
7. Kresowik TF, Khoury BV, Miller, et al. A prospective study of the incidence and natural history of femoral vascular complications after percutaneous transluminal coronary angioplasty. J Vasc Surg 1991; 13:328–336.
8. Kent KC, McArdle B, Kennedy DS, Baim E, Anninos E, Skillman JJ. A prospective study of the clinical outcome of femoral artery pseudoaneurysms and arteriovenous fistulas induced by arterial puncture. J Vasc Surg 1993; 17:125–133.

9. Perings SM, Kelm M, Jax T, Strauer BE. A prospective study on the incidence and risk factors of arteriovenous fistulae following transfemoral cardiac catheterization. Int J Cardiol 2003; 88:223–228.

10. Lumsden AB, Miller JM, Kosinski AS, Allen RC, Dodson TF, Salam AA, Smith RB 3rd. A prospective evaluation of surgically treated groin complications following percutaneous cardiac procedures. Am Surg 1994; 60(2):132–137.

11. Baltacioglu F, Cimsit NC, Cil B, Cekirge S, Ispir S. Endovascular stent-graft applications in iaterogenic vascular injuries. Cardiovasc Intervent Radiol 2003; 26(5):434–439.

12. Knight CG, Healy DA, Thomas RL. Femoral artery pseudoaneurysms: risk factors, prevalence and treatment options. Ann Vasc Surg 2003; 17:503–508.

13. Perler BA. Surgical treatment of femoral pseudoaneurysm following cardiac catheterization. Cardiovasc Surg 1993; 1(2):118–121.

14. Hughes MJ, McCall JM, Nott DM, Padley SP. Treatment of iatrogenic femoral artery pseudoaneurysms using ultrasound-guided injection of thrombin. Clin Radiol 2000; 55(10):749–751.

15. Lennox AF, Delis KT, Szendro G, Griffin MB, Nicolaides AN, Cheshire NJ. Duplex-guided thrombin injection for iatrogenic femoral artery pseudoaneurysm is effective even in anticoagulated patients. Br J Surg 2000; 87(6):796–801.

16. Sreeram S, Lumsden AB, Miller JS, Salam AA, Dodson TF, Smith RB. Retroperitoneal hematoma following femoral arterial catheterization: a serious and often fatal complication. Am Surg 1993; 59(2):94–98.

17. Wagner SC, Gonsalves CF, Eschelman DJ, Sullivan KL, Bonn J. Complications of a percutaneous suture-mediated closure device versus manual compression for arteriotopomy closure: a case controlled study. J Vasc Inter Radiol 2003; 14:735–7451.

18. Mackrell PJ, Kalbaugh CA, Langan EM, Taylor SM, Sullivan TM, Gray BH, Carsten CG, Snyder BA, Cull DL, Youkey JR. Can the Perclose suture-mediated closure system be safely used in patients undergoing diagnostic and therapeutic angiography to treat lower extremity ischemia. J Vasc Surg 2003; 38:1305–1308.

19. Whitton Hollis H, Rehring TF. Femoral Endarteriitis associated with percutaneous suture closure: new technology, challenging complications. J Vasc Surg 2003; 38:83–87.

20. Kent KC, Moscucci M, Gallagher S, DiMattia S, Skillman J. Neuropathy after cardiac catherization: incidence, clinical patterns, long term outcome. J Vasc Surg 1994; 19: 1008–1014.

21. Tsao BE, Wilbourn AJ. The medial brachial fascial compartment syndrome following axillary arteriography. Neurology 2003; 61(8):1037–1041.

22. Kennedy AM, Grocott M, Schwartz MS, Modarres H, Scott M, Schona F. Median nerve injury: an underrecognized complication of brachial artery cardiac catheterization? J Neurol Neurosurg Psychiatry 1997; 63:542–546.

23. Hoffman AI, Murphy PT. Septic arteritis causing iliac artery rupture and aneurysmal transformation of the distal aorta after iliac artery stent placement. J Vasc Interv Radiol 1997; 8:215–219.

24. Fiorani P, Speziale F, Calisti A, Misuraca M, Zaccagnini D, Rizzo L, Giannoni MF. Endovascular graft infection: preliminary results of an international inquiry. J Endovasc Therapy 2003; 10:919–927.

25. Walton KB, Hudenko K, D'Ayala M, Toursarkissian B. Aneurysmal degeneration of the superificial femoral artery following stenting: an unusual avroavropoulos infectious complication. Ann Vasc Surg 2003; 17:445–448.

26. Ashar RM, Huettl EA, Halligan R. Percutaneous retrieval of a Wallstent from the pulmonary artery following stent migration from the iliac vein. J Intervent Cardiol 2002; 15:101–106.

27. Feghaly EL, Soula P, Chaiban F, Otal P, Joffre F, Cerenee A. Endovascular retrieval of two migrated venous stents by means of balloon catheters. J Vasc Surg 1998; 28:541–546.

28. Stavropoulos SW, Itkin M, Treatola SO. In vitro study of guidewire entrapment in currently available inferior vena caval filter. J Vasc Interv Radiol 2003; 14:905–910.

3

Systemic Complications of Endovascular Therapy

Tulsidas S. Kuruvanka and Deepak L. Bhatt
Department of Cardiovascular Medicine, The Cleveland Clinic Foundation, Cleveland, Ohio, U.S.A.

Endovascular therapy has several advantages over conventional surgery, primarily due to its minimally invasive nature. However, major complications may still occur. As endovascular therapy becomes more widely applied, it has become increasingly important to recognize and treat systemic complications of endovascular therapy when they occur and prevent them altogether when possible. Major systemic complications include contrast nephropathy, atheroemboli, heparin-induced thrombocytopenia (HIT), allergic reactions, and myocardial infarction.

CONTRAST-INDUCED NEPHROPATHY

The most common cause for renal insufficiency following an endovascular procedure is due to contrast-induced nephropathy (CIN).

CIN is an important cause of hospital acquired renal failure, which can result in significant morbidity and mortality particularly in patients with underlying renal insufficiency. Acute renal failure (ARF) caused by CIN is generally non-oliguric and reversible. Various studies have used different definitions. It is generally considered if there is an increase in serum creatinine by more than 25% from baseline or an increase of more than 0.5 mg/dl (44 mmol/l) occurring within three days following IV administration of a contrast agent.

Incidence

There is wide variation in the reported incidence of CIN, due to the differences in the definition of nephropathy, patient selection, amount of contrast agent used, and the radiological procedure. Even though most studies have indicated that there is a mild impairment in renal function following exposure to contrast agents (about 0.2 mg/dl), the incidence of CIN in patients with normal renal function is relatively low. However, in patients with underlying renal insufficiency or diabetic nephropathy, the incidence could be as high as 50% or more (1–3).

Predisposing Factors

Underlying renal insufficiency with serum creatinine greater than 1.5 mg/dl, diabetic nephropathy, advanced heart failure and any other causes of renal hypoperfusion-like dehydration, high total dose of contrast agent use, concomitant use of other nephrotoxic agents like non-steroidal anti-inflammatory drugs or aminoglycosides, multiple injections of contrast agents within a 72-hour period, route of administration (the intravenous route is less nephrotoxic as compared to intra-arterial route), underlying multiple myeloma, and age greater than 60 years (because of the reduction in renal mass, function, and perfusion) have all been considered as risk factors (4).

Consequences and Sequelae

CIN is generally non-oliguric and reversible. The serum creatinine increases within 24 to 48 hours and peaks in three to five days, usually returning to baseline in one to two weeks. Proteinuria and oliguria may be observed in patients with underlying renal insufficiency. In more severe cases, CIN may develop within 24 hours with oliguria, and a peak rise in serum creatinine may occur that exceeds 5 mg/dl (440 mmol/l) occasionally requiring dialysis. In a large study, which evaluated about 1800 patients who underwent coronary intervention, the incidence of ARF was about 14%, but severe CIN requiring dialysis was rare (less than 1%). In this study, ARF was defined as any increase in serum creatinine more than 25% above the baseline value (5). However, patients who developed ARF requiring dialysis had an increased in-hospital mortality of about 36% and a poor two-year survival of 19%. In the same study, no patients with creatinine clearance of greater than 47 ml/min and total contrast volume less than 100 ml developed ARF requiring dialysis (5). In another large retrospective analysis of over 7500 patients who underwent percutaneous coronary intervention (PCI), about 3.3% experienced ARF, where ARF was defined as an increase in serum creatinine of more than 0.5 mg/dl from baseline. Risk of CIN was higher among diabetics compared to non-diabetics with serum creatinine less than 2 mg/dl. In patients with baseline serum creatinine greater than 2 mg/dl, the risk of developing CIN was significant among all patient groups. The mortality rate during the index hospitalization was 22% in patients with ARF as compared to 1.4% in patients without ARF. The one-year and five-year estimated mortality rates were about 12.1% and 44.6%, compared to 3.7% and 14.5% among patients with and without ARF, respectively (6).

Prevention and Management

The key to treatment is the prevention of CIN (Table 1). Some of the preventive measures or strategies are discussed below.

Hydration: This is one of the most important preventive measures. Most studies have incorporated a protocol of using 0.45% saline IV at 1–1.5 ml/kg/hr. It is critical to adjust hydration based on the fluid input and output. In a study by Solomon et al., 78 patients with chronic renal insufficiency (mean creatinine 2.1 ± 0.6 mg/dl) who underwent coronary angiography were included. Patients were randomized to either saline alone, saline with 25 gm mannitol or saline with 80 mg furosemide. ARF developed in 11% of the saline group as compared to 28% in mannitol and 40% in the furosomide group (7). The optimal hydration solution is not clear. Most studies have used

Table 1 Methods to Decrease Contrast-Induced Nephropathy

Pre-hydration with normal saline
Hold diuretics
Avoid non-steroidal anti-inflammatory drugs, aminoglycosides
Limit volume of contrast agent used
Iso-osmolar contrast agents—Iodixanol (Visipaque)
Avoid re-exposure to contrast agents for at least several days
Use of gadolinium, CO_2 as contrast agents

0.45% saline starting 6–12 hours prior and continuing up to 12–24 hours post-procedure. Another study also evaluated isotonic saline versus 0.45% saline. The rate of CIN was lower in patients given isotonic saline (0.7 versus 2%) and among diabetics the rate was 0 versus 5.5% (8). Oral hydration protocols have also been studied but remain unproven.

Diuretics: In the above-mentioned study by Solomon et al., patients who received furosemide along with saline had a 40% incidence of CIN as compared to 11% with saline alone. In fact, there was an increase in nephrotoxicity in this group with underlying moderate renal dysfunction (7). Diuretics are not routinely recommended in the preventive management of CIN.

Types of contrast agent: Currently available contrast agents include first generation ionic monomers, which are hyperosmolar, about 1500–1800 mosm/kg compared to plasma. Second generation agents are non-ionic monomers with a lower osmolality of about 600–850 mosm/kg, and the newest agent available is an iso-osmolar non-ionic dimer with osmolality similar to plasma, about 290 mosm/kg. In patients with normal renal function, there was no higher incidence of CIN with use of high osmolal contrast agents compared to low osmolal agents (2,9). Among patients with underlying renal insufficiency or diabetic nephropathy, the use of low osmolal agents was associated with a lower incidence of CIN, 12% versus 27% than with hyperosmolal agents (2). When the iso-osmolar agent iodixanol was compared to the low osmolar agent iohexol in a high-risk patient population in the Nephrotoxicity in High-Risk Patients Study of Iso-osmolar and Low-osmolar Contrast Media (NEPHRIC), only 3% of the patients in the iso-osmolar agent group had serum creatinine increases of greater than 0.5 mg/dl compared to 26% in the low osmolar agent group. No patients in the iso-osmolar agent group had serum creatinine rise greater than 1.0 mg/dl compared to 15% in the low-osmolar agent group. The iso-osmolar agent iodixanol (Visipaque) appears to be less nephrotoxic in high-risk patients, particularly in diabetics (10).

Fenoldopam: This is a selective dopamine (DA-1) agonist, which has been tested in the prevention of CIN. In one retrospective study of 260 patients with underlying renal insufficiency, the incidence of CIN was less than 4% with use of Fenoldopam (11). However, this particular study lacked a control group. In a more recent prospective randomized trial involving 315 patients, Fenoldopam failed to prevent any further deterioration in renal function in patients with underlying chronic renal insufficiency who were exposed to contrast agents (12).

N-Acetyl Cysteine (NAC): NAC is an antioxidant, which has been shown to offer protection against CIN in high-risk patients. Most trials have used oral NAC at 600 mg twice daily along with 0.45% saline hydration. In a study with 83 patients, the NAC group had a lower incidence of CIN, 2% compared to 21% in the saline alone group (13). In another study with 54 patients, the incidence of CIN was 8% in the NAC group, as compared to 45% in the control or placebo group (14). However, adequately powered trials of NAC versus placebo are necessary to determine whether it really is of benefit.

Gadolinium: Contrast agents used in magnetic resonance imaging are chelates of gadolinium and they appear to have very little nephrotoxicity. In a prospective, randomized, double blind, placebo-controlled study, the safety of gadolinium was evaluated in 32 patients with moderate to severe chronic renal failure (creatinine clearance ranged from 10 ml/min to 60 ml/min). None of the patients had an increase in serum creatinine greater than 0.5 mg/dl over their baseline following gadolinium exposure (15). Gadolinium has been tested as an alternative angiographic contrast agent in patients with impaired renal function and high risk for iodinated CIN. In one study of 29 patients (59% diabetics) with an average creatinine of 3.6 mg/dl, a total of 32 procedures were performed (24 diagnostic angiograms and 8 interventional procedures). Only one patient had evidence of post-procedure CIN (increase in serum creatinine >0.5 mg/dl within 72 hours), and it was thought that it was probably due to cholesterol embolism (16). Gadolinium had sufficient radiographic density to allow adequate diagnostic visualization with digital subtraction equipment in all cases. Gadolinium is an alternative and safe radiographic contrast agent for angiography and interventional procedures in patients with severe pre-existing renal impairment.

Carbon dioxide (CO_2): CO_2 has been safely and effectively used as an alternative contrast agent in vascular interventional procedures. Some of the advantages it offers are that it is not nephrotoxic, it is non-allergic, and is very inexpensive. It has also been used in the detection of minute amounts of bleeding from the gastrointestinal tract, vascular imaging of neoplasms, and during transjugular intrahepaic portosystemic shunt (TIPS) procedures. With the use of digital subtraction angiogtraphy (DSA) techniques, the images obtained with CO_2 arteriography are accurate and comparable to images obtained with use of iodinated contrast agents (17). In one study involving 21 patients who underwent 29 procedures, the efficacy of CO_2 DSA for performing renal artery angioplasty in high-risk patients was evaluated. An average dose of 114 ml of CO_2 (range of 80–200 ml) was used. There was a minimal increase in serum creatinine (<0.5 mg/dl) noted after four procedures, with no change seen after 11 procedures and a decrease in serum creatinine observed after 12 procedures (18). CO_2 should be considered in patients with a history of contrast allergy or in patients with underlying renal failure.

Hemodialysis: Studies have been undertaken to determine the efficacy of prophylactic hemodialysis in patients exposed to contrast medium, but these failed to show any benefits (19). Therefore, this strategy is currently not recommended.

Other agents like theophylline, atrial natriuretic peptide, calcium channel blockers, and endothelin antagonists have all been evaluated (20), but are not currently recommended for routine use. In general, measures to avoid dehydration, minimize contrast volume, avoid concomitant nephrotoxic agents, and use of gadolinium or CO_2 in high-risk patients should minimize or help prevent CIN.

ATHEROEMBOLIC COMPLICATIONS

Atheroembolism, also described as cholesterol crystal embolization, is perhaps an under-recognized complication of arteriography and endovascular interventions, but has significant morbidity and mortality associated with it. Given the increase in the total number of endovascular procedures, it is important to be aware of this complication. Clearly the incidence of theroembolism increases with advanced atherosclerosis and with increasing age. Most data available with regard to the incidence of atheroembolism are derived from autopsy studies. The rates have ranged from 0.79% to about 30% (21,22). In one retrospective analysis of autopsies of 71 patients who had undergone diagnostic arteriography, the incidence of cholesterol embolization was 30% compared to 4.3% of age-matched controls (21).

Predisposing Factors

Spontaneous atheroemobolization can occur; however, it is seen more often following arteriography, surgery, and following anticoagulation and thrombolytic agents. It is unclear, however, if the rigidity of the catheter or force of contrast agent injection has any role. Larger diameter catheters and catheters with angulated tips are more likely to cause atheroembolism. Using a guidewire to straighten out curved catheters while withdrawing them and using exchange-length guidewires for catheter exchanges may minimize the occurrence of embolization (23). Anticoagulation is best avoided or discontinued if atheroembolism develops, unless other clinical conditions warrant its continued use.

Clinical Manifestations

The clinical signs and symptoms of atheroembolism may be non-specific. The most common clinical findings are seen as skin changes and may be present in up to one-third of patients. Skin changes include livedo reticularis, purple or blue toe syndrome, skin ulcerations, nodules, and even frank gangrene (24). Livedo reticularis is a blue-red mottling of the skin in a net-like fashion seen on the buttocks, thighs and legs and represents the involvement of dermal blood vessels by microemboli. The livedo reticular pattern of changes may be found in other conditions like systemic vasculitis, collagen vascular disease, immune complex disorders, cryoglobulinemia or subacute bacterial endocarditis. It may also be seen in young healthy females. Purple or blue toe syndrome is acute digital ischemia secondary to microembolization from a proximal source. These changes in the presence of palpable foot pulses are highly suggestive of atheroembolic disease. It is important to note that these changes are not evident immediately and the manifestations may be delayed even up to weeks. Skin biopsy may or may not reveal cholesterol clefts and diagnosis may be presumed on the basis of fibrinous thrombosis and clinical correlation (25).

Renal Effects

The kidney is a frequently affected target organ when atheroemboli originate from suprarenal aortic disease. It can follow aortic surgery, aortic arteriography or even left heart catheterization. The interlobular and afferent arterioles of 150–200 μm in size are usually involved (26). The renal manifestations can present as uncontrolled hypertension or rapidly progressive, and fatal renal failure. It is important to differentiate the renal failure due to atheroemboli from other causes like CIN. In comparison to CIN where the serum creatinine elevation usually follows the procedure, the onset of renal failure after atheroemboli may be as late as two to six weeks after the invasive procedure. The outcome is usually poor and renal failure may progress, requiring dialysis. Certain studies have shown that some patients have stabilization or even improvement in their renal function. In one review of 221 cases of histologically proven atheroemboli, 31% of patients had at least one predisposing factor. Mortality was high (81%) and was most commonly due to multifactorial, cardiac, and renal etiologies (27). Kidney biopsy that reveals cholesterol clefts may be required for definitive diagnosis.

Other organ systems where atheroembolic changes may be evident include the central nervous system, gastrointestinal tract, and cardiovascular system. Symptoms may include transient ischemic attack, amaurosis fugax, stroke and Hollenhorst plaque, gastrointestinal bleed, bowel infarction, angina or myocardial infarction (24).

Laboratory findings are usually non-specific. Some of the changes include increased erythrocyte sedimentation rate, eosinophilia and hypocomplimentemia. Urine analysis is usually benign but may show microhematuria or eosinophiluria (28–30). The pathognomonic findings on biopsy are needle-shaped cholesterol clefts within the small vessels.

Treatment of atheroembolic disease is limited and primarily involves symptomatic care and prevention. Local skin care includes good skin hygiene, lambs wool between toes, Rooke boots and heel protectors. Surgical or chemical sympathectomy may be performed. Amputation may be required for gangrenous changes. The surgical removal of the source of emboli can be undertaken if the source is identified. If the source is the aorto-iliac region, replacement of the segment of aorta or iliac arteries is often needed. Anticoagulants are best avoided. Antiplatelet agents and statins have been used, but no controlled studies are available in terms of efficacy. Other agents such as corticosteroids and vasodilators have been used but are not currently recommended. Iloprost, a prostaglandin analogue, had been studied in a small number of patients (four), where it has shown improvement in cyanotic skin lesions, dramatic relief of pain, and, in at least one patient, stabilized and subsequently improved renal function. Even though these results appear promising, larger controlled studies are necessary to establish its efficacy in the treatment of atheroembolic disease (31).

HEPARIN-INDUCED THROMBOCYTOPENIA (HIT)

The benign form of HIT (type I) is a transient fall in platelet counts, rarely below $100,000/\mu l$, occurring within one to four days from initiation of heparin therapy. Platelet counts recover by themselves even on continued heparin therapy. The more serious form of HIT (type II) is an immune-mediated condition with formation of antibodies against the heparin platelet factor-4 (PF4) complex. This condition could be potentially lethal if not recognized, and is also termed as heparin-induced thrombocytopenia with thrombosis syndrome (HITTS) or white clot syndrome (platelet rich thrombus) (32). Type II HIT is typically seen between days 5 and 10 (the first day of heparin therapy is considered day 0). The definition of thrombocytopenia is a platelet count of less than $150,000/\mu l$ or a greater than 50% fall in platelet counts from peak levels after exposure to heparin occurring on day 5–10 (33). Platelet counts rarely fall below $20,000/\mu l$. A delayed-onset form of type II HIT is being increasingly recognized where the drop in platelet count may be delayed (median of 14 days, range 9–40 days). A rapid onset of type II HIT may be seen when patients with a prior history of HIT within the past 100 days are re-exposed to heparin. The incidence of type II HIT is about 3–5% in patients exposed to heparin. The incidence of HIT is considerably lower when low molecular weight heparin (LMWH) agents are used. In one prospective study of 665 patients receiving heparin therapy for prophylaxis following hip surgery, HIT was seen in 2.7% of patients receiving unfractionated heparin and in none of the patients who received LMWH (33). However, in patients with a history or suspicion of HIT, LMWH should not be used.

Consequences and Sequelae

Paradoxically, patients with HIT rarely have bleeding problems and the major problem or sequela of HIT is the development of thrombosis. Thrombosis could be arterial or venous in nature. Venous thrombosis can include pulmonary embolism, deep venous thrombosis, phlegmasia cerulea dolens, and cerebral sinus thrombosis. Arterial thrombosis may cause stroke, myocardial infarction or limb ischemia. Skin necrosis at the site of the heparin injection can also be a manifestation of HIT (33–36). Venous limb gangrene is a rare complication of HIT and may be seen in patients with HIT who are being treated with warfarin.

In patients with isolated type II HIT without thrombosis, even after further heparin therapy was discontinued, the 30-day thrombosis event rate was about 50% (35). Patients with type II HIT can have major adverse outcomes. In one study with 85 patients, 29% died and 18% required limb amputation. In another study involving 127 patients, 20% died during hospitalization for their acute event (35,37).

Diagnosis

HIT is primarily a clinical diagnosis. There are two types of laboratory tests available to help in diagnosing type II HIT. These laboratory studies can be divided into functional assays and immunoassays. The most widely used test (a functional assay) is the platelet aggregation test, which measures the aggregation of normal donor platelets by the patient's serum or plasma in the presence of heparin. This test is simple and inexpensive. The platelet aggregation test has a specificity of approximately 90%, but its sensitivity is reported to vary between 30% and 50%. An enzyme-linked immunosorbent assay technique for the diagnosis of type II HIT, measures IgG, IgA, or IgM that binds PF4-heparin complexes. The [^{14}C]serotonin release assay is considered to be the reference standard for the diagnosis of type II HIT. In this test, radiolabeled, washed platelets from reactive donors are incubated with heat-treated patient's serum in the presence of heparin. It is technically demanding, requires the use of radioisotopes and fresh donor platelets, is time consuming, is not readily available at all laboratories, and is primarily used to confirm type II HIT rather than for initial diagnosis of type II HIT (38,39).

Treatment

The first step in the management of type II HIT is the cessation of all heparin therapy or heparin use, including small doses of heparin used for line flushes or during dialysis. Anticoagulation with alternative agents should be undertaken if no contraindications exist for such use (Table 2). Direct thrombin inhibitors are the primary anticoagulants used in the management of type II HIT. These include argatroban, lepirudin, and bivalirudin. No agents are available to reverse the anticoagulant effects of these agents.

Argatroban is a synthetic molecule that directly binds to the thrombin catalytic site and can be monitored with the activated partial thromboplastin time (aPTT). It has been evaluated in the treatment of type II HIT in the United States and found to

Table 2 Drugs Used in the Management of Type II HIT or HITTS

Drug	Initial dose	Monitoring	Half life	Clearance
Argatroban	2 µg/kg/min intravenous drip[a]	Check aPTT 2 hr after initiation of treatment and daily. Also 2 hr after any dose adjustments	40–50 min	Hepatic
Lepirudin	0.2 mg/kg intravenous loading dose-max 44 mg. Then 0.15 mg/ kg/hr IV drip–max 16.5 mg/kg/hr	Check aPTT 4 hr after initiation of treatment and daily. Also 4 hr after any dose adjustments	1.3 hr	Renal
Bivalirudin	0.75 mg/kg intravenous bolus and 1.75 mg/kg/ hr infusion during PCI or up to 4 hr after procedure	Monitor ACT. Range: 300–350 sec	25 min	Renal
Danaparoid sodium	2250 U intravenous bolus followed by 400 U/hr for 4 hr, 300 U/ hr for 4 hr, then 150– 200 U/hr for ≥5 days aiming for a plasma anti-Xa level of 0.5–0.8 U/ml	Antithrombin levels at the beginning of therapy. Anti-Xa levels during treatment using danaparoid reference curve. Range is 0.5–0.8 anti-Xa U/ml	17–28 hr	Renal

[a]Dose adjustment needed in patients with hepatic impairment.
Abbreviations: HIT, heparin-induced thrombocytopenia; HITTS, heparin-induced thrombocytopenia with thrombosis syndrome; aPTT, activated partial thromboplastin time; PCI, percutaneous coronary intervention; ACT, activated-clotting time.

significantly reduce the risk of new thrombosis in type II HIT patients. Argatroban is currently approved for use in both the treatment and prophylaxis of patients with type II HIT (40). Caution needs to be exercised in patients with liver dysfunction. Therapy is monitored by aPTT. An aPTT ratio between 1.5 and 3.0 (42–84 seconds) of control is optimal while on argatroban therapy. Lepirudin (Refludan) is the other FDA approved agent for the treatment of HIT. Lepirudin is a recombinant form of the leech anticoagulant, hirudin. It can be monitored by the aPTT. It is predominantly metabolized by the kidney and is therefore considered relatively contraindicated in patients with renal failure. An aPTT ratio between 1.5 and 2.5 (45–60 seconds) of control is optimal while on lepirudin. In studies comparing historical controls with lepirudin, patients had a significantly lower frequency of a composite endpoint of mortality, limb amputation, or new thrombotic complications (41,42). Bivalirudin (Angiomax) is another new direct thrombin inhibitor. It has a relatively short half-life, and has been approved by the FDA in the United States for percutaneous coronary intervention. It is not yet FDA approved for the treatment of type II HIT, though it is being actively studied in that setting. A recent study by Mahaffey et al. has shown that bivalirudin was safe and provided effective anticoagulation during percutaneous coronary intervention (PCI) in patients with a history of type II HIT (43). Ecarin clotting time (ECT) is a new tool used in the monitoring of hirudin therapy. ECT is the method of choice for monitoring hirudin therapy in patients requiring a high hirudin dose (cardiopulmonary bypass). It is unclear whether ECT is more useful in patients at higher risk of bleeding, as there are no prospective trials comparing ECT and aPTT. Also at this time ECT measurement is being performed only at a few select laboratories (44). The low molecular weight heparinoid danaparoid (Orgaran) has also been used in the treatment of HIT (45). Warfarin is contraindicated if used alone in the patient with type II HIT. In addition, warfarin may precipitate venous limb gangrene in patients with deep venous thrombosis, complicating type II HIT. After initial therapy with direct thrombin inhibitors and thrombin generation has been controlled, and when platelets counts are at least 100,000/μl or greater, warfarin can be started at small doses. Warfarin therapy is monitored by the prothrombin time and international normalized ratio (INR). The target INR is 2 to 3. Lepirudin or bivalirudin does not affect the prothrombin time, whereas argatroban can falsely elevate prothrombin time. While patients are being switched to warfarin one needs to wait for the INR to be as high as 4.0 or greater before discontinuing argatroban therapy (44,46). The duration of warfarin therapy is determined by any underlying thrombotic event (three to six months), and whether thrombosis is present for at least 30–100 days. Platelet transfusions are generally not recommended, both because bleeding complications are uncommon, and because thrombotic events have been reported to follow transfusions. With the publication of the Randomized Evaluation in PCI Linking Angiomax to Reduced Clinical Events (REPLACE)-2 trial (47) of over 6000 patients undergoing PCI, half of whom were randomized to bivalirudin, the evidence supporting the use of bivalirudin in endovascular procedures is substantial. Thus, bivalirudin will likely become the treatment of choice in patients with type II HIT undergoing interventional procedures. Re-exposure to heparin is generally felt to be associated with a high risk of thrombosis and thrombocytopenia.

ALLERGIC REACTIONS

Patients undergoing endovascular procedures may experience allergic reactions secondary to either the local anesthetic agent, the contrast media, protamine sulfate, or latex.

Local Anesthetic

Reactions to local anesthetics are less likely with the use of the newer agents like lidocaine or bupivacaine. However, in patients with a prior history of reaction to a local anesthetic, preservative free agents like mepivicaine or bupivacaine may be used (48). Skin testing may also be performed if indicated prior to procedure.

Contrast Agent

Iodinated contrast agents are more often the causes of an allergic reaction, occurring in up to 1% of patients. It is an anaphylactoid reaction rather than an anaphylactic reaction. It is more often seen in patients with a history of atopic disorder, history of other allergic reactions, or history of prior reaction in whom the chances of a repeat reaction could be as high as 15–35%. It is clinically manifested as urticaria, angioedema of lips or eyelids, bronchospasm, and rarely as shock. Premedication with corticosteroids and histamine$_1$ and histamine$_2$ blockers should be used in patients with prior history, or in patients who may be at a higher risk for an allergic reaction. The availability of newer non-ionic contrast agents has also been provided, with additional safety in terms of minor contrast reactions. The incidence of cross reactivity in patients with prior history of an allergic reaction to ionic agents is less than 1% (49). In the event a severe reaction does occur, it is treated with intravenous boluses of 1 ml of dilute epinephrine (1:10,000 i.e., 0.1 mg/ml). These boluses are usually repeated until arterial pressure is restored. It is rare for patients to require more than 100 µg of epinephrine as a total dose and higher doses are best avoided.

Protamine Sulfate

Reactions to protamine sulfate may occur rarely and are more often seen in patients with diabetes mellitus, who have received NPH insulin. It is best to avoid or use it with caution in patients who are receiving NPH insulin and in patients with a history of allergy to fish (50). If protamine sulfate is administered, it is best to inject it slowly and start off with smaller doses (e.g., 5 mg or 10 mg).

Latex Allergy

Allergic reaction to latex is a problem which is being increasingly encountered. Allergy to latex could manifest as either a type IV delayed hypersensitivity reaction (which is more common) or type I immediate type hypersensitivity reaction, causing anaphylaxis or even death. Some of the important steps in the management of patients with a history of latex allergy include avoiding all direct contact with natural rubber latex products and performing the procedure in a latex safe environment (51). Care should also be taken to perform all elective cases with a history of latex allergy as the first case in the procedure room in order to avoid contamination with latex particles in the air generated by earlier procedures in the same room.

MYOCARDIAL INFARCTION

Given that most patients undergoing endovascular therapy have coexisting coronary artery disease (CAD), cardiac complications are an important cause of post-procedural morbidity and mortality. Most data regarding cardiac complications associated with endovascular procedures come from studies of endovascular abdominal aortic aneurysm (AAA) repair (EVAR).

Incidence

Open repair of AAA is associated with an operative mortality of 4–10% (52). CAD is the most important risk factor accounting for up to 60% of perioperative mortality (53). The incidence of cardiac complications following EVAR has varied in different studies. Some studies have shown event rates to be similar when compared to open AAA repair, whereas, other studies have shown the rates to be lower than open repair of AAA. In a study by May et al., 108 patients underwent EVAR with a cardiac complication rate of 7.4% and cardiac mortality of 2.7% (54). In a smaller group of patients, Moore et al. noted the rate of myocardial infarction to be 2% with no cardiac mortality (55). In a randomized study by Cuypers et al. involving 76 patients, 57 underwent EVAR and 19 underwent open AAA repair. Even though the clinical cardiac complication rates were comparable, myocardial ischemia observed by electrocardiogram (ECG) and transesophageal echocardiogram (TEE) was seen in 53% of patients who underwent open repair of AAA as compared to 26% of patients who underwent EVAR (56). The Excluder multicenter clinical trial also showed a significantly lower rate of cardiac adverse events in the EVAR group when compared to open repair (3% versus 14%) (57). The results of a meta-analysis by Adriaensen et al. have also shown lower mortality and systemic complication rates when compared to open AAA repair (58).

Eagle criteria (Q wave on ECG, diabetes mellitus, angina, history of heart failure, age >70 years and ventricular ectopy) are useful predictors of myocardial infarction (59). In a single center experience involving 365 patients, it was found that age 70 years or older, history of myocardial infarction (MI) or congestive heart failure (CHF), and lack of use of preoperative beta-blocker therapy were independent risk factors for perioperative cardiac events in patients undergoing EVAR (60). The cardiac adverse event rate was as high as 50% in patients with four of the above risk factors compared to 5.3% in patients with no risk factors (60). In addition to being responsible for the majority of periprocedural mortality, cardiac complications have an impact on long-term prognosis and survival. In a study by Aune et al. (327 patients), the 10-year survival in patients with pre-existing cardiac disease was 24% as compared to 52% in patients without cardiac disease prior to AAA repair (61). There was a nine-fold increase in cardiovascular events over a two-year period in patients who had perioperative myocardial ischemia following non-cardiac surgery (62). In a study of patients who underwent vascular surgery, McFalls et al. observed that the four-year survival was decreased from 90% to 55% in those patients who sustained a perioperative myocardial infarction (63). Though EVAR is minimally invasive and is associated with fewer adverse cardiac events, large scale randomized studies with a longer follow-up are needed to evaluate the potential extended beneficial effects of EVAR on clinical events and mortality. Patients undergoing endovascular procedures should be evaluated preoperatively and screened for risk factors in order to reduce the most common serious morbidity related to EVAR.

Carotid Stenting

Patients undergoing carotid artery stenting (CAS) might be at risk for developing non-ST elevation myocardial infarction. Potential risk factors include peri- and post procedural hypotension and/or bradycardia, as well as concomitant CAD. Although the frequency of cardiac complications is significantly lower following CAS when compared to carotid endarterectomy, MI may still occur. In the Stenting and Angioplasty with Protection in Patients at High Risk for Endarterectomy trial, the 30-day MACE (death, any stroke or MI) was significantly lower at 5.8% in the CAS group as compared to 12.6% in the endarterectomy group. This was largely driven by a difference in MI (64).

CONCLUSION

While endovascular procedures generally have a lower rate of morbidity than open surgical procedures, complications may still occur, including ones not seen in open surgical procedures. It is important to recognize the potential for these complications and try to prevent them when possible. As techniques evolve, newer strategies will be developed to make endovascular procedures even safer in the future.

REFERENCES

1. Rudnick MR, Berns JS, Cohen RM, Goldfarb S. Nephrotoxic risks of renal angiography: contrast media-associated nephrotoxicity and atheroembolism—a critical review. Am J Kidney Dis 1994 Oct; 24(4):713–727.
2. Rudnick MR, Goldfarb S, Wexler L, Ludbrook PA, Murphy MJ, Halpern EF, Hill JA, Winniford M, Cohen MB, VanFossen DB. Nephrotoxicity of ionic and nonionic contrast media in 1196 patients: a randomized trial. The Iohexol Cooperative Study. Kidney Int 1995 Jan; 47(1):254–261.
3. Lautin EM, Freeman NJ, Schoenfeld AH, Bakal CW, Haramati N, Friedman AC, Lautin JL, Braha S, Kadish EG, Sprayregen S, et al. Radiocontrast-associated renal dysfunction: incidence and risk factors. AJR Am J Roentgenol 1991; 157(1):49–58.
4. Morcos SK. Contrast media-induced nephrotoxicity—questions and answers. Br J Radiol 1998; 71(844):357–365.
5. McCullough PA, Wolyn R, Rocher LL, Levin RN, O'Neill WW. Acute renal failure after coronary intervention: incidence, risk factors, and relationship to mortality. Am J Med 1997; 103(5):368–375.
6. Rihal CS, Textor SC, Grill DE, Berger PB, Ting HH, Best PJ, Singh M, Bell MR, Barsness GW, Mathew V, Garratt KN, Holmes DR Jr. Incidence and prognostic importance of acute renal failure after percutaneous coronary intervention. Circulation 2002; 105(19):2259–2264.
7. Solomon R, Werner C, Mann D, D'Elia J, Silva P. Effects of saline, mannitol, and furosemide to prevent acute decreases in renal function induced by radiocontrast agents. N Engl J Med 1994; 331(21):1416–20.
8. Mueller C, Buerkle G, Buettner HJ, Petersen J, Perruchoud AP, Eriksson U, Marsch S, Roskamm H. Prevention of contrast media-associated nephropathy: randomized comparison of 2 hydration regimens in 1620 patients undergoing coronary angioplasty. Arch Intern Med 2002; 162(3):329–36.
9. Schwab SJ, Hlatky MA, Pieper KS, Davidson CJ, Morris KG, Skelton TN, Bashore TM. Contrast nephrotoxicity: a randomized controlled trial of a nonionic and an ionic radiographic contrast agent. N Engl J Med 1989; 320(3):149–53.
10. Aspelin P, Aubry P, Fransson SG, Strasser R, Willenbrock R, Berg KJ. Nephrotoxicity in high-risk patients study of iso-osmolar and low-osmolar non-ionic contrast media study investigators. Nephrotoxic effects in high-risk patients undergoing angiography. N Engl J Med 2003; 348(6):491–9.
11. Kini AS, Mitre CA, Kamran M, Suleman J, Kim M, Duffy ME, Marmur JD, Sharma SK. Changing trends in incidence and predictors of radiographic contrast nephropathy after percutaneous coronary intervention with use of Fenoldopam. Am J Cardiol 2002; 89(8):999–1002.
12. Stone GW, McCullough PA, Tumlin JA, Lepor NE, Madyoon H, Murray P, Wang A, Chu AA, Schaer GL, Stevens M, Wilensky RL, O'Neill WW. Contrast investigators. Fenoldopam Mesylate for the prevention of contrast induced nephropathy–a randomized controlled trial. J Am Med Assoc 2003; 290(17):2284–2291.
13. Tepel M, van der Giet M, Schwarzfeld C, Laufer U, Liermann D, Zidek W. Prevention of radiographic-contrast-agent-induced reductions in renal function by acetylcysteine. N Engl J Med 2000; 343(3):180–184.
14. Diaz-Sandoval LJ, Kosowsky BD, Losordo DW. Acetylcysteine to prevent angiography-related renal tissue injury (the APART trial). Am J Cardiol 2002; 89(3):356–358.

15. Townsend RR, Cohen DL, Katholi R, Swan SK, Davies BE, Bensel K, Lambrecht L, Parker J. Safety of intravenous gadolinium (Gd-BOPTA) infusion in patients with renal insufficiency. Am J Kidney Dis 2000; 36(6):1207–1212.

16. Rieger J, Sitter T, Toepfer M, Linsenmaier U, Pfeifer KJ, Schiffl H. Gadolinium as an alternative contrast agent for diagnostic and interventional angiographic procedures in patients with impaired renal function. Nephrol Dial Transplant 2002; 17(5):824–828.

17. Back MR, Caridi JG, Hawkins IF Jr, Seeger JM. Angiography with carbon dioxide (CO_2). Surg Clin North Am 1998; 78(4):575–591.

18. Caridi JG, Stavropoulos SW, Hawkins IF Jr. CO_2 digital subtraction angiography for renal artery angioplasty in high-risk patients. AJR Am J Roentgenol 1999; 173(6): 1551–1556.

19. Lehnert T, Keller E, Gondolf K, Schaffner T, Pavenstadt H, Schollmeyer P. Effect of haemodialysis after contrast medium administration in patients with renal insufficiency. Nephrol Dial Transplant 1998; 13(2):358–362.

20. Waybill MM, Waybill PN. Contrast media-induced nephrotoxicity: identification of patients at risk and algorithms for prevention. J Vasc Interv Radiol 2001; 12(1):3–9.

21. Ramirez G, O'Neill WM Jr, Lambert R, Bloomer HA. Cholesterol embolization: a complication of angiography. Arch Intern Med 1978; 138(9):1430–1432.

22. Kealy WF. Atheroembolism. J Clin Pathol 1978; 31:984.

23. Keeley EC, Grines CL. Scraping of aortic debris by coronary guiding catheters: a prospective evaluation of 1,000 cases. J Am Coll Cardiol 1998; 32(7):1861–1865.

24. Young JR, Olin JW, Bartholomew JR. Peripheral Vascular Diseases. 2d ed. St. Louis, MO: Mosby, 1996.

25. Colt HG, Begg RJ, Saporito JJ, Cooper WM, Shapiro AP. Cholesterol emboli after cardiac catheterization. Eight cases and a review of the literature. Medicine (Baltimore) 1988; 67(6):389–400.

26. Warren BA, Vales O. The ultrastructure of the stages of atheroembolic occlusion of renal arteries. Br J Exp Pathol 1973; 54(5):469–478.

27. Fine MJ, Kapoor W, Falanga V. Cholesterol crystal embolization: a review of 221 cases in the English literature. Angiology 1987; 38(10):769–784.

28. Kasinath BS, Lewis EJ. Eosinophilia as a clue to the diagnosis of atheroembolic renal disease. Arch Intern Med 1987; 147(8):1384–1385.

29. Kasinath BS, Corwin HL, Bidani AK, Korbet SM, Schwartz MM, Lewis EJ. Eosinophilia in the diagnosis of atheroembolic renal disease. Am J Nephrol 1987; 7(3):173–177.

30. Cosio FG, Zager RA, Sharma HM. Atheroembolic renal disease causes hypocomplementaemia. Lancet 1985; 2(8447):118–121.

31. Elinav E, Chajek-Shaul T, Stern M. Improvement in cholesterol emboli syndrome after iloprost therapy. Br Med J 2002; 324(7332):268–269.

32. Warkentin TE, Chong BH, Greinacher A. Heparin-induced thrombocytopenia: towards consensus. Thromb Haemost 1998; 79(1):1–7.

33. Warkentin TE, Levine MN, Hirsh J, Horsewood P, Roberts RS, Gent M, Kelton JG. Heparin-induced thrombocytopenia in patients treated with low-molecular-weight heparin or unfractionated heparin. N Engl J Med 1995; 332(20):1330–1335.

34. Boshkov LK, Warkentin TE, Hayward CP, Andrew M, Kelton JG. Heparin-induced thrombocytopenia and thrombosis: clinical and laboratory studies. Br J Haematol 1993; 84(2):322–328.

35. Warkentin TE, Kelton JG. A 14-year study of heparin-induced thrombocytopenia. Am J Med 1996; 101(5):502–507.

36. Fowlie J, Stanton PD, Anderson JR. Heparin-associated skin necrosis. Postgrad Med J 1990; 66(777):573–575.

37. King DJ, Kelton JG. Heparin-associated thrombocytopenia. Ann Intern Med 1984; 100:535–540.

38. Sheridan D, Carter C, Kelton JG. A diagnostic test for heparin-induced thrombocytopenia. Blood 1986; 67(1):27–30.

39. Greinacher A, Amiral J, Dummel V, Vissac A, Kiefel V, Mueller–Eckhardt C. Laboratory diagnosis of heparin-associated thrombocytopenia and comparison of platelet aggregation test, heparin-induced platelet activation test, and platelet factor 4/heparin enzyme-linked immunosorbent assay. Transfusion 1994; 34(5):381–385.

40. Lewis BE, Wallis DE, Berkowitz SD, Matthai WH, Fareed J, Walenga JM, Bartholomew J, Sham R, Lerner RG, Zeigler ZR, et al. ARG-911 Study Investigators. Argatroban anticoagulant therapy in patients with heparin-induced thrombocytopenia. Circulation 2001; 103(14):1838–1843.

41. Greinacher A, Volpel H, Janssens U, Hach–Wunderle V, Kemkes–Matthes B, Eichler P, Mueller–Velten HG, Potzsch B. Recombinant hirudin (lepirudin) provides safe and effective anticoagulation in patients with heparin–induced thrombocytopenia: a prospective study. Circulation 1999; 99(1):73–80.

42. Greinacher A, Eichler P, Lubenow N, Kwasny H, Luz M. Heparin-induced thrombocytopenia with thromboembolic complications: meta-analysis of 2 prospective trials to assess the value of parenteral treatment with lepirudin and its therapeutic aPTT range. Blood 2000; 96(3):846–851.

43. Mahaffey KW, Lewis BE, Wildermann NM, Berkowitz SD, Oliverio RM, Turco MA, Shalev Y, Ver Lee P, Traverse JH, Rodriguez AR, Ohman EM, Harrington RA, Califf RM. The anticoagulant therapy with bivalirudin to assist in the performance of percutaneous coronary intervention in patients with heparin-induced thrombocytopenia (ATBAT) study: main results. J Invasive Cardiol 2003; 15(11):611–616.

44. Warkentin TE, Greinacher. Heparin-Induced Thrombocytopenia. 2 ed. New York, NY: Marcel Dekker, 2001.

45. Chong BH, Ismail F, Cade J, Gallus AS, Gordon S, Chesterman CN. Heparin induced thrombocytopenia: studies with a new low molecular weight heparinoid, Org 10172. Blood 1989; 73:1592.

46. Sheth SB, DiCicco RA, Hursting MJ, Montague T, Jorkasky DK. Interpreting the International Normalized Ratio (INR) in individuals receiving argatroban and warfarin. Thromb Haemost 2001; 85(3):435–440. Erratum in: Thromb Haemost 2001; 86(2):727.

47. Lincoff AM, Bittl JA, Harrington RA, Feit F, Kleiman NS, Jackman JD, Sarembock IJ, Cohen DJ, Spriggs D, Ebrahimi R, et al. Bivalirudin and provisional glycoprotein IIb/IIIa blockade compared to with heparin and planned glycoprotein IIb/IIIa blockade during percutaneous coronary intervention: REPLACE-2 trial. J Am Med Assoc 2003; 289:853–863.

48. Feldman T, Moss J, Teplinsky K, Carroll JD. Cardiac catheterization in the patient with history of allergy to local anesthetics. Cathet Cardiovasc Diagn 1990; 20(3):165–167.

49. Baim DS, Grossman W. Grossman's Cardiac Catheterization, Angiography and Intervention. 6th ed. Philadelphia, PA: LWW, 2000.

50. Stewart WJ, McSweeney SM, Kellett MA, Faxon DP, Ryan TJ. Increased risk of severe protamine reactions in NPH insulin-dependent diabetics undergoing cardiac catheterization. Circulation 1984; 70(5):788–792.

51. Warshaw EM. Latex allergy. Skin Med 2003; 2(6):359–366.

52. Blankensteijn JD, Lindenburg FP, Van der Graaf Y, Eikelboom BC. Influence of study design on reported mortality and morbidity rates after abdominal aortic aneurysm repair. Br J Surg 1998; 85(12):1624–1630. Review.

53. Johnston KW. Multicenter prospective study of nonruptured abdominal aortic aneurysm. Part II. Variables predicting morbidity and mortality. J Vasc Surg 1989; 9(3): 437–447.

54. May J, White GH, Yu W, Ly CN, Waugh R, Stephen MS, Arulchelvam M, Harris JP. Concurrent comparison of endoluminal versus open repair in the treatment of abdominal aortic aneurysms: analysis of 303 patients by life table method. J Vasc Surg 1998; 27(2):213–220; discussion 220–221.

55. Moore WS, Rutherford RB. Transfemoral endovascular repair of abdominal aortic aneurysm: results of the North American EVT phase 1 trial. EVT Investigators. J Vasc Surg 1996; 23(4):543–553.

56. Cuypers PW, Gardien M, Buth J, Peels CH, Charbon JA, Hop WC. Randomized study comparing cardiac response in endovascular and open abdominal aortic aneurysm repair. Br J Surg 2001; 88(8):1059–1065..

57. Matsumura JS, Brewster DC, Makaroun MS, Naftel DC. A multicenter controlled clinical trial of open versus endovascular treatment of abdominal aortic aneurysm. J Vasc Surg 2003; 37(2):262–271.

58. Adriaensen ME, Bosch JL, Halpern EF, Myriam Hunink MG, Gazelle GS. Elective endovascular versus open surgical repair of abdominal aortic aneurysms: systematic review of short-term results. Radiology 2002; 224(3):739–747.

59. Eagle KA, Coley CM, Newell JB, Brewster DC, Darling RC, Strauss HW, Guiney TE, Boucher CA. Combining clinical and thallium data optimizes preoperative assessment of cardiac risk before major vascular surgery. Ann Intern Med 1989; 110(11):859–866.

60. Aziz IN, Lee JT, Kopchok GE, Donayre CE, White RA, de Virgilio C. Cardiac risk stratification in patients undergoing endoluminal graft repair of abdominal aortic aneurysm: a single–institution experience with 365 patients. J Vasc Surg 2003; 38(1):56–60.

61. Aune S, Amundsen SR, Evjensvold J, Trippestad A. Operative mortality and long-term relative survival of patients operated on for asymptomatic abdominal aortic aneurysm. Eur J Vasc Endovasc Surg 1995; 9(3):293–298.

62. Mangano DT, Browner WS, Hollenberg M, London MJ, Tubau JF, Tateo IM. Association of perioperative myocardial ischemia with cardiac morbidity and mortality in men undergoing noncardiac surgery. The Study of Perioperative Ischemia Research Group. N Engl J Med 1990; 323(26):1781–1788.

63. McFalls EO, Ward HB, Santilli S, Scheftel M, Chesler E, Doliszny KM. The influence of perioperative myocardial infarction on long–term prognosis following elective vascular surgery. Chest 1998; 113(3):681–686.

64. Yadav J, Wholey MH, Kuntz RE, Fayad P, Katzen BT, Mishkel GJ, Bajwa TK, Whitlow P, Strickman NE, Jaff MR, Popma JJ, Snead DB, Cutlip DE, Firth BG, Ouriel K. Stenting and Angioplasty with Protection in Patients at High Risk for Endarterectomy (SAPPHIRE) Investigators. N Engl J Med 2004; 351:1493–1501.

4

Complications in Endovascular Therapy: Access-Related Complications

Mark W. Burket
Medical University of Ohio–Toledo, Toledo, Ohio, U.S.A.

INTRODUCTION

All invasive procedures carry the risk of complications. The most common source of complications associated with endovascular procedures is the vascular access site (1). Although certain decisions and techniques may reduce this risk, it can never be completely eliminated. This chapter will address both common and unusual access-related complications, their management, and prevention.

BLOOD LOSS

Blood loss in some form accounts for most, but by no means all, vascular complications. This may range from an inconsequential ooze to fatal bleeding. In between these extremes lie various other manifestations, each with its own clinical character-istics and management.

Numerous patient and procedural characteristics may increase bleeding risk. Female gender, advanced age, hypertension, low body weight, obesity, and renal insufficiency make blood loss more likely, as do a variety of clotting disorders (2–5). Aortic insufficiency, with its "water hammer" pulse, predisposes to poor vascular closure. Procedural characteristics associated with blood loss include the use of thrombolytic (3,5) and antiplatelet drugs. Heparin, especially at high doses and when used after procedure completion, is associated with increased bleeding (3–5). As might be expected, larger access sheaths have been associated with higher bleeding risk (5), although evaluations of large numbers of patients undergoing cor-onary artery interventions failed to show an association (3,4). Likelihood of compli-cations varies with access site. Among the various arterial entry points, radial access carries the lowest risk (6). Properly performed, retrograde femoral artery puncture is also quite safe. Brachial artery entry also carries a low risk (7,8), although somewhat higher than femoral access (6,9). Risk increases with axillary access, presumably due to less ability to achieve adequate post-procedural compression (8,10). Bleeding is most likely with popliteal artery (11) and antegrade femoral artery access.

PERSISTENT BLEEDING

Some patients will demonstrate persistent blood loss from the vascular puncture, despite usual efforts at manual compression, or the use of vascular closure devices. This may occur in the absence of hematoma formation. Usually obvious immediately after the procedure, it may not develop until many hours later, often after patient movement or coughing.

Treatment consists of direct manual pressure. A vascular clamp or FemoStop device (RADI Medical System, Uppsala, Sweden) may be employed if time required for hemostasis is excessive. Blood pressure should be carefully monitored, with appropriate treatment for either hypo- or hypertension. Whenever possible and clinically appropriate, anticoagulant and antiplatelet agents should be stopped and their effects reversed. If these measures fail, surgical repair of the vessel is required. An infrequently used technique, which may be feasible in a small subset of patients, is to temporarily seal the leak by placing an angioplasty balloon in the vessel at the point of hemorrhage (12). The balloon is then inflated to a pressure just sufficient to prevent further blood loss. Use of this method for a number of minutes may result in cessation of bleeding. The obvious risk of this process is the cessation of distal blood flow and possible clot formation. Another infrequently used endovascular repair technique is the placement of a stent graft (12,13).

Much can be said about various strategies to prevent procedural blood loss. Efforts begin with patient selection. In some cases with excessive bleeding risk, for example, those with profound thrombocytopenia or a high international normalized ratio (INR), the risk of bleeding might outweigh the anticipated benefit of the procedure. Canceling the intervention may be the best treatment plan, at least until the clotting defect can be corrected. Efforts should be undertaken to regulate blood pressure in hypertensive patients. Proper access site selection mitigates risk. As an example, a superficial femoral artery angioplasty that could be performed by either ipsilateral antegrade or contralateral retrograde puncture can be performed more safely using the latter approach.

Minimizing risk with femoral arterial puncture requires a thorough understanding of anatomy at and around the common femoral artery. Taking steps to accurately locate the vessel prior to attempted puncture goes a long way toward averting complications. The common femoral artery lies directly over the femoral head (14), and can be easily located using radiographic landmarks (Fig. 1). In addition, the vessel is more anterior at this level than at the adjacent external iliac artery or superficial femoral artery. As a result, the palpable pulse is more prominent over the common femoral artery, as opposed to over these other vessels. It is vitally important to recognize that surface landmarks are notoriously unreliable as indicators of the location of the common femoral. The inguinal skin crease, which may approximate the artery early in life, becomes lower with increasing age and weight, and should not be used as a guide to vascular access (14). Failure to follow these simple steps may lead to inadvertent puncture of the external iliac artery, superficial femoral or profunda (Fig. 2), greatly increasing the risk of bleeding.

Another important technical point to prevent bleeding complications is to enter vessels using a front wall puncture only. The Seldinger technique of passing the access needle through both walls of the vessel, with lumen entry achieved upon partial withdrawal of the needle, is outdated and ill advised, increasing the risk of a complication due to bleeding from the vessel's posterior wall.

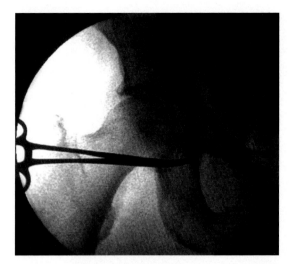

Figure 1 Radiographic image obtained by attaching a hemostat to the sterile drape at the time of angiography. This allows the operator to definitively ascertain the region of the femoral head, and thus, the common femoral artery.

Variations in anatomy at the groin are not uncommon. Most often seen is a high bifurcation of the common femoral artery (Fig. 3). Physicians would be well advised to review any previously performed angiograms, noting such variations

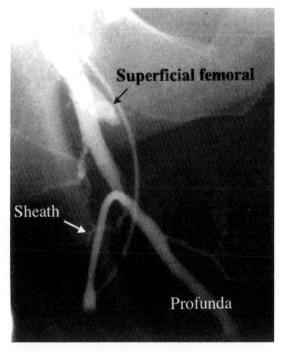

Figure 2 Angiography obtained through a vascular sheath after failed attempt to achieve antegrade common femoral artery access. From this image, it is clear that the puncture was well below the level of the femoral head.

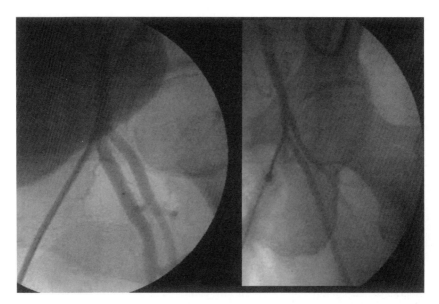

Figure 3 Unusually high bifurcations of the common femoral artery. Although sheath placement is well-centered on the femoral head, vascular entry was achieved at the bifurcation in
one instance (*left*), and in the superficial femoral artery in the other (*right*).

and taking steps to avoid punctures directly into the point of bifurcation, or into the
smaller branch vessels.

Special mention should be made regarding the management of antegrade
femoral access. Whereas the type of vascular sheath is not generally of great importance in most vessel entry sites, care must be taken with antegrade access to employ
only sheaths which are resistant to kinking under flexion. Many conventional
sheaths will kink when flexed to the degree required in antegrade puncture
(Fig. 4). Should the kink develop at the point of vessel entry, a poor seal will result,
causing ongoing blood loss for as long as the sheath remains in place. Because of the
increased bleeding risk associated with antegrade vessel entry, the operator should be
particularly cautious to avoid over anticoagulation or the use of any unnecessary
antiplatelet agents. The sheath should be removed as soon as possible after the
procedure, either by waiting for the activated clotting time to partially correct
after heparin administration, or by accelerating that process with the use of protamine
sulfate. Although commercially available closure devices are intended for retrograde
femoral access, most appear to have similar efficacy when used after antegrade puncture
(15,16). Experience with this application is much less than with retrograde access. Duda
and colleagues reported 80 consecutive patients who underwent percutaneous suture-
mediated closure after antegrade procedures (17). Hemostasis was achieved in 96%.
In this series, one patient required surgery for retroperitoneal hematoma and one had
a pseudoaneurysm which closed spontaneously.

HEMATOMA

Direct blood loss through the puncture tract to the skin surface is immediately
obvious and easily assessed. Bleeding into the subcutaneous tissues may be less

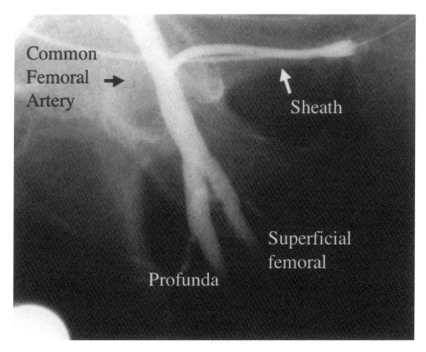

Figure 4 Antegrade access into the common femoral artery. Note the extreme angle of flexion demonstrated by the sheath in this approach.

apparent, especially with popliteal or femoral arterial entry, and particularly in obese patients. Pain reported by the patient may be an earlier manifestation of this complication than visual clues or a palpable hematoma. Eventually, most patients will develop a firm, palpable, tender hematoma. Given variations in normal anatomy from patient to patient, a simple comparison to the contralateral (non-punctured) side may help to confirm the diagnosis. It is important to recognize that blood tends to dissect along tissue planes offering the least resistance. Thus, a leak from the femoral artery will spread into the flank, thigh, and external genitalia. Men with moderate to severe blood loss may develop massive swelling of the scrotum and/or penis. Ecchymosis may be present to a variable degree. There may be extensive blood loss, an easily palpable hematoma, and yet no ecchymosis. In contrast, some bleeding episodes may only manifest themselves as ecchymosis. With time, virtually all large hematomas will develop significant ecchymosis, with extension over the lower abdomen, flank, and thigh being quite common. Occasionally discoloration may be seen below the knee after femoral artery blood loss. Brachial arterial bleeds may be followed by ecchymosis involving much of the arm.

Small- to moderate-sized hematomas result in patient discomfort, but rarely lead to serious adverse outcomes. Large hematomas may create severe complications. Blood loss may lead to anemia, hypotension, and even death. The mass effect created may cause compression of adjacent veins, leading to obstruction with or without thrombosis. Compression of nerves may lead to irreversible injury. Large hematomas may place sufficient tension on the skin so as to lead to skin necrosis.

Management

Early in the course of hematoma formation, manual pressure may serve not only to prevent further bleeding, but perhaps also to reduce the hematoma, spreading the blood throughout the surrounding tissues and decreasing the mass effect. The use of sandbags as a means of applying pressure is controversial. While there may be some benefit accrued, sandbags fail to focus pressure directly over the site of bleeding. In addition, the presence of a sandbag over the hematoma makes it impossible to assess for further enlargement. A FemoStop device (RADI Medical System, Uppsala, Sweden) allows for more focused pressure application and for better visualization of the region in question. Prolonged bed rest is advisable, with the exact duration dependent upon the severity of the bleeding episode. In rare instances, direct pressure is inadequate to limit growth of the hematoma. In this life-threatening situation, which can rapidly deteriorate into shock, urgent surgical evacuation of the hematoma and repair of the vessel are mandatory. Other indications for surgery include mass effect leading to venous obstruction, nerve injury, or potential skin necrosis. In the absence of these abnormalities even large hematomas will resolve without surgery. Patients should be informed that this process will take weeks or even months, and will be associated with discomfort which will progressively decrease. During this process extensive areas of unsightly ecchymosis will be present.

COMPARTMENT SYNDROME

Blood loss from the access site may lead to compartment syndrome, characterized by an increase in tissue pressure within an enclosed anatomic space, jeopardizing tissue function and viability.

In the condition is diagnosed by painful swelling in the affected region, followed by loss of sensory and motor function (18). Irreversible muscle and nerve injury may develop unless the condition is promptly diagnosed and treated. The diagnosis may be established by history and physical examination alone, although direct measurement of compartment pressure helps to confirm the diagnosis. To determine this pressure, a needle or small catheter is first introduced into the affected compartment. A variety of measuring tools may then be employed, from a simple fluid-filled manometer to devices specifically designed to measure compartment pressure (19).

Predisposing Factors

In order for compartment syndrome to develop as a complication of an invasive procedure, there must be both blood loss and predisposing anatomy. Whereas bleeding is not infrequent after femoral artery access, the anatomy in this region does not predispose to compartment syndrome. In contrast, the arm and lower leg are more vulnerable to this complication. Although not a frequently used access site in many interventional practices, the popliteal artery often proves useful in completing challenging femoral artery interventions. This utility comes at a cost, however: Scheinert and colleagues (11) reported a 10.7% complication rate in a series of 103 patients. Most of these were bleeding complications. This bleeding occurs in proximity to the leg's posterior compartments, and thus careful surveillance must be maintained after use of this access point. This diagnosis should also be entertained after bleeding complications develop with brachial or axillary artery access (20). The

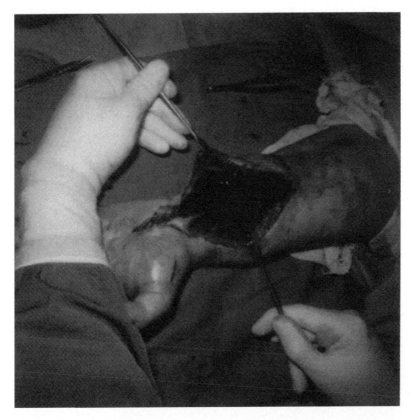

Figure 5 Surgery performed to treat compartment syndrome resulting from radial artery access. The patient had received heparin, aspirin, clopidogrel, and abciximab.

radial artery is superficial and readily compressible after sheath removal. As a result, significant blood loss at this site is rare. Nevertheless, if bleeding does occur, nearby compartments in the forearm and hand are vulnerable, with potentially serious effects (Fig. 5).

Short- and Long-Term Consequences/Sequelae

If not promptly treated, compartment syndrome leads to irreversible nerve and muscle injury. Once the diagnosis is made, surgical decompression with fasciotomy should be promptly pursued.

Prevention entails taking the steps described above which mitigate bleeding risk. Special mention should be made regarding the management of the two sites more commonly associated with this complication.

Popliteal Access

This is the deepest of all standard vascular access sites, and thus the most difficult to assess for occult bleeding. If the patient was hypertensive during the procedure, additional efforts should be made to decrease the blood pressure prior to sheath removal. Heparin should either be reversed with protamine or its effect allowed to diminish until the activated clotting time is 180 seconds or less. Closure devices are contraindicated at this location, not only due to vessel size, but also due to the fact that the popliteal vein is more superficial than the artery and could be permanently occluded and/or thrombosed by currently available equipment. An experienced staff member should be recruited for the task of sheath withdrawal, maintaining very firm pressure over the site of arterial puncture for at least 10 minutes. It is prudent to assess distal flow during compression by means of palpation or use of a hand-held Doppler device at the ankle.

Brachial Access

The brachial artery typically bifurcates into the radial and ulnar arteries just distal to the elbow joint (Fig. 6). In order to avoid this bifurcation, as well as the flexion associated with puncture over the elbow, vascular sheaths should be placed approximately 2 cm proximal to the joint. As with popliteal access, efforts should be made to

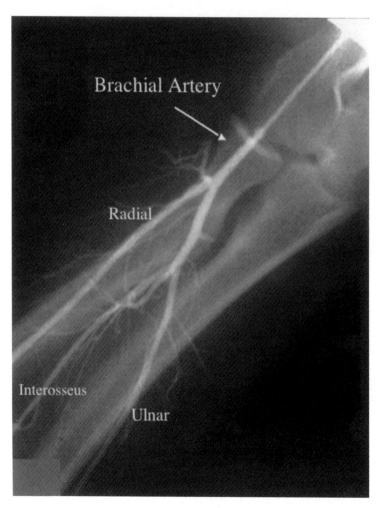

Figure 6 Normal anatomy at the level of brachial artery bifurcation.

normalize blood pressure and clotting status prior to sheath withdrawal. Unfortunately, no commercially available closure devices are designed for brachial access. This artery is relatively difficult to compress. Once again, an experienced staff member should be chosen for sheath withdrawal. Firm pressure should be applied over the puncture site for at least 10 minutes, occasionally checking the radial pulse at the wrist to ensure the presence of at least some pulsatile flow.

PSEUDOANEURYSM

Pseudoaneurysm represents the accumulation of pulsatile blood in tissues adjacent to the site of vascular entry. It is distinguished from a true aneurysm in that its borders are made up of adjacent soft tissues rather than by the vessel wall itself. This abnormality is typically apparent within 24 to 48 hours of the invasive procedure, but may not develop until several days later (21). It is diagnosed by the presence of a pulsatile mass, typically very painful and tender to palpation, and associated with a bruit. Ecchymosis may or may not be present. Diagnosis is confirmed using duplex ultrasound, in which the pseudoaneurysm cavity is identified, connected to the parent vessel with a tract, or neck, in which bi-directional blood flow is visualized (Fig. 7). Multiple cavities may be present.

The femoral artery is the vessel most commonly associated with pseudoaneurysm formation. This is to be expected, as it is the most frequently used arterial access point,

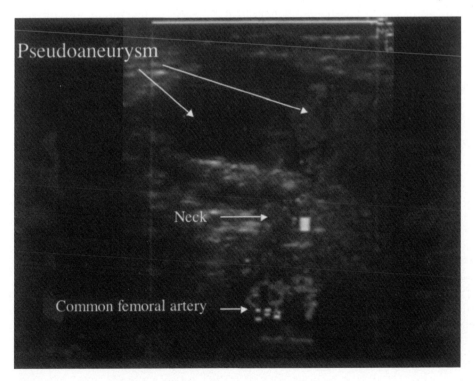

Figure 7 Duplex ultrasound image of an arterial pseudoaneurysm, demonstrating vessel of origin, neck, and pseudoaneurysm cavity.

and the anatomy in this region permits the formation of a pseudoaneurysm cavity. The incidence of this complication is 0.05–0.4% following femoral access (22,23).

Pseudoaneurysm may be seen at any location of arterial entry, including brachial (23,24) axillary, radial, and popliteal access. In the popliteal access series mentioned above, pseudoaneurysm was observed in 2.9% of patients (11).

High dose and post-procedural heparin (22), antiplatelet agents, and hypertension predispose to pseudoaneurysm formation. The location of the vascular puncture also plays an important predisposing role. Vessel entry below the femoral head, that is in the superficial femoral or profunda, has been associated with a dramatically higher rate of this complication (14,24–26) (Fig. 8). Neither vessel can be adequately compressed at the conclusion of the angiographic procedure. Puncture directly into the bifurcation of the common femoral artery into the profunda and the superficial femoral artery has been observed to predispose to this complication (27). None of the currently available closure devices has been shown to decrease the risk of this complication, and in fact when pseudoaneurysm develops after closure device use, it may be more complex and harder to treat.

From the patients' perspective, the major concern with most pseudoaneurysms is the severe associated pain. The greatest risk, however, lies in the fact that a small minority may rupture, with potentially life-threatening blood loss. Other complications relate to a mass effect, with compression of adjacent nerves or veins. This may lead to irreversible nerve injury and venous obstruction with thrombosis. Skin necrosis may develop with very large pseudoaneurysms (23).

It has been well recognized that many pseudoaneurysms thrombose spontaneously without adverse sequelae (22). As this is the natural course of many small pseudoaneurysms, a reasonable management strategy is observation without specific therapy. Repeat physical examinations and a follow-up duplex ultrasound to confirm that spontaneous closure has occurred are advisable.

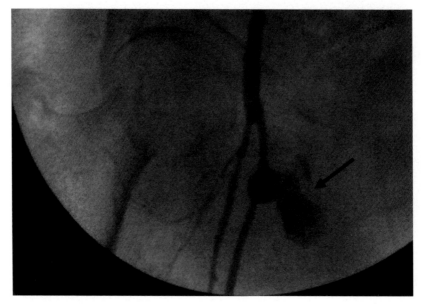

Figure 8 Angiogram demonstrating pseudoaneurysm originating from the superficial femoral artery, after puncture distal to the femoral head.

Management for larger pseudoaneurysms has undergone considerable evolution over recent years. Surgical management, once the mainstay of therapy, is now seldom required. When needed, the procedure consists of evacuation of the hematoma, and suture closure of the arterial puncture site. In the 1990s, a non-invasive approach was proposed by means of ultrasound-directed compression (27). With this technique, ultrasound imaging was used to visualize both the pseudoaneurysm, and the neck connecting it to the vessel lumen. Pressure was then applied to the pseudoaneurysm with the ultrasound probe until flow in the neck ceased. Periodic assessment was made, again using ultrasound, to determine when flow was no longer present upon release of pressure, thus indicating that the pseudoaneurysm and its neck had thrombosed. Although initial reports presented high success rates (21,27), subsequent series showed a wide variation in procedural outcome (4,12) with typical efficacy around 75% (28). In addition, direct pressure on the pseudoaneurysm produced moderate to severe pain, often requiring narcotic analgesia, and sometimes necessitating termination of the treatment attempt.

Although initially described in 1986 (29), the technique of direct injection of thrombin into pseudoaneurysms has only recently been popularized, and has now become the preferred treatment in most cases (23,24). Advantages of this approach include the avoidance of an open surgical procedure, yet with much less patient discomfort and a higher rate of success than was seen in many ultrasound compression studies. Most procedures are performed under ultrasound guidance, with small amounts (as little as 500–1000 U) of bovine thrombin introduced using a small gauge needle introduced through the skin. Ultrasound guidance allows needle introduction as far away from the neck as possible, in order to minimize the risk of embolization into the parent artery. Long, narrow necks are ideal, also presenting less risk of thrombin introduction into the vessel of origin. Needle introduction into the pseudoaneurysm cavity and subsequent cessation of blood flow can be confirmed under duplex ultrasound. This technique proved successful in 94% of patients in a recent series, using small volumes of bovine thrombin injected at a concentration of 1000 U/cc (23). This success rate occurred despite the fact that 30% of the patients were receiving anticoagulant therapy, and most were on antiplatelet drugs. A three-way stopcock allowed confirmation of entrance into the cavity by aspiration of blood and by injection of saline under ultrasound, prior to the injection of thrombin. Care must be taken not to introduce blood into the syringe containing thrombin, which would lead to clotting the syringe and needle.

Contraindications to thrombin injection include wide necks with open communication between the false aneurysm and vessel of origin, infected pseudoaneurysms, and presence of compression of the adjacent vein (30). In the latter instance, thrombosis of the cavity leaves the vein compression unaltered, setting the stage for deep venous thrombosis. Surgical evacuation is preferable. Anaphylaxis after thrombin injection has been reported in a patient who had had multiple prior exposures to this agent (31). In patients with a history of repeated exposure, skin testing prior to this form of treatment is recommended. Other allergic-type reactions of lesser severity have been reported.

Some operators have chosen to treat pseudoaneurysms in the angiographic suite instead of with the use of duplex ultrasound. After sterile skin preparation, a small needle may be introduced into the pseudoaneurysm cavity. Aspiration of blood confirms appropriate needle placement. A small volume of contrast is then injected, defining the anatomic characteristics of the cavity (Fig. 9). Thrombin is then injected, clotting the pseudoaneurysm. Although concomitant angiography is not required, the pseudoaneurysm can typically be readily identified, if desired, using

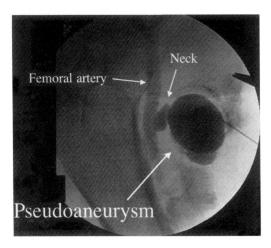

Figure 9 Radiographic image of a pseudoaneurysm obtained by direct puncture and injection of contrast. The neck and vessel of origin are also demonstrated.

digital subtraction technique. Repeat angiography after thrombin injection confirms thrombosis and obliteration of the tract and cavity. There are several reports of the use of an angioplasty balloon to temporarily occlude the vessel at the origin of the tract into the pseudoaneurysm during thrombin injection. This prevents reflux of thrombin from the cavity into the vessel, which could potentially lead to catastrophic thrombus formation and limb threat (12,32). Severe acute ischemia of both the upper and lower extremity has been reported after use of thrombin injection (33,34).

Covered stents have also been employed successfully to treat pseudoaneurysm (5,12). Although the minimally invasive nature of this strategy is appealing, the anatomy associated with many pseudoaneurysms lends itself poorly to this treatment. Covered stent placement at the common femoral artery is ill-advised as it may preclude subsequent use of this vessel for surgical bypass or vascular entry for angiography. Joint flexion may lead to metal fatigue and stent fracture. Placement of the graft material over the orifice of the profunda would obstruct flow into this vitally important vessel. Other commonly used vessel entry locations also tend to be poorly suited to covered stent placement. The brachial artery is small in diameter, near a joint, and may be near a bifurcation. The popliteal artery is subject to a large degree of flexion. Regardless of location, stent thrombosis is a potential complication. For all practical purposes, covered stents are helpful only when inadvertent puncture of the superficial femoral artery is complicated by pseudoaneurysm. Coil embolization to treat pseudoaneurysm has also been described (5,12).

Regardless of the non-surgical technique chosen to treat pseudoaneurysm, a follow-up duplex ultrasound should be performed, typically about 24 hours after closure. A small percentage will recur, making confirmation of persistent treatment efficacy advisable.

RETROPERITONEAL HEMATOMA

Special mention must be made of retroperitoneal hematoma because it is a complication which may be easily overlooked until it reaches life-threatening severity. This problem typically is associated with femoral arterial access, after which blood leaks into the retroperitoneal cavity, typically tracking along the iliopsoas muscle. A common symptom is that of back pain, which caregivers may readily dismiss as a normal concomitant of prolonged bed rest associated with femoral access procedures. The degree of back pain, however, may exceed that normally attributable to femoral procedures, requiring substantial doses of narcotic analgesia (35). Flank and/or abdominal pain may also be reported. Absence of pain does not preclude the diagnosis (13,35). Pelvic blood accumulation may compress the bladder (Fig. 10) and/or rectum, creating an urge to urinate or defecate. As blood loss continues, hypotension, tachycardia, and eventually shock may become manifest.

It is important to emphasize that the physical examination may yield no clues to this diagnosis. Retroperitoneal hematoma may develop completely independent of any visible or palpable blood loss at the groin. Ecchymosis is usually absent, especially early in the course of this complication.

Those factors described above which predispose to bleeding in general also increase the risk of retroperitoneal hematoma. Other characteristics specifically related to femoral access compound the risk. Vessel entry above the inguinal ligament creates a two-fold threat (35,36). First, since the puncture site is located cranial to the femoral head, direct compression over the entry site is impaired. Second, when bleeding does occur, it is much easier for blood to pass directly into the retroperitoneal space. Continuation of anticoagulation after the invasive procedure increases

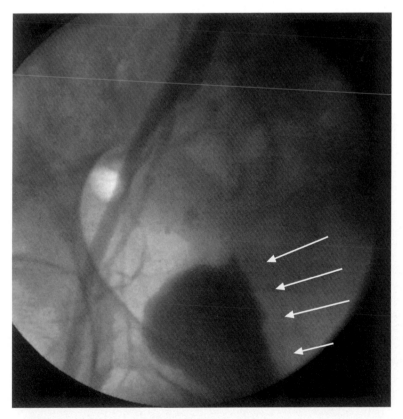

Figure 10 Radiographic demonstration of bladder compression (*arrows*) caused by a left-sided retroperitoneal hematoma.

the risk (35,36). Double arterial wall puncture, as used in the Seldinger technique, predisposes to a posterior wall bleed into the retroperitoneum. Finally, antegrade femoral access may increase the risk of this complication.

The greatest risk associated with retroperitoneal hematoma is excessive, possibly even fatal, blood loss. Additional untoward events include nerve compression which may result in both sensory and motor deficits. Retroperitoneal hematoma appears to be the most common cause of nerve injury related to arterial access. The size of the hematoma is not predictive of the presence of nerve dysfunction (37). Although the initial disability associated with nerve injury may be significant, deficits generally completely resolve over time (37). Other complications related to mass effect may also develop, such as venous obstruction with or without thrombosis.

The single most important aspect of the management of retroperitoneal hematoma is the maintenance of a high index of suspicion. It should always be considered when a patient experiences post-procedural hypotension or back, flank, or abdominal pain. As these findings are commonly encountered after angiography, obviously not every instance requires full evaluation. Rather, when they are more pronounced in terms of severity or duration, consideration should be given to further testing. The most appropriate initial step is to obtain an abdominal and pelvic computerized tomography scan, which can confirm the diagnosis in most cases (Fig. 11). Intravenous fluids and blood transfusion should be undertaken as appropriate for the degree of blood loss and hypotension. Whenever possible, anticoagulant and antiplatelet agents should be discontinued and reversed. If the patient is not already under the care of a surgeon, surgical consultation is appropriate, even though operative correction is uncommonly required (13). Most retroperitoneal bleeds are self-limited, provided the above-mentioned steps are followed. Indications for surgery include ongoing blood loss, or nerve or vein compression (36). There are also reports

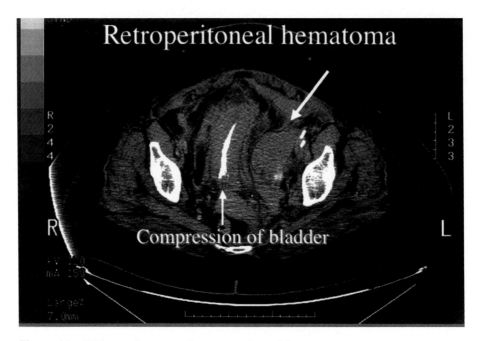

Figure 11   CT image demonstrating retroperitoneal hematoma.

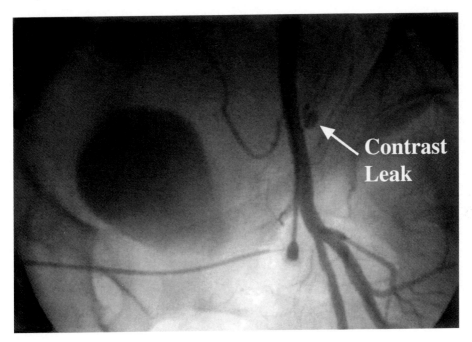

Figure 12 Left iliofemoral angiogram obtained to identify bleeding source in a patient who developed retroperitoneal hematoma after multiple left groin needle punctures during access attempts.

of angiographic identification of the leak (Fig. 12), followed by sealing using balloon tamponade (38) or placement of a covered stent (12). Whereas these techniques may prove effective in preventing additional blood loss, they do not directly impact the mass effect and compressive findings that may accompany large bleeds.

Prevention of retroperitoneal hematoma is usually accomplished by following the general steps listed earlier to avoid any type of blood loss. Special mention should be made of one situation which places the patient at particular risk of this complication, namely inadvertent puncture of the external iliac artery. Although this can occur during any procedure, it may be seen more commonly in obese patients, especially when fluoroscopic imaging of the femoral head has been used to identify the location for needle entry. If the needle is advanced at the standard angle, it will pass farther cephalad than normal due to the additional thickness of subcutaneous tissue. After sheath removal, the external iliac artery is much more difficult to compress than is the common femoral artery, especially in the obese, greatly increasing the risk of bleeding. If post-procedural angiography through the vascular sheath is not performed, this situation may be easily overlooked. If angiography is performed, external iliac artery entry is obvious (Fig. 13). Due to concerns about the inability to achieve hemostasis manually, it is the author's practice to use a mechanical vascular closure device, although at least one manufacturer warns against such an application (15).

ARTERIOVENOUS FISTULA

Arteriovenous fistula represents post-procedural direct communication between access artery and vein. Small arteriovenous fistulae may be difficult to detect

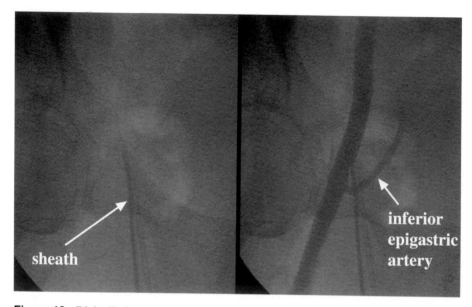

Figure 13 Right iliofemoral angiogram in a 375-pound patient demonstrating vessel entry into the distal external iliac artery. A vascular closure device was used with good hemostasis.

clinically. There may be no symptoms, and physical examination may be normal or remarkable only for a bruit over the affected site. A thrill may be present. Duplex ultrasound may be used to confirm the diagnosis (13). Larger fistulae, especially if chronic, may result in palpable vessel enlargement. A significant shunt may lead to heart failure symptoms. Ischemic limb symptoms may be present, particularly in the presence of distal arterial obstructive disease in which the flow into the low-pressure vein creates a steal phenomenon. This complication may occur at any point of vessel entry. It is seen most commonly between the femoral artery and vein, presumably because far more procedures are performed at this access point. At this location its incidence is approximately 0.9% (39). The anatomic relationships which most predispose to arteriovenous fistula, however, are found at the popliteal artery. As the popliteal vein lies posterior to the artery, it is not at all uncommon to pass through the vein on the way into the artery. An arteriovenous fistula may readily develop, whether clinically apparent or not.

Predisposing factors for arteriovenous fistula formation include excessive anticoagulation, hypertension, female gender, and accessing the left groin while standing at the patient's right side (39). The latter risk may be due to alteration of the typical angle of entry, resulting in a greater chance of puncture of both artery and vein. Overlap of artery and vein makes this complication more likely. As mentioned above, this is a common occurrence at the popliteal artery. It is less commonly observed in the region of the femoral artery, however, fistula formation between the femoral artery and underlying lateral circumflex vein has been well described (22). The use of large sheaths may increase the chance of this complication. Any procedure in which both artery and vein (whether intentional or accidental) are punctured in close proximity to each other may also make fistula formation more likely (26). Puncture below the femoral head has been associated with arteriovenous fistula (22,26) (Fig. 14).

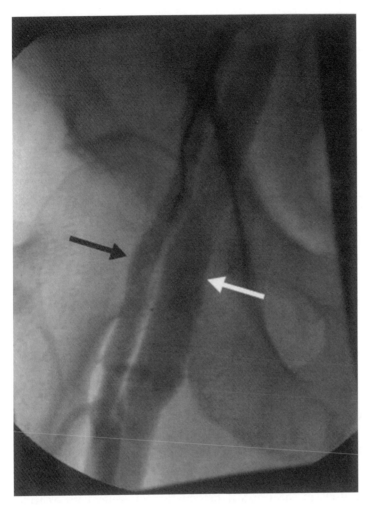

Figure 14 Angiographic demonstration of a right femoral arteriovenous fistula. Injection into the artery (*black arrow*) resulted in immediate opacification of the vein (*white arrow*) in a patient with a history of prior angiography with right-sided access. Note that the level of the fistula is well below the femoral head.

Most arteriovenous fistulae may never cause symptoms or complications. In the largest reported series to date, there were no cases of limb ischemia or heart failure among 88 patients with this disorder (39). Many close spontaneously (22,39). Although often cited as a potential complication, heart failure is infrequently seen; presumably due to the relatively low shunt volume (39). In fact, measurement of shunt volume has shown that it is typically less than that created by a dialysis access procedure (40). Other potential sequelae include aneurysmal dilatation.

Management

Most arteriovenous fistulae be observed without specific treatment. Those which have caused symptoms should be corrected. In most instances this is accomplished with surgical closure. Ultrasound-guided compression has been successfully attempted (27). An alternative approach is the placement of a covered stent at the site of arterial origin. This technique has been used with considerable success, although the limitations described above (under treatment of pseudoaneurysm) apply (5). In contrast to this percutaneous approach, open repair can be performed regardless of the proximity to joints or bifurcations.

Prevention

Effective control of hypertension in the periprocedural period may decrease the risk of arteriovenous fistula. Excessive anticoagulation, both in terms of dose and duration, should be avoided. Best avoidance strategies also include the use of small sheaths placed carefully into the intended target artery. Care should be taken post-procedure to insure adequate hemostasis. Routine screening with ultrasound to detect vessel overlap is not practical. Some studies have suggested that the popliteal vein lies somewhat lateral to the artery and that there may be benefit in directing the puncture needle from medial to lateral. This approach may be overly optimistic, however, as the vein may lie directly posterior to the artery and be impossible to avoid.

OCCLUSIVE COMPLICATIONS

As mentioned previously, most, but by no means all, access complications involve some form of bleeding. Vessel occlusion represents another type of adverse outcome which requires prompt and accurate diagnosis and appropriate treatment.

ACCESS SITE OCCLUSION

As indicated in discussions above, the common femoral artery is the most commonly employed vascular entry site, and thus accounts for most occlusive complications. Acute obstruction of the common femoral artery usually becomes immediately obvious, manifesting itself in the classical presentation of acute limb ischemia (a cool limb with pain and pallor, progressing on to sensory loss and eventually motor dysfunction). It is worth mentioning that pulse examination at the groin may be deceptive. The distal external iliac artery pulse may be palpable and may be mistaken for the common femoral pulse, which is no longer present. Since the location of occlusion prevents all flow in the superficial femoral and profunda femoris, this complication is rarely clinically unapparent. It is highly unlikely that collateral pathways have developed to a sufficient degree to provide adequate blood supply to the limb.

Obstruction at other entry sites presents in a similar fashion. Brachial, axillary, and popliteal occlusions typically produce similar acute limb ischemia manifestations. The exception to this rule lies in radial artery access. Provided the operator has shown appropriate diligence in assuring a normal Allen's test, there should be no symptoms associated with acute radial artery occlusion. Physical examination may also be unrevealing in that perfusion to the hand remains intact. Even the radial pulse may remain palpable proximal and/or distal to the point of obstruction. The only detectable problem may be the presence of an abnormal reverse Allen's test. That is, after compression of both the radial and ulnar arteries, pallor is still present in the palm after release of the radial artery, indicating that it is unable to supply adequate flow to the hand.

Predisposing Factors

Several characteristics predispose to the development of acute closure at the point of vascular entry. Atherosclerosis at the puncture site is an important factor in several respects. This disease process results in a smaller lumen, which will be less tolerant to additional reduction in area by thrombus accumulation, excessive manual pressure, or a poorly positioned vascular closure device. Plaque disruption by the entry needle, wire and/or sheath may further reduce the lumen diameter, and in addition serves as an effective nidus for clot formation.

Smaller diameter vessels are more prone to abrupt occlusion than are larger ones. As with the case of a vessel compromised by atherosclerotic disease, vessels with smaller lumens are less tolerant to further diameter reduction by thrombus, dissection, or other means.

Other factors predisposing to vessel occlusion include poor distal runoff, regardless of cause. Patients with hypercoagulable states carry a higher risk of this complication.

Several procedural factors bear mentioning. Vessel dissection at the time of entry or on subsequent catheter manipulation greatly increases risk. Inadequate anticoagulation, particularly when the access sheath is occlusive within the vessel, is another causative factor. Finally, the use of manual pressure or compressive devices that result in prolonged vessel occlusion may be followed by thrombosis of the artery.

Consequences

Without definitive treatment, acute access site closure may progress to permanent nerve injury, muscle necrosis, limb loss, and even death.

Management

Without question, one of the most crucial aspects in the management of this complication is rapid diagnosis and initiation of treatment. Early in the course of this process, there is little thrombus burden and it has not yet become organized. It responds well to thrombolytic therapy and/or mechanical thrombectomy. With delay, clot will tend to propagate and become more solidified, greatly increasing the difficulty of treatment. The permanent injuries listed above will also begin to develop.

Through one means or another, flow must be promptly restored and the obstruction treated. Specific treatment plans will vary with the nature of the vessel, the cause of the obstruction, and the equipment and skills available to the operator. Often the best strategy is to pursue prompt angiography. This allows for definitive confirmation of the diagnosis and delineation of the location of obstruction. Should mechanical thrombectomy be chosen as the initial treatment, this can be pursued at once (Fig. 15). Similarly, catheter-directed thrombolysis can be initiated in the angiographic suite.

In many instances, the use of a thrombectomy catheter such as the Possis AngioJet, may be the best initial treatment (41). It offers the advantage of being percutaneous, thus avoiding surgical access to the affected vessel. Current versions require only a six French arterial access sheath. When used in conjunction with systemic heparinization, it is effective in removing fresh thrombus (42). Residual clot may be treated with adjunctive thrombolysis and/or anticoagulation.

Catheter-directed thrombolysis without mechanical thrombectomy may be sufficient in some cases. This should generally be reserved for milder cases in which

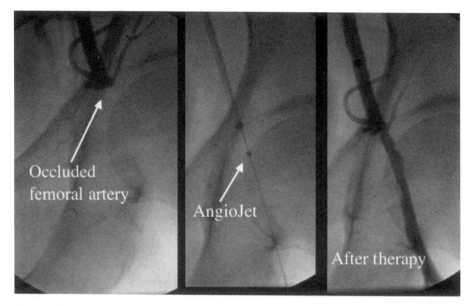

Figure 15 Images obtained in a patient who presented with acute limb ischemia shortly after left groin access. (*Left*): Complete occlusion of the common femoral artery at its origin. (*Middle*): After right femoral sheath placement and traversing the aortic bifurcation, a guide-wire is advanced into the distal vessel. The tip of the AngioJet is seen in the occluded segment. (*Right*): Patency restored after AngioJet treatment.

no nerve or motor dysfunction is evident. Once these findings are observed, more direct means of re-establishing blood flow are in order.

When effective percutaneous mechanical thrombectomy devices are unavailable, arteriotomy and the use of a balloon thrombectomy catheter may be the best option. Surgery is also indicated when dissection or atherosclerotic plaque has occluded the vessel and is not amenable to percutaneous treatment. It is important to bear in mind that stent placement, although feasible and effective to alleviate many common femoral arterial problems, should be avoided in nearly all cases. Stent placement at this location prevents or greatly complicates the later use of this vessel as an anastomotic site for vascular grafting. It may render subsequent percutaneous access impossible. Finally, stent placement over a joint is undesirable because of the repeated flexion at this location. In contrast, surgical repair of the common femoral artery is straightforward and not associated with any of these drawbacks.

Prevention

Not surprisingly, prevention of vessel occlusion is drastically easier than its treatment. Preventative steps begin well before vessel entry. When various access sites are available, those with larger diameters carry lower risk. The use of micropuncture technique may reduce vascular trauma and complications in smaller vessels. This involves the use of a 21-gauge needle (Fig. 16), through which a 0.018-inch guidewire is passed into the vessel. The two-part micropuncture introducer (Fig. 17) is then advanced into the vessel. The guidewire and inner cannula are then removed, leaving a four or five French sheath in place that can accept a 0.035 or 0.038-inch guidewire. This allows placement of a conventional vascular access sheath.

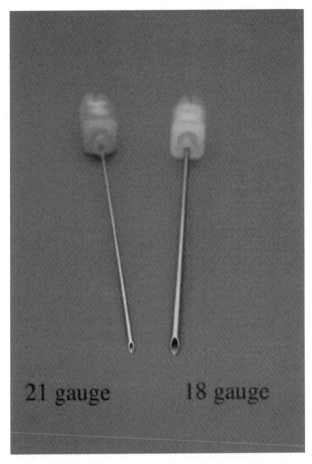

Figure 16 Comparison of the size of the 21-gauge needle used in the micropuncture technique with that of a conventional 18-gauge access needle.

Vessels with well-established atherosclerotic disease should be avoided. Sheath diameter should be limited to that which is necessary to readily complete the case. The steps of the procedure should be well thought out in advance, with equipment prepared beforehand whenever possible, in order to minimize the time that the sheath is in the vessel. This is especially important when the access sheath is of sufficient diameter so as to occlude the entry vessel. Also important in situations in which the sheath occludes the lumen is the maintenance of adequate anticoagulation throughout the case. When radial artery access is employed, the sheath typically occludes the entry vessel. Studies have demonstrated that higher doses of heparin are associated with lower rates of post-procedural radial artery occlusion.

A general rule of angiography is to never forcefully advance a guidewire. Adherence to this rule diminishes the chance of vessel dissection and access site occlusion.

Once the procedure has been completed, careful access site management is helpful in preventing subsequent occlusion. If closure is accomplished by manual compression, care should be taken to avoid prolonged pressure which completely obstructs flow. A good rule of thumb is that after initial control of bleeding has been achieved, distal limb pulses should be palpable or detectable by Doppler ultrasound

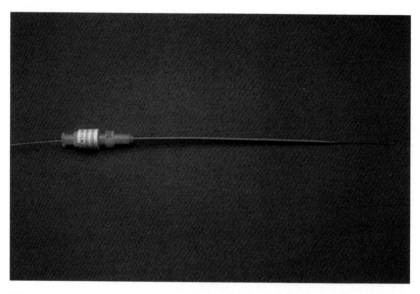

Figure 17 Micropuncture kit showing 0.018-inch guidewire and two-part introducer.

during access compression. If use of one of the commercially available closure devices is considered, angiography through the sheath should be performed to insure that sheath location, and vessel diameter and condition are suitable (Fig. 18). Most devices are not appropriate when there is advanced atherosclerosis at the entry site, and vessel diameter less than 5 mm may preclude use (16).

A brief mention should be made at this point about the incidental finding of iatrogenic arterial dissection at or near the point of vessel entry. In most cases, this situation does not call for specific therapy, provided normal flow is preserved. Some form of treatment will generally be required when there is evidence of hemodynamic impairment, such as diminished flow on angiography, a pressure gradient, or ischemic symptoms.

Special mention should also be made of vessel occlusion that occurs distal to the entry site upon withdrawal of the access sheath. There are at least two possible ways for this to occur. Thrombus may accumulate within the sheath. As it is withdrawn, if manual pressure is applied to the skin and soft tissues over the sheath, the clot may be "milked" out of the sheath and into the vessel. The clot then passes distally until it reaches a vessel of comparable diameter, where it becomes occlusive. In other instances, clot forms on the outside of the sheath. During withdrawal, this clot is stripped off the surface and into the vessel lumen, again with a similar outcome.

When such arterial occlusion occurs, it may be clinically unapparent. This could readily occur if the clot were to lodge in a well-collateralized distal vessel. In other instances, acute limb ischemia may be seen, such as when the embolus occludes the distal popliteal artery. In such cases, the tools and techniques described above may be effective. A simpler and more direct approach, however, may simply be to place an end-hole catheter, such as a six French multipurpose guide catheter, in direct contact with the clot. A 20 cc or larger syringe is then attached to the catheter and the clot aspirated. Continuous suction should be applied until the catheter tip is outside of the body. This procedure may be repeated several times until flow is restored (Figs. 19 and 20).

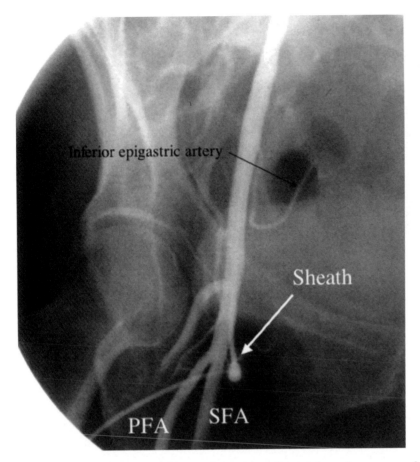

Figure 18 Right anterior oblique angiography performed through a common femoral arterial sheath. The sheath is well placed in the common femoral artery, above the bifurcation. The artery is of sufficient diameter and condition to allow use of any standard closure device.

ACCESS SITE INFECTION

Infection of the soft tissues at the point of vascular access, with or without involvement of the vessel itself, is an unusual but potentially serious complication. This may run the full spectrum from a mild superficial and self-limited problem to severe involvement requiring surgical intervention and prolonged antibiotic treatment.

Predisposing Factors

Despite ubiquitous bacterial skin colonization, infection following invasive procedures is remarkably infrequent. This low infection rate is seen in part because typical procedures are relatively brief in duration, with no prolonged placement of catheters or sheaths. Infection rates may increase if these materials are left in place, such as with overnight catheter-directed infusions of thrombolytic agents. Patient characteristics that may increase risk of infection include disorders of immunity, diabetes, obesity, or repeat procedures using the same access site over a short time period (43). Closure device use may predispose to access site infection (44). Regardless of which device is

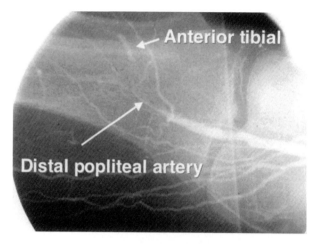

Figure 19 Embolic occlusion of the distal popliteal artery resulting in acute limb ischemia immediately after removal of a femoral arterial sheath. The anterior tibial artery is faintly visualized.

employed, some foreign material remains in the vessel wall and/or in the adjacent tissues (Fig. 21). This may serve as a nidus of infection. Because of this foreign material, infections related to closure device use may be particularly severe (43). Treatment may include surgical debridement, removal of the closure device, and repair of the vessel as needed. Prolonged antibiotic therapy is required.

Prevention

Prevention of infection starts with appropriate access site selection. Puncture should be avoided in areas of skin or soft tissue infection. A location should be chosen that

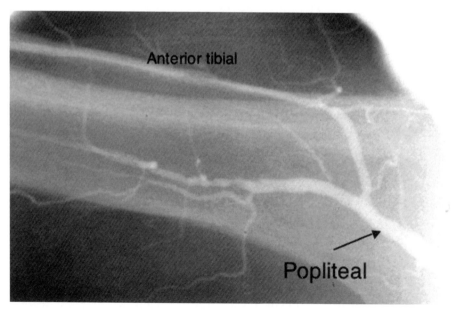

Figure 20 Same patient as seen in Figure 19, with restoration of flow after thrombus aspiration through an end-hole catheter.

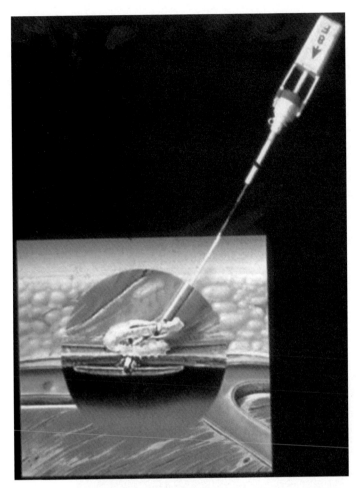

Figure 21 Detailed image of a vascular closure device demonstrating material left within the vessel lumen and adjacent tissues.

has not recently been employed for a percutaneous procedure. Sheaths and catheters should be left in place for the minimum feasible duration. When using a closure device, special care should be maintained to insure sterility in the region of the puncture. Manufacturers' instructions for use advise against closure device application in situations in which sterility cannot be maintained (15,16). The use of antibiotic prophylaxis with these devices has not been systematically evaluated.

It is important to recognize that the use of closure devices has not been associated with a decrease in access complications (5,44,45). Their unequivocal benefit lies in the facilitation of early ambulation. All of the complications cited within this chapter may be seen with these tools. In some cases, such as with infection, their use may greatly complicate management. Some authors have reported that pseudoaneurysms and bleeding complications may also be harder to manage in the presence of closure device use (13). Some adverse outcomes have been related specifically to closure device use and would not have occurred in their absence. Examples include acute vessel closure due to positioning of some portion of the device in such a way that it occludes the arterial lumen. In some instances there may be immediate complete occlusion. In other instances the device may be partially obstructive, serving as a nidus for clot, which completes the occlusion. Should partial obstruction occur without superimposed thrombus, new-onset claudication may be seen. Many of the currently available vascular closure tools involve some intravascular manipulation. During these steps plaque disruption and/or vessel dissection may occur. These events may be followed by claudication or acute limb ischemia.

Special care must be taken when arterial closure depends upon the injection of thrombin into the subcutaneous access tract. When this approach is used, the operator must be certain that there is no chance for inadvertent intravascular injection. Should this occur into the femoral artery, immediate limb-threatening ischemia may occur, which may be refractory to conventional methods of treatment. Injection into the vein may result in immediate thrombosis with substantial risk of massive pulmonary embolus. In the rare case in which the target access artery is entered via a side branch (Fig. 22), thrombin may be injected directly into such a branch and infarct the tissue supplied by it. Necrosis of the abdominal wall has been observed after injection into the inferior epigastric artery.

SUMMARY

The risk of vascular access complications must be accepted as a fact of life for those performing endovascular interventions. This chapter has outlined various strategies

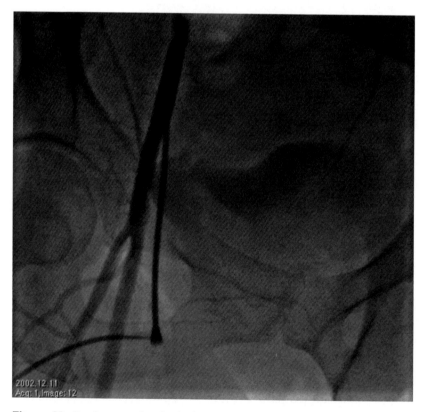

Figure 22 Inadvertent sheath placement into the inferior epigastric artery en route to the external iliac artery. The inferior epigastric artery is not opacified because the sheath occludes its lumen (compare Figs. 13 and 18).

that can be employed to minimize that risk. Through proper patient selection, and procedural timing and execution, most complications can be avoided. Through careful procedural technique and attentive post-procedural care, those which occur can be limited in duration and severity.

REFERENCES

1. TASC Working Group. Management of peripheral arterial disease. Trans Atlantic Inter-Society Consensus. J Vasc Surg 2000; 31:S110–S113.
2. Piper WD, Malenka DJ, Ryan TJ Jr, Shubrooks SJ Jr, O'Connor GT, Robb JF, Farrell KL, Corliss MS, Hearne MJ, Kellett MA Jr, et al. Predicting vascular complications in percutaneous coronary interventions. Am Heart J 2003; 145:1022–1029.
3. Popma JJ, Satler LF, Pichard AD, Kent KM, Campbell A, Chuang YC, Clark C, Merritt AJ, Bucher TA, Leon MB. Vascular complications after balloon and new device angioplasty. Circulation 1993; 88:1569–1578.
4. Waksman R, King SB III, Douglas JS, Shen Y, Ewing H, Mueller L, Ghazzal ZMB, Weintraub WS. Predictors of groin complications after balloon and new-device coronary intervention. Am J Cardiol 1995; 75:886–889.
5. Wiley JM, White CJ, Uretsky BF. Noncoronary complications of coronary intervention. Cathet Cardiovasc Interv 2002; 57:257–265.
6. Kiemeneij F, Laarman GJ, Odekerken D, Slagboom T, van der Wieken, R. A randomized comparison of percutaneous transluminal coronary angioplasty by the radial, brachial and femoral approaches: the access study. J Am Coll Cardiol 1997; 29:1269–1275.
7. Chatziioannou A, Ladopoulos C, Mourikis D, Katsenis K, Spanomihos G, Vlachos L. Complications of lower-extremity outpatient arteriography via low brachial artery. Cardiovasc Interv Radiol. 2004; 27:31–34.
8. Heenan SD, Grubnic S, Buckenham TM, Belli AM. Transbrachial arteriography: indications and complications. Clin Radiol 1996; 51:205–209.
9. Gobel FL, Stewart WJ, Campeau L, Hickey A, Herd JA, Forman S, White CW, Rosenberg Y. Safety of coronary arteriography in clinically stable patients following coronary bypass surgery. Cathet Cardiovasc Diagn 1998; 45:376–381.
10. Bettmann MA, Meyerovitz MF. Principles of angiography. In: Loscalzo J, Creager MA, Dzau VJ, eds. Vascular Medicine. Boston: Little, Brown and Company, 1996:493–517.
11. Scheinert D, Schroeder M, Braunlich S, Biamino G. Transpopliteal approach for recanalization of superficial femoral artery occlusions [abstr]. Am J Cardiol 2000; 86:32i.
12. Samal AK, White CJ. Percutaneous management of access site complications. Cathet Cardiovasc Interv 2002; 57:12–23.
13. Levine GN, Kern MJ, Berger PB, Brown DL, Klein LW, Kereiakes DJ, Sanborn TA, Jacobs AK. Management of patients undergoing percutaneous coronary revascularization. Ann Int Med 2003; 139:123–136.
14. Spijkerboer AM, Scholten FG, Mali WPTM, van Schaik JP. Antegrade puncture of the femoral artery: a morphologic study. Radiology 1990; 176:57–60.
15. Angio-Seal Instructions for Use, St. Jude Medical, Minnetonka, Minnesota.
16. Perclose Instructions for Use, Abbott Vascular, Redwood City, California.
17. Duda SH, Wiskirchen J, Erb M, Schott U, Khaligi K, Pereira PL, Albes J, Claussen CD. Suture-mediated percutaneous closure of antegrade femoral arterial access sites in patients who have full anticoagulation therapy. Radiology 1999; 210:47–52.
18. Kam JL, Hu M, Peiler LL, Yamamoto LG. Acute compartment syndrome signs and symptoms described in medical textbooks. Hawaii Med J 2003; 62:142–144.
19. Leichter RF, Barnes RW, Carabasi RA. Compartment syndrome. In: Merli GJ, Weitz HH, Carabasi RA, eds. Peripheral Vascular Disorders. Philadelphia: Saunders, 2004:143–148.

20. Smith DC, Mitchell DA, Peterson GW, Will AD, Mera SS, Smith LL. Medial brachial fascial compartment syndrome: anatomic basis of neuropathy after transaxillary arteriography. Radiology 1989; 173:149–154.

21. Fellmeth BD, Baron SB, Brown PR, Ang JGP, Clayson KR, Morrison SL, Low RI. Repair of postcatheterization femoral pseudoaneurysms by color flow ultrasound guided compression. Am Heart J 1992; 123:547–551.

22. Kresowik TF, Khoury MD, Miller BV, Winniford MD, Shamma AR, Sharp WJ, Blecha MB, Corson JD. A prospective study of the incidence and natural history of femoral vascular complications after percutaneous transluminal coronary angioplasty. J Vasc Surg 1991; 13:328–336.

23. La Perna L, Olin JW, Goines D, Childs MB, Ouriel K. Ultrasound-guided thrombin injection for the treatment of postcatheterization pseudoaneurysms. Circulation 2000; 102:2391–2395.

24. Ghersin E, Karram T, Gaitini D, Ofer A, Nitecki S, Schwarz H, Hoffman A, Engel A. Percutaneous ultrasonographically guided thrombin injection of iatrogenic pseudoaneurysms in unusual sites. J Ultrasound Med 2003; 22:809–816.

25. Rapoport S, Sniderman KW, Morse SS, Proto MH, Ross GR. Pseudoaneurysm: a complication of faulty technique in femoral arterial puncture. Radiology 1985; 154:529–530.

26. Altin RS, Flicker S, Naidech HJ. Pseudoaneurysm and arteriovenous fistula after femoral artery catheterization: association with low femoral punctures. AJR 1989; 152:629–631.

27. Fellmeth BD, Roberts AC, Bookstein JJ, Freischlag JA, Forsythe JR, Buckner NK, Hye RJ. Postangiographic femoral artery injuries: nonsurgical repair with US-guided compression. Radiology 1991; 178:671–675.

28. Paulson EK, Sheafor DH, Kliewer MA, Nelson RC, Eisenberg LB, Sebastian MW, Sketch MH Jr. Treatment of iatrogenic femoral arterial pseudoaneurysms: comparison of US-guided thrombin injection with compression repair. Radiology 2000; 215:403–408.

29. Cope C, Zeit R. Coagulation of aneurysms by direct percutaneous thrombin injection. Am J Roentgenol 1986; 147:383–387.

30. Hung B, Gallet B, Hodges TC. Ipsilateral femoral vein compression: a contraindication to thrombin injection of femoral pseudoaneurysms. J Vasc Surg 2002; 35:1280–1283.

31. Pope M, Johnston KW. Anaphylaxis after thrombin injection of a femoral pseudoaneurysm: recommendations for prevention. J Vasc Surg 2000; 32:190–191.

32. Samal AK, White CJ, Collins TJ, Ramee SR, Jenkins JS. Treatment of femoral artery pseudoaneurysm with percutaneous thrombin injection. Cathet Cardiovasc Interv 2001; 53:259–263.

33. Lennox A, Griffin M, Nicolaides A, Mansfield A. Regarding "percutaneous ultrasound guided thrombin injection: a new method for treating postcatheterization femoral pseudoaneurysms." J Vasc Surg 1998; 28:1120–1121.

34. Forbes TL, Millward SF. Femoral artery thrombosis after percutaneous thrombin injection of an external iliac artery pseudoaneurysm. J Vasc Surg 2001; 33:1093–1096.

35. Kent KC, Moscucci M, Mansour KA, DiMattia S, Gallagher S, Kuntz R, Skillman JJ. Retroperitoneal hematoma after cardiac catheterization: prevalence, risk factors, and optimal management. J Vasc Surg 1994; 20:905–913.

36. Sreeram S, Lumsden AB, Miller JS, Salam AA, Dodson TF, Smith RB. Retroperitoneal hematoma following femoral arterial catheterization: a serious and often fatal complication. Am Surg 1993; 59:94–98.

37. Kent KC, Moscucci M, Gallagher SG, DiMattia ST, Skillman JJ. Neuropathy after cardiac catheterization: incidence, clinical patterns, and long-term outcome. J Vasc Surg 1994; 19:1008–1014.

38. Mak GY, Daly B, Chan W, Tse KK, Chung HK, Woo KS. Percutaneous treatment of post catheterization massive retroperitoneal hemorrhage. Cathet Cardiovasc Diagn 1993; 29:40–43.

39. Kelm M, Perings SM, Jax T, Lauer T, Schoebel FC, Heintzen MP, Perings C, Strauer BE. Incidence and clinical outcome of iatrogenic femoral arteriovenous fistulas. J Am Coll Cardiol 2002; 40:291–297.

40. Perings SM, Kelm M, Lauer T, Strauer BE. Duplex ultrasound determination of shunt volume in iatrogenic arteriovenous fistulas after heart catheterization. Z Kardiol 2002; 91:481–486.

41. Silva JA, Ramee SR, Collins TJ, Jenkins JS, Lansky AJ, Ansel GM, Dolmatch BL, Glickman MH, Stainken B, Ramee E, White CJ. Rheolytic thrombectomy in the treatment of acute limb-threatening ischemia: immediate results and six-month follow-up of the Multicenter AngioJet Registry. Cathet Cardiovasc Diagn 1998; 45:386–393.

42. Ansel GM, George BS, Botti CF, McNamara TO, Jenkins JS, Ramee SR, Rosenfield K, Noethen AA, Mehta T. Rheolytic thrombectomy in the management of limb ischemia: 30-day results from a multicenter registry. J Endovasc Ther 2002; 9:395–402.

43. Hollis HW, Rehring TF. Femoral endarteritis associated with percutaneous suture closure: new technology, challenging complications. J Vasc Surg 2003; 38:83–87.

44. Carey D, Martin JR, Moore CA, Valentine MC, Nygaard TW. Complications of femoral artery closure devices. Catheteriz Cardiovasc Interv 2001; 52:3–7.

45. Amin FR, Yousufuddin M, Stables R, Shammim W, Al-Nasser F, Coats AJS, Clague J, Sigwart U. Femoral haemostasis after transcatheter therapeutic intervention: a prospective randomized study of the angio-seal device vs. the femostop device. Int J Cardiol 2000; 76:235–240.

5

Complications of Femoral Artery Access

David A. Phillips and Krishna Kandarpa
Department of Radiology, UMass Memorial Health Care, University Campus,
North Worcester, Massachusetts, U.S.A.

COMPLICATIONS OF FEMORAL ARTERY ACCESS

The common femoral artery (CFA) is the access of choice for diagnostic arteriography and arterial interventions. Ever since Seldinger (1) first published his technique of percutaneous needle cannulation of an artery followed by passage of a wire through a hollow needle, the CFA has been used for the introduction of flexible catheters into the arterial system. Other access sites, such as the brachial and radial artery, are useful when there is aorto-iliac or femoral artery occlusive disease (2–10). Proponents of radial artery access for diagnostic and interventional procedures within the coronary arteries cite safety, decreased cost and patient preference as compelling arguments to pursue this access route. Proponents have also stated that radial artery access has a steeper learning curve before one feels comfortable with the procedure.

Although the placement of catheters within the CFA using the Seldinger technique is successful and safe, in a majority of instances, complications do occur. Puncture of the CFA where it overlies the distal/medial third of the head of the femoral bone, allows optimal positioning for its compression below the inguinal ligament upon removal of the catheter. In this chapter, we discuss the most common severe complications (requiring medical, surgical, or some other corrective intervention), comment on the mechanisms of injury, the short-term and long-term sequelae, and the prevention and management of these complications (11–19). Retroperitoneal hematoma is the most severe of these with a reported incidence of 0.5% (20). Hessel et al. (14) cite incidences of arterial obstruction at 0.14%, pseudoaneurysm (PSA) formation at 0.05%, and arteriovenous fistula (AVF) formation at 0.01%.

RETROPERITONEAL HEMATOMA

Pathogenesis

Hemorrhage from the access site in the CFA, its branches or immediately adjacent arterial structures have been reported to produce retroperitoneal hematoma by tracking retrograde along the iliacus and psoas muscle (20,21). Predisposing factors for severe hemorrhage of this nature include ineffective compression secondary to high puncture (external iliac artery), damage to the arteriotomy, or anticoagulation.

Diagnosis

Hypotension occurring in a patient during or after femoral artery access should alert the interventionist to the possibility of retroperitoneal hematoma formation. Symptoms are often delayed and vague (backache, nausea) and several units of blood may be lost in the extravascular space before their onset. Physical examination of the groin is likely to reveal tenderness to palpation at and above the inguinal ligament (20). On rare occasions, this type of hemorrhage may lead to femoral nerve palsy due to compression within a confined space under the inguinal ligament (20,21). Femoral nerve palsy usually begins with heralded groin pain (with or without apparent hematoma formation) followed by sensory and motor deficits. Computer tomography of the abdomen and pelvis to include the femoral head is very helpful when this complication is suspected but not confirmed on physical examination (20) (Fig. 1).

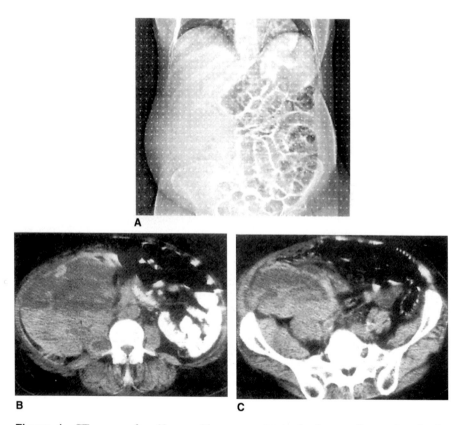

Figure 1 CT scans of a 65-year-old woman obtained after cardiac catheterization and streptokinase infusion. (**A**) CT topogram shows a large abdominal mass on the right. (**B**) Abdominal and (**C**) pelvic CT scans demonstrate a massive retroperitoneal hematoma with fluid–fluid level involving the right anterior and posterior pararenal spaces.

Management

Management of this type of hemorrhage should include stopping anticoagulation, close clinical observation for signs/symptoms of continued or accelerated hemorrhage, and closure/repair of the arteriotomy in those instances of uncontrolled hemorrhage. Hematoma evacuation may or may not be beneficial in prevention of femoral nerve palsy (20,21).

It is imperative to aggressively replace volume/blood loss from retroperitoneal hematoma.

PSEUDOANEURYSM

Pathogenesis

The incidence of pseudoaneunysn (PSA) formation after CFA access has been reported to be as low as 0.07% and as high as 0.38% (22,17).

PSA formation results from severe arterial hemorrhage that pools in a confined space and develops a wall of thrombus that remains liquid centrally. The blood moves to-and-fro from the artery into this pool of confined thrombosis. As with retroperitoneal hematoma and anticoagulation, atypical access sites leading to insufficient arterial compression (the CFA, its branches or immediately adjacent arterial structures) have been identified as predisposing factors (15,17). There is an increased association of superficial femoral artery puncture with PSA formation because of the lack of a sufficient compression site over a boney structure when such low punctures are made (17).

The majority of small PSAs are thought to close spontaneously (20).

Diagnosis

Clinically PSAs may present as a tender area over the groin or upper thigh with a pulsatile sensation to palpation. Auscultation may reveal a soft bruit. Duplex ultrasound may show characteristic features such as expansile pulsation, internal turbulent flow (described as a "swirl" or ying-yang sign), antegrade systolic flow into the PSA, and retrograde diastolic flow from the PSA to the artery of origin (23) (Fig. 2).

Retrograde diastolic flow is due to the high potential energy in the PSA sac secondary to the systolic input; the potential energy in diastole is higher than that downstream in the native circulation (24). The swirl pattern within the PSA is due to the flow pathway created by systolic input and diastolic output. The PSA neck resulting from a needle/catheter puncture is usually a thin track several millimeters to 1–2 cm in length (Fig. 2).

Conventional duplex Doppler may be equally as accurate as color Doppler flow imaging in diagnosing PSA. Color Doppler flow imaging is thought to be advantageous in its ability to clearly demonstrate the neck as well as the swirl pattern within the PSA (24).

Management

Ultrasound-guided compression (25–27) or thrombin injection (28–31) will cause resolution of the PSA in most cases. Hajarizadeh et al. (26) cited an overall success rate of 95% using ultrasound-guided compression to thrombose femoral PSAs. The diameter

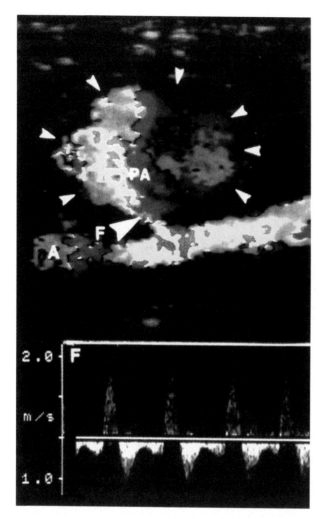

Figure 2 Color-coded duplex scan (shown here in gray scale) shows longitudinal section of pseudoaneurysm (*PA*, *small arrowheads*) near the CFA. In the fistula (*F*, *large arrowhead*s), communication of the pseudoaneurysm with an artery (A), the typical "to-and-fro" flow is seen.

of the PSAs ranged from 1 cm to 5.2 cm. Multivariate analysis of 14 variables revealed heparin anticoagulation as the only significant risk factor ($p = 0.001$) for failure of ultrasound-guided compression. PSAs recurred in 2 of 57 patients in this study. Both patients underwent repeat ultrasound-guided compression with success. Operator arm fatigue during compression and patient discomfort were common occurrences. Patient discomfort was managed with analgesics and periodic pressure release. Arm fatigue was managed by having more than one individual available to perform ultrasound-guided compression. Cox et al. (25) reported on 100 PSA ultrasound-guided compressions in 86 patients. Their overall success rate was 94%. PSA diameter ranged from 0.5 cm to 5.2 cm. PSA duration ranged from 1 day to 80 days, median four days. Factors such as PSA size and duration, the presence of a large surrounding hematoma, associated AVF, the size of the arterial sheath used, the site of arterial injury, and the presence of underlying femoral artery disease did not affect outcome. Hood et al. (27) reported similar results; they found that with the exception of anticoagulation, sheath size, PSA diameter, and duration before compression were not significantly different between lesions that were successfully compressed and those that were not.

Several proponents of percutaneous thrombin injection to occlude femoral artery PSAs cite simplicity, high success rate (100%, 96%, and 77%, respectively), low complication and recurrence rate (28–30). Sackett et al. (31) reported a 3% occurrence of femoral artery embolic complications and a 7% failure rate after thrombin injection to occlude PSAs. Surgery to correct PSA is usually reserved for those that fail to thrombose when treated with one of the less invasive techniques. A PSA may lead to distal emboli and may be life-threatening if it ruptures (32).

ARTERIOVENOUS FISTULA (AVF)

Pathogenesis

In the present context, AVF represents abnormal communication between an artery and vein resulting from penetrating injury or rupture of an aneurysm. The description by Robbins et al. on the pathogenesis of AVF may explain the formation of most AVF resulting from femoral arterial puncture (33). Conceivably a PSA rupturing into an adjacent vein or needle puncture/catheterization of an artery and adjacent vein may lead to an AVF. The occurrence of AVF resulting from attempted femoral artery puncture is less than the occurrence of PSA (34).

Diagnosis

Large hematoma formation should alert one to the possibility of AVF formation. A continuous murmur heard at auscultation over the site of hematoma formation and color duplex ultrasonography is diagnostic (Fig. 3). Characteristic findings on color duplex show continuous antegrade arterial systolic and diastolic flow cephalad to the fistula site, perivascular tissue vibration at the fistula site, most marked during systole, and turbulence with arterial flow characteristics in the draining vein. In the artery immediately caudal to the fistula site, there will be retrograde diastolic flow to the fistula (36).

Management

AVF is usually asymptomatic and mostly spontaneous within the first two months (35). If undetected, however, it may increase in size and become symptomatic. Patients with myocardial compromise and AVF may experience heart failure and those with severe peripheral vascular disease may claudicate in the ipsilateral extremity due to arterial steal. Velocity has been used to quantify the magnitude of AVF. Kent et al. reported on six AVF resulting from femoral artery access (35). Velocity within the fistula ranged from 30 cm/sec to 150 cm/sec, but it was not a reliable predictor of closure. They concluded that many AVFs close spontaneously, and repair is not required unless symptoms or signs of progressive enlargement develop.

Today surgical management of AVF may be reserved for those instances of failure to spontaneously close or respond to ultrasound-guided compression.

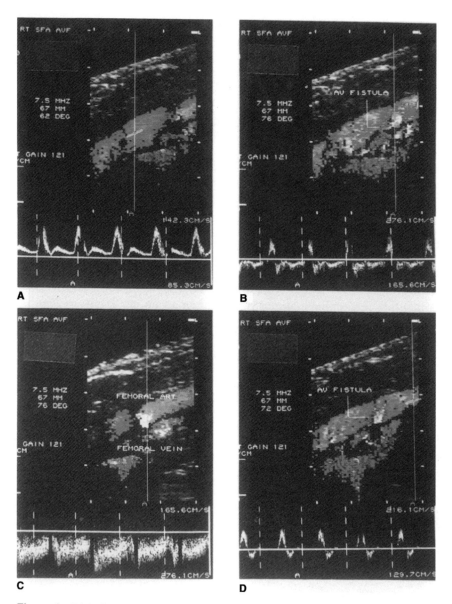

Figure 3   Right femoral arteriovenous fistula. Selective waveform analysis (**A**) above the fistula, (**B**) at the fistula site, (**C**) in the draining vein , and (**D**) in the artery to the fistula. Note continuous antegrade flow with modified triphasic waveform proximal to the fistula (**A**), bi-directional arterial flow at the fistula site (**B**), arterialized venous flow from the fistula (**C**), and normal triphasic arterial flow distal to the fistula (**D**). There is perivascular tissue vibration, most marked during systole (**B,D**). Retrograde diastolic flow is demonstrated only in color distal to the fistula (shown here in gray scale) (**A,C**).

OCCLUSION

Pathogenesis

Bouhoutsos and Morris reporting on 25 patients with arterial occlusions after femoral artery access listed five factors which seem to predispose to hemorrhage or occlusion after arterial puncture: (1) the condition of the artery, (2) the size of the artery, (3) the cardiac output, (4) the position of the puncture, and (5) polycythemia (11). Of the 25 patients with arterial occlusions, 16 (64%) were cardiac invalids without atheroma; one was a young woman with small arteries and Raynaud's phenomenon. Seven of the thirteen known puncture sites associated with occlusion were in the external iliac artery. They concluded that a high puncture, soft arteries, and a low cardiac output predispose to thrombosis after arterial puncture. Soft arteries are easy to occlude with compression, high punctures lead to excessive pressure to control hemorrhage, and low cardiac output leads to stagnation of blood flow, all of which facilitate thrombosis. Gaspar and Yellin identified two mechanisms of femoral artery occlusion associated with access: (1) occlusion of the femoral artery due to stripping off of thrombus formed on the intra-arterial catheter, and (2) subintimal dissection of an atherosclerotic plaque with secondary thrombosis (13).

Diagnosis

Acute occlusion of the femoral artery secondary to access may or may not produce symptoms. Physical exam usually reveals a cool pale extremity with absent or subdued femoral pulse. Absent popliteal and tibial pulses suggest thrombo-emboli. Patients may complain of pain, numbness or coldness in the affected extremity. These signs and symptoms should prompt one to suspect acute occlusion. The diagnosis of arterial spasm should only be considered after occlusion has been ruled out.

Management

Immediate anticoagulation with heparin followed by thrombectomy to remove the acute thrombus is advised. Endarterectomy of a plaque or surgical repair of the femoral artery may be performed at the time of thrombectomy.

PREVENTION OF COMPLICATIONS ASSOCIATED WITH FEMORAL ARTERY PUNCTURE

Today the interventionist has an array of techniques at his/her disposal to prevent complications that may arise from femoral artery access. As our knowledge regarding the pathogenesis of these complications has increased, so have techniques of circumvention. A good clinical evaluation paying close attention to the patients' cardiac status, coagulation state, and peripheral vascular system, will aid greatly in reducing complications of femoral artery access.

Adhering to good technique while puncturing the femoral artery will likely reduce hemorrhagic and occlusive complications associated with femoral artery access (11,15,17). Strict attention to needle puncture of the CFA near the medial distal third of the head of femoral bone will allow optimal puncture site compression. Palpation of the superior pubic ramus along which the inguinal ligament lies will mark the upper boundary below which the needle puncture is to be made to assure an optimal compression site.

Also, taking care to align the needle puncture over the femoral artery and parallel to the course of the CFA will reduce the likelihood of entering the adjacent common femoral vein, avoiding an AVF (Fig. 4). In obese patients palpation of this bony landmark may not be possible, therefore, fluoroscopic or ultrasonic guidance of the

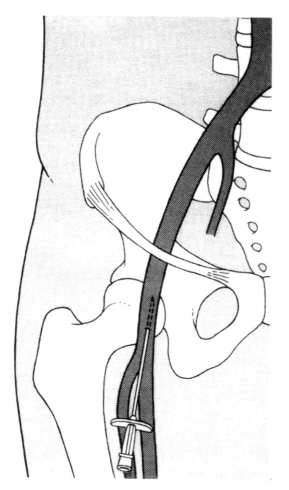

Figure 4 Note needle entrance into femoral artery over the distal third of the femoral bonehead below the inguinal ligament. Note also the alignment of the needle parallel to the course of the femoral artery.

needle puncture may be performed. In instances where reversal of anticoagulants may put the patient at an inordinate amount of risk, one of the closure devices may be used.

There have been significant breakthroughs at the equipment level. Although the 18-gauge needle is the standard, a smaller needle (21-gauge) (Cook Micropuncture Kit, Cook Incorporated, Bloomington, Indiana; www.cookgroup.com) may be used to reduce puncture size and facilitate cannulation of the artery. Femoral artery access occlusions, thrombus formation or emboli secondary to intimal dissection during guidewire insertion have been virtually eliminated with the use of exceedingly floppy tip guidewires.

Heparin remains the gold standard for anticoagulation, however, combinations of heparin and newer agents such as GP IIb IIIa inhibitors are coming into vogue. More recently, the REPLACE-2 trial suggests that bivalirudin, a direct thrombin inhibitor, is superior to heparin and as effective as heparin plus planned GP IIb IIIa inhibition in suppressing acute ischemic events, while producing significantly less bleeding than heparin plus GP IIb IIIa inhibition (37). Assuming others are able to duplicate the experience of the REPLACE-2 trial, bivalirudin or similar drugs may be used routinely to help reduce hemorrhage and occlusion complications resulting from femoral artery access.

Recently, closure techniques designed to decrease the likelihood of CFA hemorrhage and facilitate mobilization after catheter removal have come into vogue. Closure techniques may include collagen plugs (38,39) or a mechanical suturing device (40,41).

Touted advantages of these closure devices are uninterrupted coagulation, faster hemostasis, earlier mobilization and decreased manpower, which may reduce medical costs. Reported severe complication rates associated with the use of collagen plug closure devices range from 0.1% to 30.5% and include vascular obstruction, thromboembolism, groin infection and bleeding (38,41,42). Severe complications from mechanical closure devices being used to close femoral artery access sites have been reported to range from 0% to 5% (43–45). Infection, as well as occlusions and hemorrhage, are the common complications reported. The results of efficacy and safety of closure devices are mixed (38–49).

CONCLUSION

Severe complications resulting from percutaneous access in the femoral artery are low. Adhering to good technique and exercising good clinical judgment in the use of anticoagulants may further control hemorrhage and occlusion complications. Immediate treatment of these complications will minimize morbidity for the patient and prevent long-term sequela.

REFERENCES

1. Seldinger IS. Catheter replacement of the needle in percutaneous arteriography: a new technique. Acta Radiologica 1953; 39:368–376.
2. Ziakas A, Klinke P, Mildenberger R, Fretz E, Williams M, Della Siega A, Kinloch D, Hilton D. Comparison of the radial and the femoral approaches in percutaneous coronary intervention for acute myocardial infarction. Am J Cardiol 2003; 91:598–600.
3. Galli M, Taratantino F, Mameli S, Zerboni S, Butti E, Sagone A, Passerini F, Cappucci A, Ferrari G. Transradial approach for renal percutaneous transluminal angioplasty and stenting: a feasibility pilot study. J Invasive Cardiol 2002; 14:386–390.
4. Scheinert D, Braunlich S, Nonnast-Daniel B, Schroeder M, Schmidt A, Biamino G, Daniel WG, Ludwig J. Transradial approach for renal artery stenting. Catheteriz Cardiovasc Interv 2001; 54:442–447.
5. Shuck J, Khan A, Cavros N, Galanakis S, Patel V. Transradial renal angioplasty: initial experience. Catheteriz Cardiovasc Interv 2001; 54:346–349.
6. Kim MH, Cha KS, Kim HJ, Kim JS. Bilateral selective internal mammary artery angiography via right radial approach: clinical experience with newly designed Yumiko catheter. Catheter Cardiovasc Interv 2001; 54:19–24.
7. Matsumoto Y, Hongo K, Toriyama T, Nagashima H, Kobayashi S. Transradial approach for diagnostic selective cerebral angiography: results of a consecutive series of 166 cases. Am J Neuroradiol 2001; 22:704–708.
8. Campeau L. Entry sites for coronary angiography and therapeutic interventions: from the proximal to the distal radial artery. Can J Cardiol 2001; 17:319–325.
9. Mann T, Cubeddu G, Schneider J, Arrowood M. Left internal mammary artery intervention: the left radial approach with a new guide catheter. J Invasive Cardiol 2000; 12:298–302.

10. Mann JT 3ʳᵈ, Cubeddu MG, Schneider JE, Arrowood M. Right radial access for PTCA: a prospective study demonstrates reduced complications and hospital charges. J Invasive Cardiol 1996; 8(suppl D):40D–44D.

11. Bouhoutsos J, Morris T. Femoral artery complications after diagnostic procedures. Br Med J 1973; 3:396–399.

12. Morris T, Bouhoutsos J. The dangers of femoral artery puncture and catheterization. Am Heart J 1975; 8:260–261.

13. Gaspar MR, Yellin AE. Femoral artery occlusion caused by percutaneous angiography: mechanisms and management. Acta Chirurgica Belgica 1977; 3:323–328.

14. Hessel SJ, Adams DF, Abrams HL. Complications of angiography. Radiology 1981; 138:273–281.

15. Rapoport S, Sniderman KW, Proto MH, Ross GR. Pseudoaneurysm: a complication of faulty technique in femoral arterial puncture. Radiology 1985; 154:529–530.

16. Lilly MP, Reichmann W, Sarazen AA Jr, Carney WI Jr. Anatomic and clinical factors associated with complications of transfemoral arteriography. Ann Vasc Surg 1990; 4:264–269.

17. Kim D, Orron DE, Skillman JJ, Kent CK, Porter DH, Schlam BW, Carrozza J, Reis GJ, Baim DS. Role of superficial femoral artery puncture in the development of pseudoaneurysm and arteriovenous fistula complicating percutaneous transfemoral cardiac catheterization. Catheteriz Cardiovasc Diag 1992; 25:91–97.

18. Ray CE Jr, Kaufman JA. Complications of diagnostic angiography. Complications in Diagnostic Imaging and Interventional Radiology. 3d ed. Blackwell Science, 1996:303.

19. Spies JB, Berlin L. Complications of femoral artery puncture. AJR 1998; 170:9–11.

20. Kent KC, Moscucci M, Mansour KA, Dimattia S, Gallagher S, Kuntz R, Skillman JJ. Retroperitoneal hematoma after cardiac catheterization: prevalence, risk factors, and optimal management. J Vasc Surg 1994; 20:905–913.

21. Cadman PJ. Case report: femoral nerve palsy complicating femoral artery puncture and intra-arterial thrombolysis. Clin Radiol 1995; 50:345–346.

22. Babu SC, Piccorelli GO, Shah PPM, Atein JH, Clauss RH. Incidence and results of arterial complications among 16350 patients undergoing cardiac catheterization. J Vasc Surg 1989; 10:113–116.

23. Mitchell DG, Needleman L, Bezzi M, Goldberg BB, Kurtz AB, Pennell RG, Rifkin MD, Vilaro M, Baltorowich OH. Femoral artery pseudoaneurysm: diagnosis with conventional duplex and color Doppler ultrasound. Radiology 1987; 165(3):687–690.

24. Foley DW, Mewissen MW. Extremity arterial disease. Color Doppler Flow Imaging. Andover Medical Publishers, Inc., 1991:113.

25. Cox GS, Young JR, Gray BR, Grubb MW, Hertzer NR. Ultrasound-guided compression repair of postcatheterization pseudoaneurysms: results of treatment in one hundred cases. J Vasc Surg 1994; 19:683–686.

26. Hajarizadeh H, LaRosa CR, Cardullo P, Rohrer MJ, Cutler BS. Ultrasound-guided compression of iatrogenic femoral pseudoaneurysm failure, recurrence, and long-term results. J Vasc Surg 1995; 22(4):425–430; discussion 430–433.

27. Hood DB, Mattos MA, Douglas MG, Barkmeier LD, Hodgson KJ, Ramsey DE, Summer DS. Determinants of success of color-flow duplex-guided compression repair of femoral pseudoaneurysms. Surgery 1996; 120:585–590.

28. Liau CS, Ho FM, Chen MF, Lee YT. Treatment of iatrogenic femoral artery pseudoaneurysm with percutaneous thrombin injection. J Vasc Surg 1997; 26:18–23.

29. Kang SS, Labropoulos N, Mansour MA, Baker WH. Percutaneous ultrasound guided thrombin injection: a new method for treating postcatheterization femoral pseudoaneurysms. J Vasc Surg 1998; 27:1032–1038.

30. McCoy D, Scharfstein B, Walker W, Evans J. Ultrasound-guided percutaneous thrombin injection for femoral artery pseudoaneurysms. Am Surgeon 2000; 66:975–977.

31. Sackett WR, Taylor SM, Coffey CB, Viers KD, Langan EM III, Cull DL, Snyder BA, Sullivan TM. Ultrasound-guided thrombin injection of iatrogenic femoral pseudoaneurysms: a prospective analysis. Am Surgeon 2000; 66:937–942.

32. McCann Rl, Schwartz LB, Pieper KS. Vascular complications of cardiac catheterization. J Vasc Surg 1991; 14:375–381.
33. Robbins SL, Cotran RS, Kumar V. Pathologic Basis of Disease. 3rd ed. W.B. Saunders Company, 1984;502–546.
34. Ansell G, Bettman MA, Kaufman JA. Complications in Diagnostic Imaging and Interventional Radiology. 3d ed. Blackwell Science, Inc., YEAR:336.
35. Kent KC, Colin R, McArdle MD, Kennedy B, Baim DS, Anninos E, Skillman JJ. A prospective study of the clinical outcome of femoral pseudoaneurysms and arteriovenous fistulas induced by arterial puncture. J Vasc Surg 1993; 17:125–133.
36. Igidbashian VN, Mitchell DG, Middleton WD, Schwartz RA, Goldberg BB. Iatrogenic femoral arteriovenous fistula: diagnosis with color Doppler imaging. Radiology 1989; 170:749–752.
37. Becker R, Butenas S, Carr M Jr, Jaffer F, Kleiman NS, Mamur JD, Schneider DJ, Spiess BD, Steinhubl SR, Weitz JI. Bivalirudin, thrombin and platlets: clinical implications and future directions. J Invasive Cardiol 2003; 15(suppl):1–15.
38. Carere RG, Webb JG, Miyagishima R, Djurdev O, Ahmed T, Dodek A. Groin complications associated with collagen plug closure of femoral arterial puncture sites in anticoagulated patients. Catheteriz Cardiovasc Diagn 1998; 43:124–129.
39. Mooney MR, Ellis SG, Gershony G, Yehyawi KJ, Kummer B, Lowrie M. Immediate sealing of arterial puncture sites after cardiac catheterization and coronary interventions: initial U.S. feasibility trial using the duet vascular closure device. Catheteriz Cardiovasc Diagn 2000; 50:96–102.
40. Mann T, Cowper PA, Peterson ED, Cubeddu G, Bowen J, Giron L, Cantor WJ, Newman WN, Schneider JE, Jobe RL, Zellinger MJ, Rose GC. Transradial coronary stenting: comparison with femoral access closed with an arterial suture device. Catheteriz Cardiovasc Interv 2000; 49:150–156.
41. Dangas G, Meharan R, Kokolis S, Feldman D, Satler L Pichard AD, Kent KM, Lansky AJ, Stone GW, Leon MB. Vascular complications after percutaneous coronary interventions following hemostasis with manual compression versus arteriotomy closure devices. J Am Coll Cardiol 2001; 38:638–644.
42. Goyen M, Mariz S, Kroger K, Massalha K, Haude M, Rudofsky G. Interventional therapy of vascular complications caused by the hemostatic puncture closure device angio seal. Catheteriz Cardiovasc Interv 2000; 49:142–147.
43. Tron C, Koning R, Eltchaninoff H, Douillet R, Chassaing S, Sanchez-Giron C. A randomized comparison of a percutaneous suture device versus manual compression for femoral artery hemostasis after PTCA. J Interv Cardiol 2003; 16(3):217–221.
44. Starnes BW, O'Donnell SD, Gillespie DL, Goff JM, Rosa P, Parker MV, Chang A. Percutaneous arterial closure in peripheral vascular disease: a prospective randomized evaluation of the perclose device. J Vasc Surg 2003; 38:263–271.
45. Wagner SC, Gonsalves CF, Eschelman DJ, Sullivan KL, Bonn J. Complications of a percutaneous suture-mediated closure device versus manual compression for arteriotomy closure: a case-controlled study. J Vasc Interv Radiol 2003; 14:735–741.
46. Whitton HH Jr, Rehring TF. Femoral endarteritis associated with percutaneous suture closure: new technology, challenging complications. J Vasc Surg 2003; 38:83–87.
47. Hoffer EK, Bloch RD. Percutaneous arterial closure devices. J Vasc Interv Radiol 2003; 14:865–885.
48. MacDonald LA, Beohar N, Wang NC, Nee L, Chandwaney R, Ricciardi MJ, Benzuly KH, Meyers SN, Gheorghiada M, Davidson CJ. A comparison of arterial closure devices to manual compression in liver transplantation candidates undergoing coronary angiography. J Invasive Cardiol 2003; 15:68–70.
49. Rickli H, Unterweger M, Sutsch G, Brunner-La Rocca HP, Sagmeister M, Ammann P, Amann FW. Comparison of costs and safety of a suture-mediated closure device with conventional manual compression after coronary artery interventions. Catheteriz Cardiovasc Interv 2002; 57:297–302.

6

Complications of Brachial Artery Catheterization

Hilde Jerius, Gregory S. Domer, and Frank J. Criado
Center for Vascular Intervention and Division of Vascular Surgery, Union Memorial Hospital-MedStar Health, Baltimore, Maryland, U.S.A.

The transbrachial route for cardiovascular intervention was described in 1962 by Sones and Shirley (1). In spite of this, the transfemoral catheterization technique became the preferred approach for vascular access. The small size of the brachial artery, combined with the availability of only bulky and relatively non-flexible devices limited its use. In addition, several large series cited consistently lower complication rates for femoral catheterization, though it was recognized that complications of brachial access were far less likely to be life-threatening than their femoral counterparts (2–4). Contemporary studies demonstrate brachial complication rates that are essentially equivalent or lower than those for femoral access (5,6). Refined techniques, improvement and downsizing of device technology, and routine use of anticoagulants are responsible for this encouraging trend.

INDICATIONS

Brachial artery catheterization (BAC) is the preferred route in patients with hostile scarred groins, femoral synthetic vascular grafts (i.e., aorto-femoral and femoro-popliteal bypass grafts), advanced atherosclerotic disease in the aorto-iliac and femoro-popliteal segments, and transfemoral arterial lines (such as intra-aortic balloon pumps). BAC is also an attractive option in markedly or morbidly obese patients whose groin anatomy is obscured by the large "fat apron," and where the achievement of hemostasis (through external compression) after sheath pull can be difficult and uncertain (7).

Retrograde access to the subclavian and brachiocephalic vessels through the brachial artery can be achieved when the femoral approach fails, or by preference in certain situations. The brachial approach has been used effectively to place covered stents in injured subclavian and axillary arteries (8,9). It is ideally suited to engage the origin of the superior mesenteric artery and other similarly oriented aortic branches. Renal artery and lower extremity interventions are also performed using this approach (10); in fact, the transbrachial technique is a very sound access strategy in a significant number of patients with renal artery stenosis. Additionally, BAC has been reported as a useful adjunct during endovascular repair of abdominal aortic aneurysms in some cases (11).

TECHNIQUE

The left arm is fully extended, and maintained at 60–70° abduction and supinated. This position allows for patient comfort and easy access for the interventionist. After performing an Allen's test and documenting distal pulses, the left brachial artery is punctured at the antecubital fossa (or immediately above it) where it becomes more superficial and—very importantly—where it can be easily compressed against the humerus for hemostasis after pulling the sheath. The left brachial approach provides a more direct course to the visceral aorta, and avoids crossing the cerebral flow-path and performing manipulations through the brachiocephalic trunk that are required when using the right brachial artery. The latter implies a theoretical increase in risk of cerebral embolization. However, at times, the right brachial artery may be the best or only access option for vascular intervention, and one should not hesitate to use it.

A micropuncture introducer set is routinely used; it consists of a 21-gauge 7 cm long needle, a 0.018 stainless steel guidewire, and a 5F 10 cm long coaxial catheter. This set is also available with the option of a stiffened 15 cm coaxial catheter and a 0.018-inch nitinol Cope mandril guidewire that allows penetration through dense and scirrhous tissue. The 5F catheter accepts 0.035 and 0.038 wires. A standard 5F sheath can then be placed over a 0.035 Bentson (or similar) access wire. Systemic heparin is administered immediately after guidewire placement into the brachial artery. The choice of additional catheters, wires and other devices is dictated by the requirements of the specific diagnostic or interventional procedure being performed.

Up to 6F and 7F systems are well tolerated by the brachial artery with little risk of significant complications. With rare exceptions, the use of sheaths larger than 7F should be avoided, as should those with a corrugated surface (i.e., ArrowFlex). The introducer sheath is removed after normalization (<180 seconds) of the activated clotting time (ACT), with hemostasis being achieved by careful external manual compression against the humerous for 15 to 20 minutes. We have not used closure devices for brachial punctures.

CLINICAL EXPERIENCE AND RESULTS

BAC was used in 434 patients over a recent 6.5-year period (ending 7/31/03). The indications included diagnostic angiography (5.0F sheath) in 221, technical adjunct during aortic stent grafting (5.0–6.0F sheath) in 97, renal/visceral artery intervention (6.0–7.0F sheath) in 80, and endovascular treatment of subclavian or innominate artery stenosis (7.0F sheath) in 36. In 419 patients (97%), the left brachial artery was used, and the right in 15 (3%).

Successful BAC was achieved in 431/434 (99.3%). Complications included a significant hematoma in 14 (3.2%), brachial artery occlusion requiring operative intervention in 2 (0.4%). One patient developed compressive neuropathy that improved partially after three months, and 10 others showed evidence of transient motor and/or sensory nerve dysfunction. Duplex scan-confirmed brachial artery pseudoaneuryms were diagnosed in 3 (0.6%), with one of these requiring surgical repair. There were no strokes or cerebrovascular events of any kind.

COMPLICATIONS OF BAC—PREVENTION AND MANAGEMENT

Contemporary studies have demonstrated that complications following BAC tend to be self-limited, rarely requiring surgical intervention. In the present series, only one patient required surgical intervention for brachial artery occlusion. The incidence of brachial artery occlusion following BAC ranges from 0.06% to 1.5% (12). It is easily recognized on physical examination and may be the result of entry site complications, inadequate anticoagulation, or pre-existing occlusive disease. If unrecognized or treated late, it can result in significant forearm claudication (13), tissue loss resulting in amputation, and permanent neuropathy (14). The results of surgical treatment of brachial artery injuries have been described in several publications; they all emphasize prompt operative intervention (<24 hours), and standard vascular techniques depending on the mechanism of occlusion. These range from simple transverse closure in larger arteries to interposition grafts using arm or greater saphenous vein (12,15,16). The incidence of brachial artery occlusion following BAC is very low in the hands of experienced operators using meticulous technique. Attention to detail, use of a micropuncture set to gain entry into the vessel, systemic heparinization, and routine use of a relatively small (4–6F) arterial sheath go a long way in limiting the occurrence of this complication (17).

Transient nerve dysfunction with complete recovery was noted in 2.3% of the study population. This reversible nerve deficit appeared to be related most frequently to the local infiltration of an anesthetic agent, and more rarely reflected neuropraxia secondary to hand compression of the nerve following sheath removal. The incidence of permanent median nerve injury ranges from 0.2% to 1.4%; there have been occasional case reports of reflex sympathetic dystrophy following BAC (18,19). Permanent nerve injuries are felt to be the result of direct nerve trauma, prolonged compression of the neurovascular bundle by a large intra-sheath hematoma, or ischemic neuropathy secondary to brachial artery occlusion.

Meticulous access technique as well as limiting the amount of compressive force used after sheath removal may all reduce the occurrence of such nerve injuries.

Gagliardi et al. reported a 3.8% incidence of central neurological events after brachial catheterization, 0.7% of which were permanent (20). Age >80, previous transient ischemic attacks (TIA), critical carotid stenosis, and antecedent angina pectoris were associated with significantly increased risk of neurological events. Anecdotal reports of vertebrobasilar events during angiography have been reported (B.R. Hopkinson, oral communication, Feb. 1999). These may result from embolization of platelet aggregates or small clots (forming on the catheter) into the ipsilateral vertebral artery. Thus, the institution of prompt anticoagulation immediately after successful vessel entry, and gentle retrograde flushing through the side-port of the sheath, are felt to be important preventive measures.

Finally, hematoma formation accounted for 3.2% of complications following brachial access. Measures aimed at minimizing its occurrence include placement of the puncture site at the antecubital fossa where secure hemostasis can be achieved, correct angulation of the entry needle into the artery to prevent tenting of the guidewire, and ensuring that normal coagulability (ACT <180 seconds) has been restored before removing the introducer sheath. Bruising and ecchymoses, on the other hand, are essentially inevitable in a relatively large number of patients. They can be extensive, but are always self-limited and inconsequential.

OVERVIEW AND CONCLUSIONS

BAC can be described as a very useful and must-have technique in the armamentarium of all endovascular specialists. It can serve as the optimal access tool in a wide range of diagnostic and interventional vascular procedures. Meticulous technique with a micropuncture set, limiting the size of the introducer sheath to 6F or smaller, and instituting prompt anticoagulation after successful vessel entry permit its use in a safe and essentially complication-free manner. BAC is underutilized at present, largely because of fears of morbidity and technical difficulty. Neither is well founded.

REFERENCES

1. Sones FM, Shirey EK. Cine coronary angiography. Mod Concepts Cardiovasc Dis 1962; 31:735–738.
2. Grollman JH, Marcus R. Transbrachial arteriography: techniques and complications. Cardiovasc Interv Radiol 1988; 11:32–35.
3. Babu SC, Piccorelli GO, Shah PM, Stein JH, Clauss RH. Incidence and results of arterial complications among 16,350 patients undergoing cardiac catheterization. J Vasc Surg 1989; 10:113–116.
4. Khoury M, Batra S, Berg R, Rama K, Kozul V. Influence of arterial access sites and interventional procedures on vascular complications after cardiac catheterizations. Am J Surg 1992; 164:205–209.
5. Armstrong PJ, Han DC, Baxter JA, Elmore JR, Franklin DP. Complication rates of brachial artery access in peripheral vascular angiography. Ann Vasc Surg 2003; 17: 107–110.
6. Kiemeneij F, Laarman GJ, Odekerken D, Slagboom T, van der Wieken R. A randomized comparison of percutaneous transluminal coronary angioplasty by the radial, brachial and femoral approaches: the access study. J Am Coll Cardiol 1997; 29:1269–1275.
7. Johnson LW, Esente P, Giambartolomei A, Grant WD, Loin M, Reger MJ, et al. Peripheral vascular complications of coronary angioplasty by the femoral and brachial techniques. Cathet Cardiovasc Diagn 1994; 31:165–172.
8. Schoder M, Cejna M, Hoetzenbein T, Bischof G, Lomoschitz F, Funovics M, et al. Elective and emergent endovascular treatment of subclavian artery aneurysms and injuries. J Endovasc Ther 2003; 10:58–65.
9. Bartorelli AL, Trabattoni D, Agrifoglio M, Galli S, Granacini L, Spirito R. Endovascular repair of iatrogenic subclavian artery perforations using the Hemobahn stent-graft. J Endovasc Ther 2002; 8:417–421.
10. Kaukanen ET, Manninen HI, Matsi PJ, Soder HK. Brachial artery access for percutaneous renal interventions. Cardiovasc Interv Radiol 1997; 20(5):353–358.
11. Criado F, Wilson EP, Abul-Khoudoud O, Barker C, Carpenter J, Fairman R. Brachial artery catheterization to facilitate endovascular grafting of abdominal aortic aneurysm: safety and rationale. J Vasc Surg 2000; 32:1137–1141.
12. Kline RM, Hertzer NR, Beven EG, Krajewski LP, O'Hara PJ. Surgical treatment of brachial artery injuries after cardiac catheterization. J Vasc Surg 1990; 12:20–24.
13. Karmody AM, Lempert N, Jarmolych J. The pathology of post-catheterization brachial artery occlusion. J Surg Res 1976; 20:601–606.
14. Waller DA, Sivananthan UM, Diament RH, Dester RC, Rees MR. Iatrogenic vascular injury following arterial cannulation: the importance of early surgery. Cardiovasc Surg 1993; 1:251–253.
15. McCollum CH, Mavor E. Brachial artery injury after cardiac catheterization. J Vasc Surg 1986; 4:355–359.

16. Mann JW 3rd, Davidson JT 3rd. Vein patch angioplasty for brachial arterial occlusion after cardiac catheterization. Am Surg 1990; 56:520–522.
17. Watkinson AF, Hartnell GG. Complications of direct brachial artery puncture for arteriography: a comparison of techniques. Clin Radiol 1991; 44:189–191.
18. Kennedy AM, Grocott M, Schwartz MS, Modarres H, Scott M, Schon F. Median nerve injury: an under-recognized complication of brachial artery cardia catheterization? J Neurol Neurosurg Psychiatry 1997; 63:542–546.
19. Inoue T, Yaguchi I, Mizoguchi K, Iwasaki Y, Takayanagi K, Morooka S, Asano S. Reflex sympathetic dystrophy following transbrachial cardiac catheterization. J Invasive Cardiol 2000; 12:481–483.
20. Gagliardi JM, Batt M, Avril G, Declemy S, Hassen-Khodja R, Daune B, et al. Neurological complications of axillary and brachial catheter arteriography in atherosclerotic patients: predictive factors. Ann Vasc Surg 1990; 4:546–549.

7

Complications Associated with the Use of Percutaneous Arterial Closure Devices

Daniel G. Clair
Department of Vascular Surgery, The Cleveland Clinic Foundation, Cleveland, Ohio, U.S.A.

Despite the fact that manual pressure has proven effective in sealing arterial access sites, percutaneous closure device use has steadily increased over time. Increasing anticoagulation regimens, increasing diameters of devices being used, and an increasing need to free-up interventional recovery room beds have combined to create a situation which now more than ever favors the use of a device to seal large bore arterial access sites quickly and reliably. Percutaneous closure devices fulfill this role well, but this has not been without some problems. While numerous complications, some of which are exceedingly rare, have occurred with these devices, emphasis here will be placed upon defining those complications which have been noted more commonly with these devices, and attempting to clarify the methods by which these complications can be dealt with or, preferably, averted.

Closure devices come in two basic forms. The initial devices developed use the deposition of a bioresorbable material within the tract of the sheath to obtain hemostasis. These devices remain the largest number of available devices for treatment of arterial access sites. Included in this group of closure systems are Vasoseal (Datascope, Montvale, New Jersey), Angioseal (St. Jude Medical, Minnetonka, Minnesota), and more recently the Duett system (Vascular Solutions, Minneapolis, Minnesota). The other major category of devices utilize some mechanism to achieve mechanical closure of the arterial wall, utilizing either sutures or clips to physically seal the defect. The devices available with this type of closure technique include the Closer and Prostar made by Perclose (Perclose, Abbott, Redwood City, California), the X-press device (X-site Medical, Blue Bell, Pennsylvania) and the SuperStitch (Sutura, Fountain Valley, California); however, the SuperStitch device is approved for vascular stitching in general surgery including endoscopic procedures and not for "blind-closure" of arteries. Additionally, there is limited data available for the two latter mentioned suture-mediated closure systems, and the majority of data for this chapter does not include information on these devices.

Some complications encountered relate directly to the type of closure device used and some are obviously very similar to the problems which can develop with the use of manual pressure. First, a brief description of all the closure devices will be presented. This will be followed by a presentation of the different types of complications. It will be easier to address these issues by complication type, and to further categorize this by device type, if the type of device affects the occurrence of the problem or the ways in which it can be dealt with or avoided.

DEVICES

Devices depositing material extraluminally at the arterial entry site depend upon precise localization of the arterial wall in order to deposit the material extrinsic to the lumen.

The Vasoseal® device (Datascope, Montvale, New Jersey) deposits a bovine collagen plug just outside the vessel wall. The initial version of the Vasoseal device used a physical measuring technique to determine the depth at which to deploy the plug. However, the newer device, Vasoseal ES, utilizes a flow channel to identify when the sheath is within the arterial lumen and, in addition, a wire that exits the device at an acute angle directed opposite to the angle of entry to allow passage into the prograde channel of flow in the femoral artery. The collagen delivery sheath is advanced to the point at which it is limited by the wire and is left in place upon removal of the lumen-identifying system to allow for delivery of the collagen plug to achieve hemostasis. With this system, the intraluminal portion of the device is removed prior to the release of material outside the arterial wall (Fig. 1).

The Angioseal system (St. Jude Medical, Minnetonka, Minnesota) utilizes a mechanical anchor to localize the anterior vessel wall. Unlike the Vasoseal, the Angioseal vessel wall localization system utilizes an anchor, which stays within the vessel against the intraluminal surface of the anterior vessel wall. This anchor is made of a bioresorbable copolymer of polylactic and polyglycolic acids. The device anchor is introduced through a sheath, which utilizes a parallel lumen for initial localization of the vessel lumen. After advancing the sheath to 1 cm within the vessel lumen, the anchor is delivered within the vessel through a system introducer sheath. The collagen plug is attached to the anchor via a resorbable suture and a tamper is used to push the collagen plug to the level of the anterior vessel wall, pinching the plug down on top of the anchor and tamponading the exit of blood from the vessel access site. Once again, with this device, vessel access is abandoned prior to delivery of the closure system (Fig. 2).

The Duett device (Vascular Solutions, Minneapolis, Minnesota) utilizes a 3F compliant balloon inserted through a standard sheath. The balloon is then inflated within the lumen of the vessel beyond the sheath and withdrawn until resistance is encountered. Here the device tamponades the arterial entry site. Through the standard sheath, a procoagulant mixture of bovine collagen and thrombin is introduced as the sheath is removed. Manual pressure is then held as the occlusion balloon is removed via its 3F introducer for two to five minutes. As with the other devices, access to the vessel is abandoned upon deployment of the pro-coagulant (Fig. 3).

Having completed the discussion for systems deploying material outside the arterial access site, we will now address mechanical closure systems. The most widely used of these devices are the devices made by Perclose (Perclose, Abbott, Redwood City, California). The initial device design (Techstar 6F) had a single suture attached to two needles positioned within a catheter, which was advanced over a wire. A needle capture barrel was bluntly dissected through the soft tissue and through a parallel lumen-identifying port; back bleeding from the vessel could be noted when

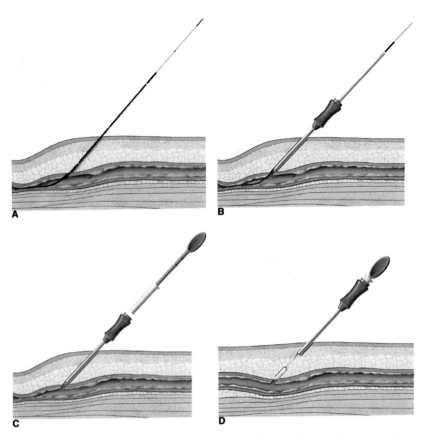

Figure 1 (**A**) Identifying position of the anterior luminal wall with the Vasoseal device. (**B**) Advancing delivery sheath to tissue external to vessel wall. (**C**) Insertion of collagen plug into Vasoseal delivery sheath. (**D**) Collagen plug in position.

the barrel was adjacent to the exterior of the artery. The needles with attached sutures were then pulled into the barrel and identified externally at the outer end of the barrel. These were then extricated from the barrel and the attached suture was used to tie a slipknot, which slid down and fastened the anterior surface of the artery. The device allows the user to assess adequacy of closure prior to removing wire access to the lumen. The Prostar XL (8F and 10F) devices utilize similar technology with four needles attached to two sutures arranged in a crossed fashion to close larger arteriotomy sites. The newer Closer (6F) system positions the needles outside the vessel lumen and utilizes a footplate, which is opened within the vessel, to locate the anterior wall. Suture is located in the anterior and posterior wells of the footplate and the needles are pushed through the artery wall "grasping" the suture and pulling it out to the skin surface. From here closure is similar to what it had been with the previous 6F device and access can be maintained to the lumen while assessing closure (Fig. 4).

The X-press device (X-site Medical, Blue Bell, Pennsylvania) has been reported in one major trial (1). This device is advanced over a wire and contains a gap that is located over the arterial wall layer when back bleeding through a side-port identifies the correct position of the device. A needle attached to one end of a suture is advanced through the wall into the distal aspect of the device. The device is then rotated 180° and a second needle attached to the opposite end of the same suture is

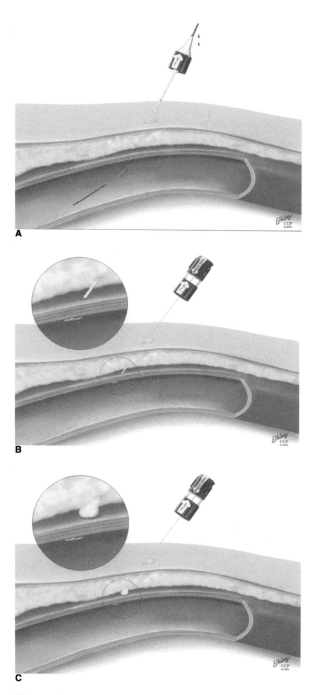

Figure 2 (**A**) Insertion of Angioseal device sheath. (**B**) Footplate deployment against anterior arterial wall. (**C**) Collagen deployment outside of vessel.

advanced into the shaft of the device as well. The needles and ends of the sutures are then brought out and the suture tied with a slipknot. The device allows maintenance of arterial access, and as well allowing more than one suture to be placed prior to complete removal of the device.

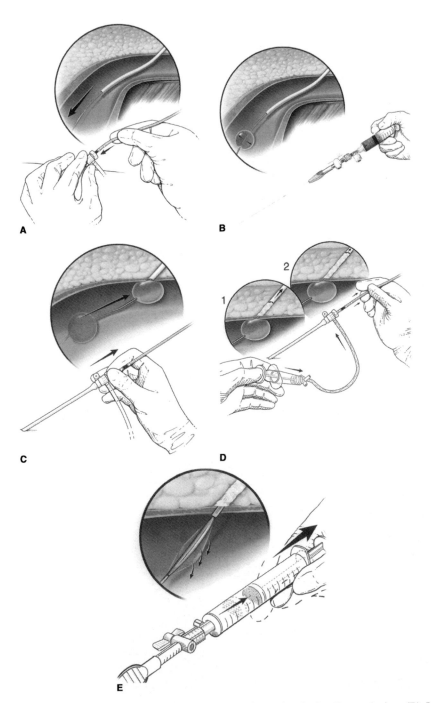

Figure 3 (**A**) Insertion of balloon catheter into sheath for Duett device. (**B**) Inflation of balloon catheter within vessel lumen. (**C**) Retraction of balloon catheter to identify anterior vessel wall. (**D**) Delivery of Duett device sealing mixture with retraction of sheath. (**E**) Deflation and removal of Duett balloon.

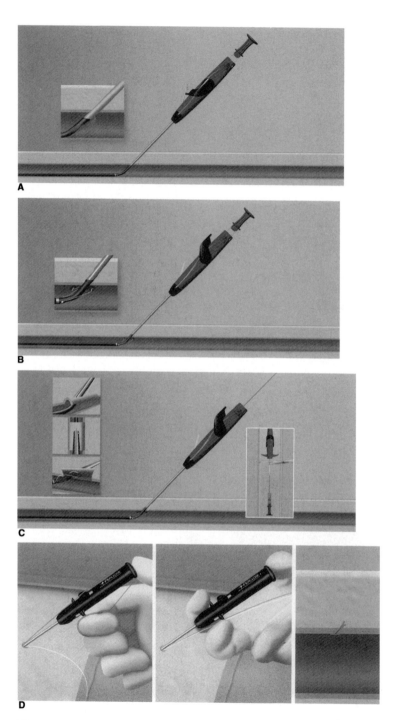

Figure 4 (**A**) Confirming intra-arterial position of the Perclose device. (**B**) Deployment of footplate of Perclose device. (**C**) Needles of Perclose device capturing suture ends. (**D**) Knot-pushing device for cinching suture and clipping ends.

TYPES OF COMPLICATIONS

Device Failure

The most common type of complication encountered is that referred to as "device failure." This is reported as occurring anywhere from 0% to 10% with various devices, although some trials have reported larger failure rates than those noted in Hoffer and Block's review (2,3) and can represent a number of different occurrences, from failure to achieve hemostasis at the puncture site to inability to deploy the device because of a technical difficulty. As technical difficulty is the most common event in reported series using these devices, it is relevant that this be discussed in a description of the complications occurring with these devices.

It is helpful to divide the devices into deposition devices and mechanical closure devices. Technical failure with the Vasoseal device has been reported to occur anywhere from 0% to 10% (3–10). Utilizing the Vasoseal device, difficulties can be had in advancing the additional wire and in retrieving the luminal identification system completely. Standard instructions for use of this device call for up to two minutes of pressure to be applied after deposition of the collagen plug. Failure of the device to achieve hemostasis within this time frame has been viewed in some studies as device failure. Achieving success with the device mandates adequate entry above the femoral bifurcation and adequate luminal diameter of the vessel caudal to the access site so that the wire placed for localization can be used to identify the anterior wall. It is also imperative that the sheath location be fixed carefully during delivery of the collagen as motion in either direction (withdrawal or advancement) can result in either hemorrhage or vessel occlusion.

The Angioseal system has similar deployment failure rates to the Vasoseal system in randomized trials comparing these two systems (4,5). Difficulties can be encountered identifying an intraluminal position secondary to either sheath angulation such as can be seen in obesity and tortuous vasculature, patient motion, or diseased femoral arteries (10,11). The anchor should not be deployed unless successful identification of the lumen is achieved. Deployment of the anchor in an extraluminal position can result in inadequate hemostasis and difficulty in controlling hemorrhage secondary to the device impairing the ability to achieve adequate closure with compression. Deployment of the device in a position further into the vessel than recommended can result in the anchor inadvertently becoming "hung-up" on the posterior wall, and occluding the vessel with the tension placed upon the device to tamponade the collagen plug onto the anterior surface of the artery.

The Duett device has a variable rate of success. Deployment failure rates have varied from 0% to 12% (4,12,13) with the causes of device or deployment failure poorly elucidated in reported series. Deployment difficulties have been related to device malfunction (balloon-related) and inability to introduce the liquid through the standard sheath, according to the report of the SEAL study trial group (9). In this study, failure of the device occurred in 6.9% of cases and was most often due to balloon leakage.

Evidence from several trials assessing the Perclose device reveals failure rates of 0–12% (7,14–20). An advantage of this device however, is that the success can be evaluated prior to giving up wire access to the vessel, and if necessary, a sheath can be reinserted over the wire and left in place until the coagulation profile of the patient has returned to normal. Subsequent to this, manual pressure can be held.

The majority of device failures with the Perclose devices were related to continued bleeding from the site after completion of successful deployment of the device.

However, problems with breakage of the suture, inability to have the knot slide appropriately, failure to locate the arterial lumen adequately via the port, and failure of the needles to capture tissue were also significant problems. This device has been associated with a need for surgical removal of the device in a limited number of cases as well.

A recent report by Mackrell et al. documents the reasons for failure of the device in a large population with ischemic lower extremity disease in whom the device was utilized (19). These authors documented device failure in 25 of 500 patients (5%) displaying in whom the device was used. Of the failures, 15 were due to inability to deliver the device into the artery secondary to scar tissue (12), or heavy calcification (3). Four patients had devices that did not deploy as expected, difficulty in needle deployment or questionable device fracture. The final six failures had unsuccessful hemostasis after successful deployment of the device, necessitating manual compression.

The other suture-mediated closure devices, Sutura Superstitch and X-site X-press, have not had enough published experience to give adequate information regarding rates of failure.

Predisposing Factors

With any of these devices, significant patient motion while trying to maintain the delivery sheath in its position can lead to loss of position and inability to achieve precise deposition. Additionally, there can be problems in attempting to assure that the arterial identification system is within the lumen of the artery. Access either too high (above the inguinal ligament) or too low (close to the common femoral bifurcation) can make it difficult to localize the lumen with the use of the lumen localization wire, or make it impossible to deliver the hemostatic agent to the area just outside the arterial wall. Significant disease in the artery can make identifying the lumen difficult, which can result in misplacement of the occlusion device. For mechanical closure devices, as with the deposition devices, the access site is important in assuring successful closure. Access either too high or too low in the femoral artery can make successful closure impossible. Disease in the access vessel can make localization of the vessel wall difficult, and calcification in the vessel wall can make it difficult to allow the needles to pass through the vessel wall or to be returned into the barrel of the device for the larger diameter devices. Unusual angulation to the access or significant scar in the area of the access can also make the devices less likely to be successful. Some alternative methods to deliver the device to the arterial wall have been utilized specifically in patients with severe scar (21).

Short-/Long-Term Sequelae

In most instances, the inability to deploy the device will lead to the need to either replace a standard sheath or to convert to manual compression. There is little by way of significant sequelae other than these.

Management

Dealing with device failures for all of these devices requires either sheath replacement, conversion to standard compression closure, or in some cases, conversion to surgical closure. In particular, regarding the Perclose devices, several authors have documented the need for surgical extraction of the device in the setting of deployment failure (7,21,22). If one is unable to adequately identify the arterial lumen and does not proceed to an attempt to deploy the material, wire access can be maintained, and the delivery system replaced with a standard sheath to allow normalization of the anticoagulation, and conversion to manual compression. With all of the devices utilizing deployment of material outside the arterial lumen, access to the artery is abandoned during the deployment procedure. With the mechanical closure systems, access can sometimes be maintained until assessment of the closure is completed. Abandoning vessel access in the setting of device failure requires the conversion of a closure device-mediated access site repair, most often to pressure-mediated repair that can be done with either manual compression or a mechanical compression device. In most instances, device deployment failure may lead to additional early complications (15,17), and it clearly will lengthen the time to achieve vessel sealing and ambulation. Normally, there are no long-term sequelae of converting to compression-mediated closure.

Prevention

Preventing the failure of these devices often requires the access to be precisely placed and the vessel and access site to be assessed fluoroscopically prior to an attempt at device deployment. One must be sure that defining the precise location of the arterial wall is easily accomplished prior to deployment. The interventionalist as well must make sure the patient is comfortable and maintains a steady position during device deployment. In certain situations where there is uncertainty regarding access and closure, in order to maintain access with thrombosis-inducing material deposition devices, dual wire access can be utilized through the initial sheath access and the device deployed over one of the wires, maintaining access alongside the deployed device in case the deployment is unsuccessful (17).

Thrombosis (Vessel Occlusion)

Thrombosis or vessel occlusion is a relatively rare event with manual compression and does not often occur with closure devices. Eidt et al. in their review of surgical complications noted vessel occlusion to be the most common complication they encountered with the Angioseal device (23). In 425 patients having deployment of this device, the authors noted six (1.4%) having vessel occlusion as a complication. All of these patients required operative intervention to treat the resultant extremity ischemia. In this same paper, an assessment was made of the FDA MAUDE database to record adverse events related to devices; in evaluating the last 100 medical device reports (MDR) for these devices, the authors noted vessel obstruction to be the most common adverse event recorded for the Angioseal (65/100). Evaluation of the MAUDE database for the Vasoseal and Perclose device at the same time revealed occlusion was a much less frequent reason for filing an MDR for these devices. In nearly all series reviewed using various devices, the incidence of this complication was rarely greater than 1% (1–22). The occurrence with manual compression is likewise uncommon from studies done comparing devices with manual pressure (3,7,11,13,15–18).

Predisposing Factors

The majority of descriptions of this problem occurring relate to either deployment of the device too far into the vessel (6), or occlusion of the artery from a portion of the system itself (23). It would seem from descriptions of the problem that the most significant factor related to this occurrence is the inability to adequately identify the access point into the femoral artery. Significant patient obesity and disease of the artery in which the device is being deployed are probably the most important factors leading to this type of problem.

Short- and Long-Term Sequelae

For the majority of patients, the treatment of vessel occlusion will mandate operative repair of the vessel in question. Often this is done via local groin exploration, with thrombectomy if necessary. There have been descriptions of techniques to remove portions of a device occluding a femoral artery following maldeployment, as that of Stein and Tierstein (24); however, this is the unusual scenario. In certain situations, there is the possibility of mechanical thrombectomy, local thrombolytics (4), or snare of intra-arterial material (25); however, one must be sure the limb is viable and that the additional time to try and arrange a novel removal of the intraluminal problem is not going to cost the limb. For the majority of patients, this additional local procedure will add to the hospital length of stay, but should cause few other sequela.

Management of the Complication

As noted above, the majority of these problems are dealt with using surgical intervention. If access is still maintained, it is possible that visualization of the defect by angiography may identify the exact location and nature of the occlusion. A mechanical thrombectomy device and potentially angioplasty can be used in limited circumstances. Clearly, here, a vascular surgeon should be involved in the decision-making process. One should also remember that the procedure to deal with this problem is usually not debilitating and can be performed under local anesthesia with little morbidity to the patient, and the earlier the revascularization is performed, the better the long-term outcome.

Prevention

The important point in preventing this complication is the correct identification of the site for deployment of the foreign body or the correct positioning of the device prior to suture deployment. If there is any question regarding this point, the attempt at percutaneous closure should be abandoned and the sheath replaced. Another attempt at closure device placement can then be made or the patient can have manual pressure applied after normalization of the coagulation studies. In almost all reports involving occlusion-utilizing devices deploying a procoagulant outside the vessel wall, a portion of the collagen plug has been deployed endoluminally, or the device anchor or sutures have interacted with a plaque, causing occlusion. Efforts to limit these problems have focused on assuring the device is deployed extraluminally. Despite the reported safety as well in patients with peripheral vascular devices for some of the devices (19), most would recommend avoiding closure devices in the setting of severe occlusive disease in the vessel accessed. These patients are likely best treated with manual pressure.

Infection

Infection with closure devices has the potential to be a life-threatening, severe infection. All devices currently in use require the deposition of a foreign body in the area accessed. Infection in the setting of the foreign body can be difficult if not impossible to eradicate.

Thankfully, the incidence of this is extremely small in those treated with closure devices, ranging from 0% to 1.6% (3–22). It appears to be remarkably uncommon with the Angioseal device, yet comprised almost one-third of the most recent MDRs reported in the paper by Eidt and colleagues (23). In Hoffer's recent review of closure devices (2), the number of trials documenting infection appeared to be higher for the suture-mediated Perclose system (8 of 13) than for the Angioseal device (2 of 10). Additionally, three of the trials cited by Hoffer that included the use of the Perclose device noted statistically significant increases in infectious complications in patients having closure with the Perclose device.

Predisposing Factors

In many of the trials performed evaluating these devices, access sheaths left in for prolonged periods of time have not been treated with closure devices because of concerns of the increased risk of infection. None of the devices are recommended for use in extended access sheaths (e.g., sheaths left for extended lysis). Additionally, those things that predispose a person to an increased risk of infection, which are host factors, are likely to increase the risk of infection in the access site. These would include such things as diabetes, ongoing systemic infection and those patients with ipsilateral lower leg infections, especially ascending lymphangitis. Obviously, any infections within the groin such as fungal infection in the groin crease of the obese patient can predispose to this problem as well. While the use of these devices is more difficult in the obese patient, it is precisely in this patient population that the benefit will be the greatest. There is currently no evidence that obesity bears any relationship to infection in the area of device deployment. Prior surgeries in the groin may be a predisposing factor as a number of the reported complications of this nature have been noted in patients with prosthetic grafts in the femoral region. This can obviously have catastrophic consequences.

Short-/Long-Term Sequelae

The sequelae of infection are normally limited to the short-term issues related to dealing with the infection of a vascular structure, which can lead to rupture of the blood vessel and severe hemorrhage. All of these patients will need to be dealt with surgically, and often debridement of the arterial wall will be necessary, in addition to long-term intravenous antibiotic management. Ideally, culture-directed therapy could be initiated.

Management

The management of this problem is essentially always surgical. Attempts to temporize with intravenous antibiotic therapy or local wound dressing changes only exposes the patient to the potential for vessel rupture and death. The earlier and more aggressively these problems are dealt with, the less dramatic the operation that needs to be performed, and the sooner the patient can begin the road to recovery. In repairing this problem, the patient will require debridement of the involved arterial wall and if there is question regarding the extent of the infection, a frozen section of the arterial wall can be used to assess the presence of bacteria in the wall. Any and all material related to the closure device (suture, collagen, or fragments of the device) should be removed. Once healthy arterial tissue is remaining, the defect should be repaired with autogenous tissue. This is often performed with adjacent vein, if possible preserving the saphenous vein. If inadequate local vein is present, the saphenous vein or alternative vein sources can be used to repair the defect. One method of reinforcing the vein is to invert the venous segment and create a "double-walled" patch to repair the defect. Upon completion of the arterial repair, attention should be placed upon assuring that the artery is covered with viable tissue. There may be the need to aggressively debride the subcutaneous tissues to assure all infection is removed from this area as well. In some situations, if the infection is extensive, one may need to utilize the sartorius muscle for arterial coverage. If there were to be extensive arterial involvement, and there was concern for directly repairing the artery, an extra-anatomic bypass could be performed and the ends of the vessel ligated. In all cases, the skin should be left open for the wound to granulate so that all infected fluid can freely drain from the wound. Vigorous and extended dosing of intravenous antibiotics should be undertaken. Dressing changes should be started early to the region. Close monitoring of the area should ensue over the first five to seven days to assure the infection is completely under control.

Prevention

The best way to prevent this problem is to avoid the use of these devices in patients with any evidence of ipsilateral groin infection or significant evidence of ipsilateral leg infection. Clearly these devices should not be used in patients with systemic infections, and those patients having extended sheath dwell times are likely better treated with manual compression rather than these devices. In the event that there is any potential for infection, systemic dosing with intravenous antibiotics should be given prior to device placement. One might potentially add antibiotics in the case of all percutaneous closure devices. It is of obvious importance that sterile technique is adhered to during all percutaneous procedures; this should be maintained during closure device placement as well.

Pseudoaneurysm

Arterial flow outside the full vessel lumen is a potential complication of any form of access site treatment. It would seem obvious as well that this complication would represent a failure of the device to achieve acceptable lumen closure of the vessel. In the studies reviewed, the incidence of this complication is between 0% and 1.5% for all devices (3–22). It does not appear to be more commonly associated with one type of device compared with the others.

Predisposing Factors

As with the complications of bleeding above, the most significant factor that would appear to be associated with pseudoaneurysm formation is the inability to easily identify the exact depth of the artery within the access site, making deployment of the material or sutures less effective and subject to the possibility of the formation of a pseudoaneurysm. This can be affected by the amount of patient motion during use of the device, the obesity of the patient, and the disease of the artery itself. In access sites where there is some question regarding the placement of the device, either the attempt should be abandoned or a new device should be utilized.

Short-/Long-Term Sequelae

The outcomes from this problem are often very good with little significance for the patients long-term; however, in the short term this will often require additional interventions to deal with this problem and it is often associated with a groin hematoma, which can be uncomfortable for the patient. In some instances, it may prolong hospitalization and may in rare instances necessitate operative intervention to correct the problem when less invasive measures prove unsuccessful.

Management

The current management of arterial pseudoaneurysms typically involves one of the three methods of repair. The size of the communication with the artery can determine the success of less invasive methods to treat the problem. Most patients currently are managed by initial attempts at thrombosis with either ultrasound-guided thrombin injection (26,27) or ultrasound-guided compression (28,29). In each of these techniques, the operator will attempt to perform this either in the neck of the pseudoaneurysm or as close to the neck as possible within the collection. In the majority of instances, because these access sites are small, one of these techniques will be successful. In the situation where one cannot achieve obliteration of the pseudoaneurysm by these means, surgical repair is indicated. In the setting of a very small pseudoaneurysm (<2 cm), it may be reasonable to wait prior to surgical intervention as a significant percentage of these may thrombose without any intervention being performed (30).

Operative intervention is fairly straightforward, with direct approach to the vessel with proximal control if possible and usually a simple suture or two on the anterior surface of the artery. However, in some series evaluating the risks associated with surgical repair of these problems, an subject of post-surgical complications was noted in as many as 21% of patients (31). For this reason, attempts at percutaneous closure are clearly the first line of therapy. In cases where hematoma and patient habitus prevents proximal control, an assistant can compress the artery proximally while a suture closing the defect is placed. Any debris from the device should be removed and a layered closure of the superficial tissues ensues. Several authors have recently reported other innovative ways to percutaneously treat pseudoaneurysms to achieve thrombosis when the standard methods above have failed. Given the potential risks and discomfort associated with surgical repair, one might potentially find the use of para-aneurysmal saline injections, percutaneous coil placement, or even transluminal delivery of thrombin into the pseudoaneurysm, a useful alternative to standard surgical repair of these problems (32–34).

Prevention

Prevention of this complication is predicated on precise deployment of the device at the arterial entry site. Adequate anesthesia to keep the patient comfortable, easy visualization of the lumen identifying port, and minimizing operator and patient motion during the procedure are key. In the setting where adequate identification of the anterior of the vessel cannot be performed, the sheath should be replaced and manual pressure held after normalization of the anticoagulation profile.

Device-Specific Complications

Given the distinct differences between the various devices, it is important that users understand there are complications that appear either more frequently with one device or one class of device. The most significant of these complications is the risk of embolization, which can be seen with the devices deploying material outside the vessel wall, and the risk of needing surgical removal of the device which is seen more commonly with the suture-mediated closure system made by Perclose. Embolization of the collagen system can be seen anywhere from 0.2% to 1.6% of patients closed with deposition devices (4,6,7,11,13,23). These problems can be related to the material deployed or the anchor used to fix this material. Similarly, in a small number of patients, the need for surgical removal of the Perclose device has been noted (11,16). While these issues are different for each of the devices, they are unique to the specific type of device and in particular, are not seen with the other type of device.

Predisposing Factors

It is the deployment of material within the vessel itself that gives rise to the potential embolization that can be seen with deposition devices. Since the Angioseal purposefully leaves material behind in the vessel lumen, it is not surprising that one can see this problem with this device. For the other deposition devices, the depth of deployment determines the risk of this complication occurring. With obesity, difficult access, and trouble with motion during advancement, the collagen material can easily be deployed intra-arterially, ultimately leading to occlusion or embolization.

Severe scar, calcification, and difficult advancement of the device can lead to trouble in removing the device, ultimately leading to the need for surgical removal. With severe scarring or significant vessel calcification, one may be better off utilizing manual pressure rather than trying to extend the use of these devices.

Short-/Long-Term Sequelae

Embolization ultimately leads to the need for surgical removal of the deposited material. This can lead to long-term intimal hyperplasia in the vessel and vascular compromise. It is the short-term need for surgical exploration that exposes the patient to the largest risk.

Entrapment of the Perclose device within the vessel obviously mandates emergent exploration and repair of the vessel. This can pose the threat of groin infection, healing problems, and vessel damage in the area of the need for repair and removal. Long-term, this can lead to difficulties with repeat access in the area and the problems attendant with repair of the femoral artery, although in most instances, this is not a significant problem.

Management

As noted above, a number of different approaches have been used to treat maldeployment of the collagen plug or embolization of the Angioseal anchor; in most instances, this problem will lead to the need for surgical exploration and removal of the foreign body (24,25). This may require surgical embolectomy and perhaps even wire-directed catheter thrombectomy. Additionally, if the embolus cannot be reached from the groin, it may be necessary to more directly approach the embolus. While this is likely no more risky than approaching the vessel in the groin, it can often be more challenging to repair, and may at times necessitate two surgical incisions to remove all the debris. If approaching the procedure from the groin, all foreign material should be removed and the artery repaired directly at the same time.

Removal of the Perclose device requires direct surgical exposure of the femoral artery to repair the arteriotomy. The device should be left in place and an oblique incision placed to include the access site incision. Dissection can be carried down along the shaft of the device, and once the artery is identified, either a purse string suture can be placed and the device removed or proximal and distal control achieved and the vessel removed prior to more extensive vessel repair. The suture should be fully removed. If necessary, a patch of prosthetic material can be used to perform a surgical angioplasty of the femoral artery.

Prevention

In order to prevent embolization, the surgeon should assure the material is being deployed outside the vessel lumen. It is likely that with the Angioseal device, since a portion of the device is deployed endoluminally, there will be a fixed small number of patients who may develop embolization of the anchor. This problem, however, should be of less significance with the other devices by assuring the point of deployment of the procoagulant.

Prevention of the need for surgical removal of the Perclose device may require the willingness to abandon the use of it in severe scar or problematic deployment. In addition, this problem may be more common with the larger Perclose devices. With these devices, the operator should assure all four returning needles are visualized at the outer aspect of the hub prior to beginning to remove the needles and sutures. Maintaining wire access, as this device allows, also tends to make abandoning the closure device for replacement with another closure device a more palatable option.

CONCLUSION

Manual compression has been proven to be a safe and effective method of sealing percutaneous arterial access sites; however, as the size of devices and the need for faster patient throughput increases, there is increasingly a need to close these access sites rapidly and securely. The use of percutaneous closure devices fulfills the requirement of rapid closure, however, the use of these devices is not completely without drawbacks. These drawbacks include device failure, vessel thrombosis, hematoma formation (sometimes large enough to warrant transfusion), pseudoaneurysm formation, and infection.

Each of the devices has been shown to have a certain failure rate and in a number of instances, when these devices fail, the risk of complications can increase. The goal of the interventionalists remains the application of newer, minimally invasive technologies with limited morbidity. Closure devices, when they function well, significantly decrease the time needed for patients to remain supine, and they can clearly increase the opportunity for hospitals and physicians to treat more patients. By understanding the potential complications related to device usage and avoiding situations where they will have a higher risk of failure, one can improve device efficacy and at the same time offer the largest benefit to patients. It is important in the setting of questionable anatomy to utilize a device or a technique that maintains the ability for sheath access, should the device fail. Here the suture-mediated Perclose devices appear to have a distinct advantage, although modifications of the technique of device deployment can allow the maintenance of wire access with nearly all of the devices. As these technologies continue to evolve, it is likely that the risk of all these complications will continue to decrease and as informed users of these devices, interventionalists can aid in the decreasing numbers of patients suffering complications from the use of closure devices.

REFERENCES

1. Sanborn TA, Obilby JD, Ritt JM, Stone GW, Klugherz BD, Fields RH, White CC, Wilensky RL. Reduced vascular complications after percutaneous coronary interventions with a non-mechanical suture device: results from the randomized rapid ambulations after closure (RACE). Am J Cardiol 2002; 90:172h.
2. Hoffer EK, Bloch RD. Percutaneous arterial closure devices. J Vasc Interv Radiol 2003; 14:865–885.
3. Silber S, Bjorvik A, Muhling H, Rosch A. Usefulness of collagen plugging with VasoSeal after PTCA as compared to manual compression with identical sheath dwell times. Catheteriz Cardiovasc Diagn 1998; 43:421–427.
4. Michalis LK, Rees MR, Patsouras D, Katsouras CS, Goudevenos J, Pappas S, Sourla E, Koettis T, Sioros L, Zotou P, Gartzou-Matsouka P, Sideris DA. A prospective randomized trial comparing the safety and efficacy of three commercially available closure devices (Angioseal, Vasoseal and Duett). CVIR 2002; 25:423–429.
5. Shammas NW, Rajendran VR, Alldredge SG, Witcik WJ, Robken JA, Lewis JR, McKinney D, Hansen CA, Kabel ME, Harris M, Jerin MJ, Bontu PR, Dippel EJ, Labroo A. Randomized comparison of Vasoseal and Angioseal closure devices in patients undergoing coronary angiography and angioplasty. Catheteriz Cardiovasc Interv 2002; 55(4):421–425.
6. Carere RG, Webb JG, Miyagishima R, Djurdev O, Ahmed T, Dodek A. Groin complications associated with collagen plug closure of femoral arterial puncture sites in anticoagulated patients. Catheteriz Cardiovasc Diagn 1998; 43:124–129.
7. Carey D, Martin JR, Moore CA, Valentine MC, Nygaard TW. Complications of femoral artery closure devices. Catheteriz Cardiovasc Interv 2001; 52:3–7.
8. Lunney L, Darim K, Little T. Vasoseal hemostasis following coronary interventions with Abciximab. Catheteriz Cardiovasc Diagn 1998; 44:405–406.
9. Foran JP, Patel D, Brookes J, Wainwright RJ. Early mobilization after percutaneous cardiac catheterizations using collagen plug (Vasoseal) hemostasis. Br Heart J 1993; 69:424–429.
10. Ward SR, Casale P, Raymond R, Dussmaul WG III, Simpfendorfer C. Efficacy and safety of a hemostatic puncture closure device with early ambulation after coronary angiography. Angio-Seal Investigators.. Am J Cardiol 1998; 81:569–572.
11. Duffin DC, Muhlestein JB, Allisson SB, Horne BD, Foweles RE, Sorensen SG, Revenaugh JR, Bair TL, Lappe DL. Femoral arterial puncture management after percutaneous coronary procedures: a comparison of clinical outcomes and patient satisfaction between manual compression and two different vascular closure devices. J Invasive Cardiol 2001; 13:354–362.
12. Heyer G, Atzenhofer K, Meixl G, Lampersberger C, Gershony G. Arterial access site closure with a novel-sealing device: Duett. Vasc Surg 2001; 35:199–201.
13. The SEAL Trial Study Team. Assessment of the safety and efficacy of the Duett vascular hemostasis device: final results of the safe and effective vascular hemostasis (SEAL) trial. Am Heart J 2002; 143:612–619.
14. Sesana M, Vaghetti M, Albiero R, Corvaja N, Martini G, Sivieri G, Colombo A. Effectiveness and complications of vascular access closure devices after interventional procedures. J Invasive Cardiol 2000; 12:395–399.

15. Assali AR, Sdringola S, Moustapha A, Ghani M, Salloum J, Schroth G, Fujise K, Anderson HV, Smalling RW, Rosales OR. Outcome of access site in patients treated with platelet glycoprotein IIb/IIIa inhibitors in the era of closure devices. Catheteriz Cardiovasc Interv 2003; 58:1–5.
16. Chamberlin JR, Lardi AB, McKeever LS, Wang MH, Ramadurai G, Grunenwald P, Towne WP, Grassman ED, Leya FS, Lewis BE, Stein LH. Use of vascular sealing devices (VasoSeal and Perclose) versus assisted manual compression (Femostop) in transcatheter coronary interventions requiring abciximab (ReoPro). Catheteriz Cardiovasc Interv 1999; 47:143–147.
17. Applegate RJ, Grabarczyk MA, Little WC, Craven T, Walkup M, Kahl FR, Braden GA, Rankin KM, Kutcher MA. Vascular closure devices in patients treated with anticoagulation and IIb/IIIa receptor inhibitors during percutaneous revascularization. J Am Coll Cardiol 2002; 40:78–83.
18. Starnes BW, O'Donnell SD, Gillespie DL, Goff JM, Rosa P, Parker MV, Chang A. Percutaneous arterial closure in peripheral vascular disease: a prospective randomized evaluation of the Perclose device. J Vasc Surg 2003; 38(2):263–271.
19. Mackrell PJ, Kalbaugh CA, Langan EM 3rd, Taylor SM, Sullivan TM, Gray BH, Carsten CG 3rd, Snyder BA, Cull DL, Youkey JR. Can the Perclose suture-mediated closure system be used safely in patients undergoing diagnostic and therapeutic angiography to treat chronic lower extremity ischemia? J Vasc Surg 2003; 37:1305–1308.
20. Morice MC, Dumas P, Lefevre T, Loubeyre C, Louvard Y, Piechaud JF. Systematic use of transradial approach or suture of the femoral artery after angioplasty: attempt at achieving zero access site complications. Catheteriz Cardiovasc Interv 2000; 51:417–421.
21. Winter K, Khalighi K, Claussen CD, Duda SH. Percutaneous arterial closure in severely scarred groins: a technical note. Catheteriz Cardiovasc Diagn 1998; 45:315–317.
22. Cura FA, Kapadia SR, L'Allier PL, Schneider JP, Kreindel MS, Silver MJ, Yadav JS, Simpfendorfer CC, Raymond RR, Tuzcu EM, et al. Safety of femoral closure devices after percutaneous coronary interventions in the era of glycoprotein IIb/IIIa platelet blockade. Am J Cardiol 2000; 86:780–782.
23. Eidt JF, Habibipour S, Saucedo JF, McKee J, Southern F, Barone GW, Talley D. Surgical complications from hemostatic puncture closure devices. Am J Surg 1999; 178: 511–516.
24. Stein BC, Teirstein PS. Nonsurgical removal of angio-seal device after intra-arterial deposition of collagen plug. Catheteriz Cardiovasc Interv 2000; 50:340–342.
25. Shaw JA, Gravereaux EC, Winters GL, Eisenhauer AC. An unusual cause of claudication. Catheterization & Cardiovascular Interv 2003; 60:562–565.
26. Cope C, Zeit R. Coagulation of aneurysms by direct percutaneous thrombin injection. American Journal of Roentgenology 1986; 147:383–387.
27. Wixon CL, Philpott JM, Bogey WM Jr, et al. Duplex-directed thrombin injection as a method to treat femoral artery pseudoaneurysm. Journal American college of Surgeons 1998; 187:464–466.
28. Fellmeth BD, Roberts AC, Bookstein JJ, et al. Postangiographic femoral artery injuries: non-surgical repair with US-guided compression. Radiology 1991; 178:671–675.
29. Chatterjee T, Do DD, Kaufmann U, Mahler F, Meier B. Ultrasound-guided compression repair for treatment of femoral artery pseudoaneurysm: acute and follow-up results. Catheterization & Cardiovascular Diagnosis 1996; 38(4):335–340.
30. Kresowik T, Khoury M, Miller B, et al. A prospective study of the incidence and natural history of femoral vascular complications after percutaneous transluminal coronary angioplasty. Journal of Vascular Surgery 1991; 13:328–336.
31. Lumsden AB, Miller JM, Kosinski AS, et al. A prospective evaluation of surgically treated groin complications following percutaneous cardiac procedures. American Surgeon 1994; 60:132–137.

32. Gehling G, Ludwig J, Schmidt A, Daniel WG, Werner D. Percutaneous occlusion of a femoral artery pseudoaneurysm by para-aneurysmal saline injection. Catheterization & Cardiovascular Interv 2003; 58(4):500–504.
33. Kobeiter H, Lapeyre M, Becquemin JP, Mathieu D, Melliere D, Desgranges P. Percutaneous coil embolization of postcatheterization arterial femoral pseudoaneurysms. Journal of Vascular Surgery 2002; 35(5):1280–1283.
34. Badran MF, Gould DA, Sampson C, Harris PL, Hewitt H, Stables R, Rashid A. Transluminal occlusion of a pseudoaneurysm arising from a thoracic aortic graft patch using catheter delivery of thrombin. J Vasc Interv Radiol 2003; 14(9 Pt 1):1201–1205.

8

Complications of Vascular Access Procedures

Mark J. Sands
Section of Vascular and Interventional Radiology, The Cleveland Clinic Foundation, Cleveland, Ohio, U.S.A.

OVERVIEW

Image-guided placement of vascular access devices has evolved to become the method of choice in many institutions as a result of safety, economic, and practical considerations. While previously within the exclusive domain of surgical practitioners, percutaneous venous access for the purposes of placing tunneled catheters and ports is now widely performed by interventional radiology services. Current practice has resulted in a demonstrable decrease in procedure-related complications (1–3).

Generally, these procedure-related complications can be categorized into those arising in the early period—within 30 days—following the placement of the indicated access device and those occurring later than this time period. Early complications can be further subdivided into those that occur at the time of or within 24 hours of the procedure, and those occurring beyond 24 hours.

Immediate procedure-related complications commonly originate from direct injury of the target vein, neighboring arterial vessels and nearby tissues and include vascular laceration, hemorrhage (including hemothorax and mediastinal hematoma), pneumothorax, and device misplacement into arterial or mediastinal structures. Additionally, during the course of venous vascular access, air may be aspirated through the placement sheath intravascularly resulting in a symptomatic air embolism. Procedure-induced sepsis may also occur.

Beyond the first 24 hours following the establishment of venous vascular access, delayed hematoma formation (most commonly within the catheter tunnel or port-pocket), thrombotic complications affecting the catheter or the underlying vein, and early infection may be seen. Infectious complications of venous access device placement occurring in the first two to five days after placement may be ascribed to a violation of meticulous barrier technique at the time of the procedure. Device-related malfunctions such as catheter migration, kinking, and flow compromise may also occur.

Late or delayed complications include the aforementioned items and may be more likely to involve device failure or fracture. Catheters placed via the subclavian route may "pinch off" if the entry point into the vein is medial to the space formed by the clavicle, first rib and the costo-clavicular ligament. Occluded or thrombosed catheters can rupture upon forceful attempts to clear the catheter lumen. Repeated use of a portacath may contribute to skin and subcutaneous tissue erosion. Similarly, hubs of frequently accessed dialysis catheters have been seen to crack and leak. Infection by *Staph aureus*, *Staph epidermidis*, *or Candida albicans* may signify line maintenance issues. Thrombotic issues may become more significant over time as injury and the response to injury of the underlying vein contribute to the development of a relative stenosis along the venous course of the catheter. Thrombosis, involving both the catheter and the underlying vein, is acknowledged to play a role in the generation of further infectious complications.

Guidelines for quality improvement and thresholds levels for the occurrence of these events were established by the standards and practice committee of the Society of Cardiovascular & Interventional Radiology in 1997 (4).

PROCEDURAL COMPLICATIONS

Image-guided vascular access has a low incidence of non-target vascular or tissue injury (5–7). Carotid artery puncture was noted to be roughly seven times more common in one prospective, randomized trial of sonographic-guided access compared with landmark-guided puncture (6). A second comparison performed in the cardiac catheterization laboratory demonstrated complications of carotid puncture, brachial plexus irritation, and hematoma to be 8.3%, 1.7%, and 3.3%, respectively, with landmark guidance compared with 2.6%, 0.3%, and 0%, respectively, with sonographic guidance (7).

While an inadvertent carotid artery puncture recognized early in the procedure may simply result in hematoma formation, following dilatation to allow peel-away sheath insertion, arterial dissection, thrombosis and stroke may result (Figs. 1 and 2). Complications may be further minimized by the use of a 21-gauge "mini-stick," access needles, and access kits (1).

Access procedures utilizing the subclavian vein may similarly traumatize the subclavian artery. Hematoma or pseudoaneurysm formation may result. Bleeding from the latter may occur in a delayed fashion. Internal jugular vein access procedures resulting in traumatic laceration of the subclavian artery have also been described (8,9). The somewhat variable course of ascension of the subclavian arteries into the neck, particularly on the right side may be a predisposing factor (8,9).

Collectively, the risk of precipitating a pneumothorax, air embolism or hemothorax during vascular access device placement, particularly from the jugular approach is less than 2% (3). This injury appears more common with the subclavian access route, particularly with multiple puncture attempts. Patients with COPD are at higher risk. It may be more common in children than adults when internal jugular access cannulation is performed (10,11). Most pneumothoraces resulting from injury with a 21-gauge needle tend to be small and asymptomatic. They typically resolve over a few hours and require no further treatment. Continued patient complaint of sharp chest or shoulder girdle pain should necessitate the procurement of a chest radiograph (Fig. 3). Enlarging or symptomatic pneumothoraces may be treated with an apical small bore chest tube or Heimlich valve placement usually via the second anterior interspace. Aspiration of air through a "peel-away" introducer sheath during central venous access device placement may be life-threatening.

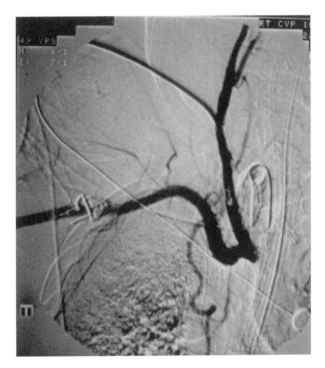

Figure 1 Inadvertent carotid artery puncture.

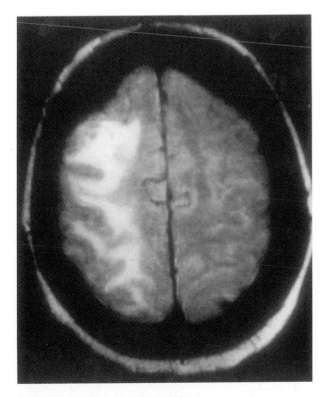

Figure 2 Right hemispheric infarct.

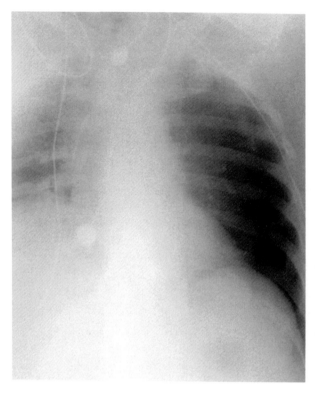

Figure 3 Post-line placement pneumothorax.

Trendelenberg positioning (head down), or having the patient perform a
Valsalva maneuver may be helpful in avoiding this complication (12). However, as
patient compliance with breathing instructions during the procedure may be poor,
particularly when sedated, efforts must be made to crimp or otherwise occlude the
sheath during catheter insertion. It is estimated that approximately 100 ml/min of
air can pass through a 14-gauge needle, and that 300–500 ml of aspirated air may
be fatal (13,14). Traditional teaching mandates prompt placement of the patient in
a left lateral decubitus position in order to "trap" air in the right atrium. Careful
monitoring and administration of supplemental oxygen should be performed while
awaiting air resorption.

Vascular perforation during catheter placement may result in the development
of hemothorax or hemomediastinum (Fig. 4) (15). The former may be rapidly life-
threatening. After establishment of initial access, attempts at advancing a tapered
dilator or "peel-away" sheath, if not observed carefully under fluoroscopy, may
result in the formation of a kink in the angiographic guidewire which in turn may
become a stiletto-like point, and with continued operator pressure directed centrally,
may lead to vascular perforation. If suspected, contrast injection through the dilator
or catheter may confirm the injury (Fig. 5). The pleural space, usually a vacuum, will
accommodate a large amount of circulating blood in such an injury and will rapidly
lead to hypovolemia. If only a result of venous injury, mediastinal hematomas may
remain stable as the space of the mediastinum is more confined and under higher
pressure than the pleural space. These may require treatment if circulatory embar-
rassment occurs (16). An example of right innominate vein injury incurred during

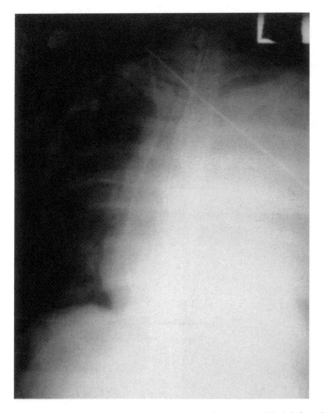

Figure 4 Hemothorax after unsuccessful non-guided left subclavian vein access attempt.

an attempt at subclavian venous access for triple-lumen venous catheter placement resulting in injury to the mediastinum and the thoracic aortic arch is illustrated below (Fig. 5).

While there is no definite consensus among practitioners, many prefer to place the tips of the central venous access catheter within the right atrium. Perforation of the right atrial wall with stiffer, larger diameter catheters more commonly placed in the past for hemodialysis has been described (16). This appears relatively infrequently with the softer, more pliable catheter tip designs currently available. Where possible, it has been recommended to place the tip of central venous catheters not intended for hemodialysis above the flexure of the visceral and parietal pericardial layer (17).

Neurologic injury other than stroke may occur during central venous access procedures. Specifically, brachial plexus irritation following subclavian vein central venous catheter placement may be seen. Patients may experience mild discomfort and tingling in the utilized upper extremity. Symptoms are usually of short duration (18). More serious injuries to the brachial plexus and phrenic nerve have also been described (19).

PERIPROCEDURAL COMPLICATIONS

Infection, device malposition/malfunction, and catheter thrombotic issues mark the periprocedural period after the placement of central venous access catheters and ports.

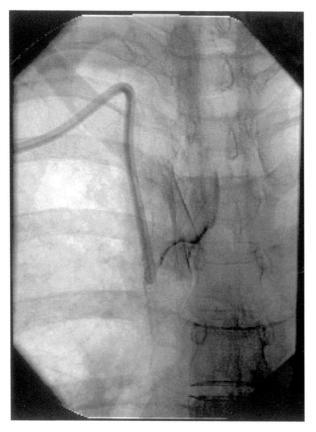

Figure 5 Contrast injection through triple-lumen catheter that was not able to aspirate blood immediately after placement. Contrast is seen in medial recess of right pleural space.

Infection that develops in the immediate post-procedural period within the first three to five days following the procedure is most probably caused by intra-operative contamination (20). While the use of prophylactic antibiotic coverage remains controversial, careful preventive measures such as pre-procedural hair removal, full-field surgical scrub, and meticulous use of barrier technique can mitigate this potential complication. The majority of patients present with local symptoms of pain, erythema, warmth, tenderness, and swelling. These may be followed by fever and the development of significant cellulitis. Failure to remove the infected catheter or port may result in abscess formation. The removed infected device, tip of the attached catheter, wound, and peripheral blood should be cultured. The patient should be started on broad-spectrum antibiotics, which may be later adjusted to the culture results. In the case of an infected portacath, the wound should be irrigated and a wick of regular or iodoform gauze should be placed in the wound to prevent premature closure before complete wound drainage. The wound should be repacked daily for several days until drainage has diminished and then left to heal by secondary intention (21).

Mechanical catheter-related issues such as catheter migration, malposition and fragmentation are common periprocedurally. Catheter malposition is much less frequently encountered in procedures performed under fluoroscopic guidance, however, even in the best of circumstances catheters have been seen to "flip" from the intended position to lie in neighboring veins upon vigorous thoracic exertions such as valsalva

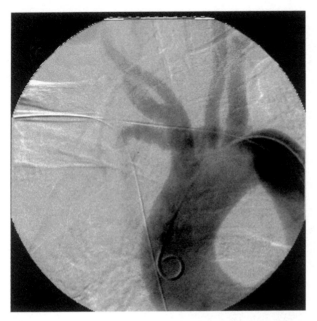

Figure 6 Inadvertent right innominate vein and aortic perforation via right subclavian access. Injury resulted in an aortic to right innominate vein fistula which likely averted fatal mediastinal hematoma development. Injury required open surgical repair.

and coughing. Catheters tips may thus come to rest in the contralateral subclavian vein, the azygous vein, and the ipsilateral internal jugular vein if placed via the subclavian route. When necessary, the catheter may be re-positioned with the use on an intravascular snare. If the catheter length is inappropriate, predisposing to migration and/or poor function, over guidewire exchange for a better-sized catheter may be performed. This is more difficult for portacaths; however, catheters may be snared through a neighboring access sheath, trimmed to a more appropriate length, and re-inserted.

Occasionally, access devices thought to have been placed within the vein lumen may be found to demonstrate pulsatile flow, suggesting inadvertent arterial placement (Fig. 6). Contrast injection was performed to confirm the intra-arterial position (Fig. 7). As the catheter had been indwelling for several weeks, a transesophageal echocardiogram was performed to exclude the presence of a vegetation on the catheter tip. CT-scan obtained prior to catheter removal demonstrated that the 15 French outer diameter catheter was nearly occlusive in the subclavian artery and that supraclavicular access would permit removal and repair of the arteriotomy (Figs. 8 and 9). This was performed uneventfully.

Thrombosis of central venous catheters is a significant issue both in the periprocedural period and extended catheter dwell times. The rate has been estimated at 0.23 per 1000 catheter days in an outcome analysis study of over 50,000 patients (22). This will be addressed in the next section.

DELAYED COMPLICATIONS

Catheters placed via the subclavian route are vulnerable to "pinch off." An incidence of 1.1% was noted in a retrospective review of 1457 subclavian tunneled venous

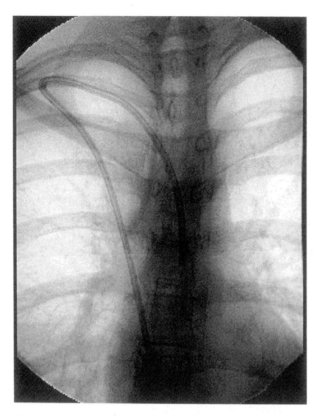

Figure 7 Catheter inadvertently placed via right subclavian artery in patient whose access was thought to be through the right internal jugular vein.

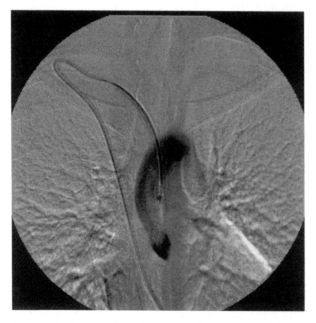

Figure 8 Contrast injection confirming intra-arterial catheter position.

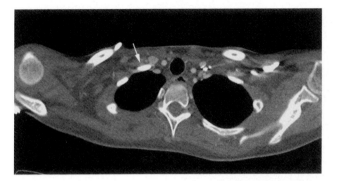

Figure 9 Fifteen French triple-lumen catheter shown entering the right subclavian artery.

percutaneous catheter placements conducted by Andris et al. (23). This occurs when the catheter enters the vein medial to the space formed by the border of the first rib, clavicle and the costo-clavicular ligament. External pressure in this space initially compresses and subsequently may fracture the distal portion of the catheter (Fig. 10). The fractured portion typically embolizes centrally to the right ventricle or the pulmonary arterial tree (Fig. 11).

Transjugular or transfemoral venous endovascular snare retrieval techniques may then be applied to extract the embolized fragment (Figs. 12 and 13).

Catheter-related thrombotic complications may occur in 3.7–10% of patients (20,24). Underlying hypercoagulable states, venous stasis and venous irritation, induced by infused hyperalimentation and chemotherapeutic drugs as well as the irritation produced by the catheter itself, are likely contributing factors (25). Difficulty in aspirating from the catheter lumen which is not relieved by changes in patient positioning likely signify the development of a thrombus or fibrin sheath

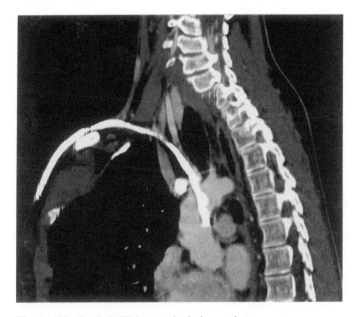

Figure 10 Sagital CT-image depicting catheter course.

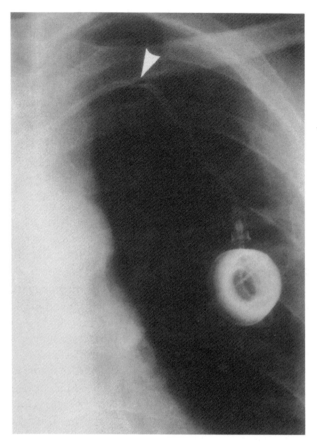

Figure 11 Compression of subclavian venous catheter at site marked by arrowhead. Failure to recognize and explant the device may result in catheter fracture and embolization.

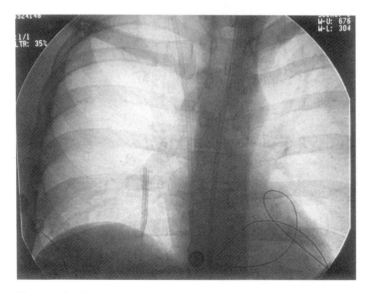

Figure 12 Embolized double lumen hemodialysis catheter tip.

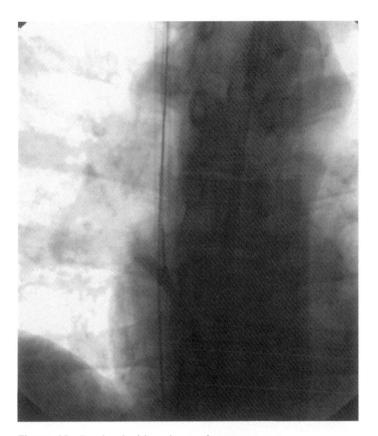

Figure 13 Retrieval with endovascular snare.

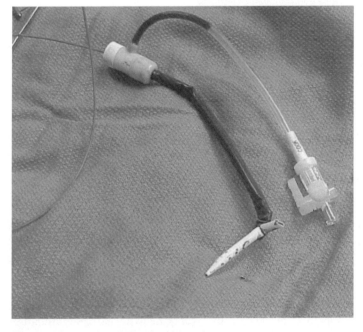

Figure 14 Retrieved distal catheter fragment.

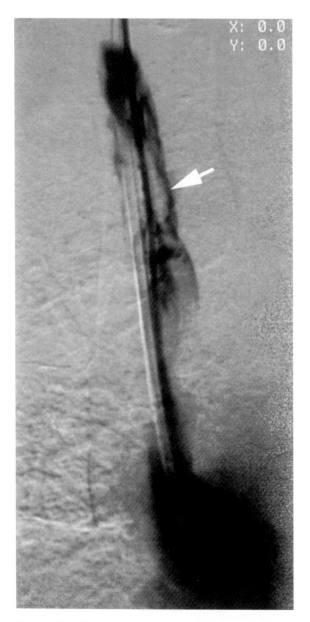

Figure 15 Contrast injection through the arterial limb of a Tessio hemodialsysis catheter lumen demonstrating the presence of a prominent fibrin sheath (*arrow*).

at the catheter tip. The presence of a fibrin sheath may be confirmed by injection of contrast through the catheter lumen with digital subtraction angiography. Initial fluoroscopy will confirm adequate catheter position and, upon injection, contrast should be seen to stream freely away from the catheter tip. Contrast seen tracking back along the catheter is abnormal and denotes the presence of a fibrin sheath (Fig. 14). This can be managed by infusion of a thrombolytic agent, physical stripping of the fibrin sheath (Fig. 15) or by over guidewire catheter exchange performed with balloon disruption of the putative fibrin sheath (26–28). Low-dose

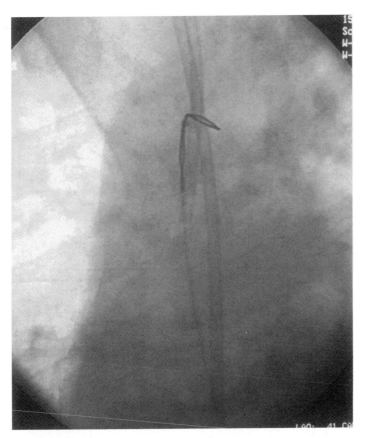

Figure 16 Fibrin sheath stripping performed via transfemoral approach with an Amplatz Gooseneck snare.

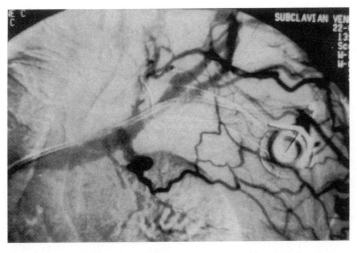

Figure 17 Left upper extremity venogram demonstrating thrombosis of the axillary and subclavian veins in this patient with a long-term indwelling subclavian portacath.

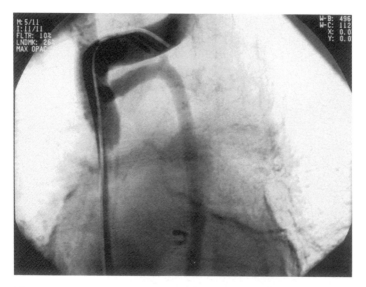

Figure 18 Distal SVC stenosis secondary to multiple hemodialysis access catheters. Patient became symptomatic when new left arm AV fistula was created. Note the prominent azygous vein serving as a collateral upper body venous drainage route.

coumadin therapy (1 mg/day) has been shown to be of benefit in preventing or forestalling catheter-related thrombosis in a prospective, randomized trial (29).

Venous stenoses and occlusions can develop surrounding the intravascular catheter course. Thrombosis in the central veins may be seen in 35–67% of patients

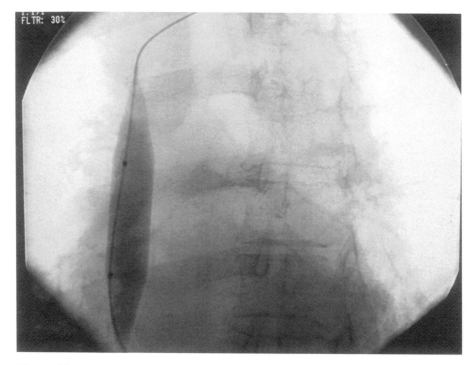

Figure 19 Failed angioplasty attempt. The stenosis exhibited elastic recoil after balloon deflation and stent placement was performed.

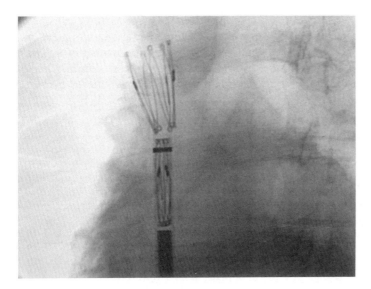

Figure 20 Gianturco stent deployment.

with long-term indwelling central catheters (16,30). Depending upon location, this may be independent of catheter function (Fig. 16). Patients may present with significant arm swelling and discomfort. Treatment is determined by the extent of the symptoms and the remaining suitable venous access sites; conservative measures such as elevation and anticoagulation may be employed initially, however, catheter removal may be required if symptoms persist. In instances where central venous access sites are limited, catheter-directed thrombolytic administration may be useful

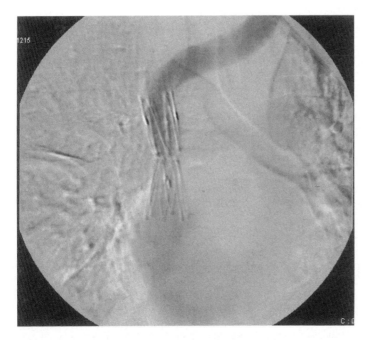

Figure 21 SVC after Gianturco stent deployment.

in preserving the existing access site (31). Catheter-related stenosis and occlusion of the superior vena cava has also been described. Gradual stricture development and the presence of collateral pathways generally prevents the development of an overt superior vena caval syndrome, however, subsequent venous access sites and hemodialysis grafts and fistulae may require recanalization of the stenotic or occluded vessel (32,33). A variety of methods and materials may be employed (Figs. 17–21).

REFERENCES

1. Mauro M, Jaques P. Radiologic placement of long-term central venous catheters: a review. J Vasc Interv Radiol 1993; 4(1):127–137.
2. Lund GB, Trerotola SO, Scheel PFJ, et al. Outcome of tunneled hemodialysis catheters placed by radiologists. Radiology 1996; 198(2):467–472.
3. Mauro MA. Interventional radiologic placement of central venous catheters. Hospital Physician 1996:55–59.
4. Lewis CA, Allen TE, Burke DR, Cardella JF, Citron SJ, et al. Quality improvement guidelines for central venous access. J Vasc Interv Radiol 1997; 8(3):475–479.
5. Skolnick M. The role of sonography in the placement of and management of jugular and subclavian cetral venous catheters. Am J Roentgenol 1994; 163:291–295.
6. Troianos C, Jobes D, Ellison N. Ultrasound-guided cannulation of the internal jugular vein: a prospective, randomized study. Anesth Analg 1991; 72:823–826.
7. Denys B, Uretsky B, Reddy P. Ultrasound-assisted cannulation of the internal jugular vein: a prospective comparison to external landmark-guided technique. Circulation 1993; 87:1557–1562.
8. Farmery AD, Shlugman D, Anslow P. How high do the subclavian arteries ascend into the neck? A population study using magnetic resonance imaging. Br J Anaesth 2003; 90(4):452–456.
9. Kulvatunyou N, Heard SO, Bankey PE. A subclavian artery injury, secondary to internal jugular vein cannulation, is a predictable right-sided phenomenon [see comment]. Anesth Anal 2002; 95(3):564–566, table of contents.
10. Lorenz J, Funaki B, Van Ha T, Leef A. Radiologic placement of implatable chest ports in pediatric patients. Am J Roentgenol 2001; 176:991–994.
11. Bagwell C, Salzberg A, Sonnino R, Haynes J. Potentially lethal complications of central venous catheter placement. J Pediatric Surg 2000; 35:709–713.
12. Vesely T. Air embolism during insertion of central venous catheters. J Vasc Interv Radiol 2001; 12:1291–1295.
13. Orebaugh S. Venous air embolism: clinical and experimental considerations. Crit Care Med 1992; 20:1169–1177.
14. Breaux E, Dupont J, Albert H, Bryant L, Schecter F. Cardiac tamponade following penetrating mediastinal injuries: improved survival with early pericardiocentesis. J Trauma 1979; 19:461–466.
15. Robinson J, Robinson W, Cohn A, Garg K, Armstrong J. Perforation of the great vessels during central venous line placement. Arch Intern Med 1995; 155:1225–1228.
16. Teichgraber UK, Gebauer B, Benter T, Wagner HJ. Central venous access catheters: radiological management of complications. Cardiovasc Interv Radiol 2003; 26(4): 321–333.
17. Schuster M, Nave H, Piepenbrock S, Pabst R, Panning B. The carina as a landmark in central venous catheter placement. Br J Anaesth 2000; 85:192–194.
18. Karakaya D, Baris H, Guldogus F, Incesu L, Sarihasan B, Tur A. Brachial plexus injury during subclavian vein catheterization for hemodialysis. J Clin Anesth 2000; 12:220–223.
19. Hadeed H, Braun T. Paralysis of the hemidiaphragm as a complication of internal jugular vein cannulation: report of a case. J Oral Maxillofac Surg 1988; 46:409–411.

20. Denny DFJ. Placement and management of long-term central venous access catheters and ports. Am J Roentgenol 1993; 161:385–393.

21. Simpson KR, Hovsepian DM, Picus D. Interventional radiologic placement of chest wall ports: results and complications in 161 consecutive placements. J Vasc Interv Radiol 1997; 8:189–195.

22. Moureau N, Poole S, Murdock M, Gray S, Semba C. Central venous catheters in home infusion care: outcomes analysis in 50,470 patients. J Vasc Interv Radiol 2002; 13:1099–1102.

23. Andris D, Krzywda E, Schulte W, Ausman R, Quebbeman E. Pinch-off syndrome: a rare etiology for central venous catheter occlusion. J Parenter Enteral Nutr 1994; 18:531–533.

24. Moss J, Wagman L, Riihimaki D, et al. Central venous thrombosis related to the silastic Hickman–Broviac catheters in an oncologic population. J Parenter Enteral Nutr 1989; 13:397–400.

25. Forauer AR, Theoharis C. Histologic changes in the human vein wall adjacent to indwelling central venous catheters. J Vasc Interv Radiol 2003; 14(9 Pt 1):1163–1168.

26. Merport M, Murphy TP, Egglin TK, Dubel GJ. Fibrin sheath stripping versus catheter exchange for the treatment of failed tunneled hemodialysis catheters: randomized clinical trial. J Vasc Interv Radiol 2000; 11(9):1115–1120.

27. Gray RJ, Levitin A, Buck D, et al. Percutaneous fibrin sheath stripping versus transcatheter urokinase infusion for malfunctioning well-positioned tunneled central venous dialysis catheters: a prospective, randomized trial. J Vasc Interv Radiol 2000; 11(9): 1121–1129.

28. Savader SJ, Haikal LC, Ehrman KO, Porter DJ, Oteham AC. Hemodialysis catheter-associated fibrin sheaths: treatment with a low-dose rt-PA infusion. J Vasc Interv Radiol 2000; 11(9):1131–1136.

29. Bern M, Lokich J, Wallach S, et al. Very low doses of warfarin can prevent thrombosis in central venous catheters: a randomized prospective trial. Ann Intern Med 1990; 112: 423–428.

30. Valerio D, Hussey J, Smith F. Central vein thrombosis associated with intravenous feeding—a prospective study. J Parenter Enteral Nutr 1981; 5:240–242.

31. Burkart D, Borsa J, Anthony J, Thurlo S. Thrombolysis of occluded peripheral arteries and veins with tenecteplase: a pilot study. J Vasc Interv Radiol 2002; 13:1099–1102.

32. Patel TM, Shah SC, Ranjan A, Malhotra H, Patel R, Gupta AK. Stenting through a portacath for totally occluded superior vena cava in a case of non-Hodgkin's lymphoma. J Invasive Cardiol 2003; 15(2):86–88.

33. de Gregorio Ariza MA, Gamboa P, Gimeno MJ, et al. Percutaneous treatment of superior vena cava syndrome using metallic stents. Eur Radiol 2003; 13(4):853–862.

9

Complications of Endovascular Carotid Artery Stenting

Jacqueline Saw
Cardiac Catheterization Laboratory, Vancouver General Hospital, University of British Columbia, Vancouver, British Columbia, Canada and Department of Cardiovascular Medicine, The Cleveland Clinic Foundation, Cleveland, Ohio, U.S.A.

Jay S. Yadav
Department of Cardiovascular Medicine, The Cleveland Clinic Foundation, Cleveland, Ohio, U.S.A.

INTRODUCTION

Carotid revascularization has evolved as an important tool to prevent thromboembolic strokes and deaths over the past five decades. In the United States, stroke is the leading cause of disability and the third leading cause of death (1). The recognition that the majority of strokes have an ischemic basis from embolism (24%) or thrombosis (61%) fueled the development of effective preventive strategies (1). Medical therapies with antiplatelet, antihypertensive and lipid-lowering agents play vital roles in reducing ischemic strokes. Atherosclerotic preventive strategies including smoking cessation and optimal diabetic treatment are also effective. In addition, surgical revascularization with carotid endarterectomy (CEA) has long been established as the gold standard procedure for preventing strokes with benefit in patients with >50% symptomatic, or >60% asymptomatic carotid stenosis (2–4). This modality, however, may soon be supplanted by percutaneous carotid artery stenting (CAS), at least in high surgical risk patients. CAS was recently proven to be superior to CEA in the Stenting and Angioplasty with Protection in Patients at High Risk for Endarterectomy (SAPPHIRE) trial in patients at high-risk for CEA (5). Further randomized data involving low-risk patients currently in progress are expected to propel the upsurge in CAS. It is important to appreciate that CAS is a technically challenging procedure, requiring meticulous technique to reduce procedural complications. Before embarking on this procedure, operators should have a thorough understanding of the prevention and management of complications.

Several known complications may occur with CAS, stroke and death being the most significant. With the advancement in technology and equipment for performance of CAS, the peri procedural complications have shifted downwards. This is particularly true with the use of emboli protection devices (EPD), whereby the combined 30-day stroke and death rate was 1.8% in those with EPD use compared to 5.5% without EPD in a meta-analysis of 3196 patients (6). In the global experience of 5210 procedures reported by Wholey et al., the combined incidence of 30-day death and stroke (major and minor) was 6.29% (7). The incidence of individual endpoints were as follows: transient ischemic attacks (TIA) 2.82%, minor strokes 2.72%, major strokes 1.49%, and death 0.86% (7). Stroke can be a devastating complication of CAS, and is about 2.5 times more frequent in patients with symptomatic, as opposed to asymptomatic carotid stenosis (8). Other clinical predictors of stroke complicating CAS are advanced age and the presence of long lesions (>10 mm) or multiple stenoses (9). Although involving a different vascular bed, the incidence of peri procedural myocardial infarction (MI) is not trivial, ranging from 0.9% to 2.6% (5,10,11). Nonetheless, CAS was safer than CEA in the SAPPHIRE trial which randomized 307 high-risk patients, with peri procedural death, stroke or MI rates of 5.8% for CAS and 12.6% for CEA ($p = 0.047$) (5).

While the majority of ischemic complications tend to occur during the procedure, clinicians still need to be vigilant of post-procedural delayed complications. The incidence of neurologic events and deaths after the initial 30 days was 1.39% in 3924 patients at up to one-year follow-up (7). We have categorized potential complications accordingly (Table 1): procedural which can be subdivided into three stages: during access of the common carotid artery, during placement of EPD, or during angiopiasty or stenting of the target lesion early post-procedural, and late post-procedural (1–3,12).

PROCEDURAL COMPLICATIONS

Complications During Access of the Common Carotid Artery

Arterial Access Complications

The transfemoral retrograde approach is most frequently used for CAS. However, transbrachial or transradial approaches are also feasible for contralateral carotid interventions. Direct carotid puncture was performed previously but has been abandoned due to higher complications (carotid dissection and thrombosis; neck hematoma that

Table 1 Complications of CAS

Procedural complications	
Access of common carotid artery	Arterial access complications
	Carotid access complications
Placement of EPD	Embolization
	Dissection
	Ischemia
Angioplasty/stent of carotid stenosis	Cerebral ischemia
	Distal embolization
	Acute vessel closure
	Reflex bradycardia and hypotension
Early post-procedural complications	Cerebral hyperperfusion syndrome
	Stent thrombosis
	Late distal embolization
Late post-procedural complications	Stent deformation
	In-stent restenosis

Abbreviations: EPD, emboli protection devices; CAS, carotid artery stenting.

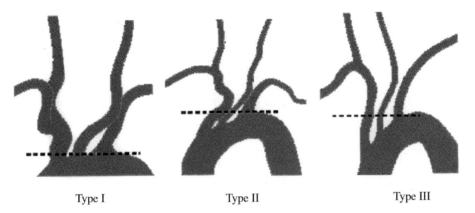

Type I   Type II   Type III

Figure 1 Aortic arch classification.

may compromise airway) and lack of necessity given the improvements in guide cathe-ter and angioplasty/stent devices. With such advances in equipments, the requirements of access site sizes have also decreased with most procedures accomplished via 6 French sheaths or 8 French guides. The complications associated with femoral, brachial and radial arterial access sites and their managements are well described in numerous cathe-terization textbooks, and will not be further discussed in this chapter.

Carotid Access Complications

Difficulties in accessing the common carotid arteries may arise depending upon the aortic arch anatomy. Type I arch generally allows straightforward access to all great vessels, whereas Type II and III arches (where the origins of the innominate or left common carotid artery are inferiorly displaced) portend more difficult access (Fig. 1), often requiring more complex catheters (Vitek or Simmons). Complications during guide engagements include plaque embolization or dissection of the common carotid artery. The development of new carotid guide catheters (Fig. 2) lowered such compli-cations and also contributed to improvement in technical success rates to >98% (7). Several techniques of carotid artery access have been described, including the popu-lar "telescoping approach" that is currently favored at the Cleveland Clinic (Table 2). In our experience, a meticulous strategy of performing complete pre-intervention diagnostic cerebral angiography (including an aortic arch angiogram) (Table 3) and utilizing appropriate guide catheters or telescoping apparatus with minimal catheter manipulation, allows carotid artery access with minimal complications.

Complications During Placement of EPD

The demonstration of microembolization with transcranial Doppler during carotid angiopiasty fueled the development and utilization of a wide selection of EPDs (13). Even though these devices reduce the risk of brain embolizations and are essen-tially mandatory in all CAS, they are not benign. First, challenging and complicated (such as tight and tortuous) carotid stenoses may preclude successful delivery and deployment of these devices. Second, crossing with these devices may roughen up the intimal surface and shear off debris distally, although with proper technique we have found this to be an exceedingly rare event. Third, the EPD may not be well opposed to the arterial wall, thus allowing microemboli to escape downstream

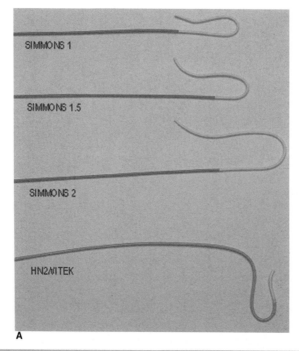

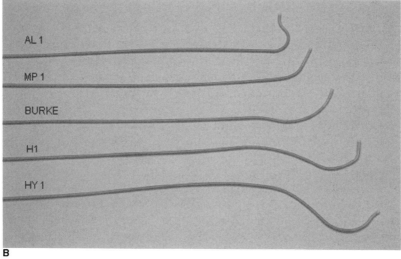

Figure 2 Carotid (**A**) diagnostic and (**B**) guide catheters.

around the devices; this is particularly true for filters with an eccentric guidewire location. Fourth, inadvertent displacement of the deployed devices (especially the occlusive EPD) could injure the vessel wall and cause major dissection and emboliza-tion. Lastly, prolonged balloon inflation with the occlusive devices, or complete fill-ing of filter baskets can protract cerebral ischemia with its attended complications (see section "Complications during angioplasty or stenting of the target lesion"). Therefore, like all steps in the CAS procedure, placement and retrieval of EPDs requires planning and meticulous technique to reduce complications.

Table 2   The Cleveland Clinic Foundation Protocol for Carotid Stenting

Patients lightly sedated with short-acting intravenous sedation; arterial sheath inserted in
  femoral artery
Aortic arch angiographic study (LAO 30° projection) performed to determine origin of great
  vessels to choose an appropriate catheter for selective angiography
Baseline angiography performed of bilateral vertebral and carotid arteries to determine extent
  of vascular disease and presence of collateral circulation
Unfractionated heparin 60 units/kg with target ACT >250 s
125 cm 5 French JR4 diagnostic catheter (Cordis Corporation, Miami, Florida) placed inside
  a 100 cm 8 French H1 Guide (Cordis)
Origin of common carotid artery intubated with JR4 catheter and 0.035 angled stiff glide wire
  (Boston Scientific) guidewire advanced into the external carotid artery
H1 advanced into common carotid artery over the JR4 catheter
JR4 catheter withdrawn and diagnostic angiograms performed in the ipsilateral 30° oblique
  and left lateral projections
Lesion in the carotid artery traversed with an Angioguard (Cordis) or other EPD
4.0 × 20 mm Monorail Aviator (Cordis) angioplasty balloon catheter or Viatrac (Guidant)
  used to predilate lesion to allow subsequent passage of self-expanding stent
Stenting performed with a nitinol stent
Stent postdilated with 5.5 to 6.0 × 20 mm Aviator or Viatrac
Patients receive 325 mg aspirin and 300 mg clopidogrel prior to procedure and are discharged
  home the following day on clopidogrel (75 mg po qd) for 4 wk and on aspirin (325 mg po
  qd) indefinitely

Abbreviations: ACT, activated clotting time; LAO, left anterior oblique; EPD, emboli protection devices.
Source: From Ref. 33.

Complications During Angioplasty or Stenting of the Target Lesion

Cerebral Ischemia

Transient obstructions of cerebral blood flow occur frequently during CAS,
especially during balloon inflation and stent deployment. The utilization of EPDs
can also contribute to cerebral ischemia during prolonged inflation of occlusive balloon devices. Patients normally tolerate short ischemic episodes relatively well unless
the collateral circulation is compromised, such as an incomplete circle of Willis with
hypoplastic anterior communicating or posterior communicating arteries, or if multiple stenoses are present in the contralateral arterial supply. Thus, symptom presentations vary among patients, from none to loss of consciousness, seizures, or TIA.

Table 3   Diagnostic Cerebral Angiogram Views

Aortic arch with 45° LAO, 30 cc non-ionic contrast, large field of view
Ipsilateral oblique and lateral of both carotid arteries
PA and lateral intracranial views of both carotids with particular attention
  to the carotid siphons
Selective injections of both subclavian arteries in contralateral oblique projections
  to adequately visualize the vertebral artery ostia
Non-selective injection of the dominant vertebral with intracranial views
  of the vertebrobasilar system in lateral and steep cranial PA projections

Abbreviations: LAO, left anterior oblique; PA, posteroanterior.
Source: From Ref. 20.

In a report by Yadav et al., the four patients (of 107 CAS patients) who transiently lost consciousness during angioplasty balloon inflation had contralateral carotid occlusions (8). TIA can occur in ~3% of CAS procedures, manifesting as either amaurosis fugax or transient motor-sensory deficits (7). There are no long-term sequelae from these transient ischemic episodes. Prevention and management includes short angioplasty balloon inflation, and expeditious but meticulous techniques to limit occlusive EPD balloon inflation times. With non-occlusive EPDs, if the filters are coated with debris leading to decreased flow distally, it is crucial to prevent embolization by suctioning the stagnant column of blood proximal to the filter basket with either a 5 French multipurpose catheter or an Export catheter of the PercuSurge® GuardWire™ (Medtronic, Minneapolis, Minnesota) device prior to retrieval of the filter. The stagnant column of blood contains suspended debris, which will go to the brain if the filter is collapsed and retrieved with aspiration of the internal carotid.

Distal Embolization

Monitoring with transcranial Doppler during carotid angioplasty has demonstrated that microembolization occurs in virtually all procedural phases, even with guide and wire manipulations (14,15). However, the significant embolization occurs with stent deployment and balloon dilatation (Fig. 3) (14–16). Despite these inevitable embolizations that occur with CAS (Fig. 4), the brain has an amazing tolerance to smaller size particles, with much lower clinical neurologic complications compared with embolization rates. In 301 patients undergoing surgical CEA, adverse clinical events occurred in only 5.7% of patients despite the occurrence of detected embolization in the majority of patients (17). Nevertheless, the quantity and size of embolic particles do correlate with the incidence of neurologic deficits and infarcts after CEA (17–19). To address this prevalent problem, numerous EPDs have been developed which can

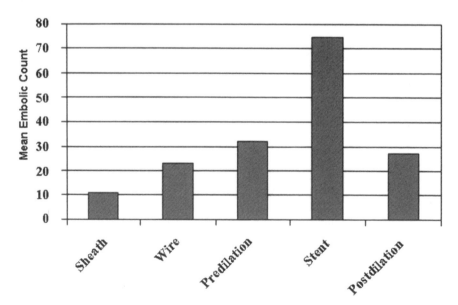

Figure 3 Detection of microemboli with transcranial Doppler during percutaneous carotid interventions.

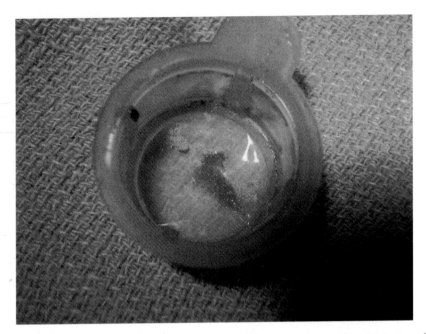

Figure 4 Embolic material collected from the Export catheter of the PercuSurge® device.

be divided into occlusive (distal or proximal balloon occlusions) and non-occlusive devices. None of these devices are currently approved by the FDA for use in the carotid, the PercuSurge GuardWire (Medtronic, Minneapolis, Minnesota) and the FilterWire EX™ (Boston Scientific/Medi-tech, Natick, Massachusetts) are currently approved for use in SVGs. A number of EPD devices are in CAS clinical trials (Table 4). In fact, all modern CAS trials necessitate the adjunctive use of EPDs (6). There have been no studies to date that compare the safety and efficacy of different devices. Despite the obvious advantages, it is important to be aware of potential problems that may arise with EPD use (see Complications during placement of EPD). In addition, not all embolic materials may be captured by these devices, which may result in procedural strokes (typically atherosclerotic fragments as opposed to thrombotic materials). Management in such a circumstance would depend on the significance of the intracranial arterial occlusion. If no occlusion is identified, medical management with fluid resuscitation and maintenance of blood pressure is recommended. However, if the M1 or M2 segment of the middle cerebral artery (MCA) is occluded, a mechanical approach is recommended (using a hydrophilic wire to cross the blockage and dislodge the embolus, with or without a small 1.5 mm coronary angioplasty balloon; alternatively, a small snare can be used to capture the embolus) (20). Although intra-arterial tPA or glycoprotein (GP) llb/llla antagonists (specifically abciximab) have been used successfully in refractory cases, it is important to weigh the benefits against the risk of intracranial hemorrhage (21). Occlusions beyond the M2 segment of the MCA generally have a good prognosis.

Acute Vessel Closure

Abrupt closure of the vessel during CAS is very uncommon with current techniques and equipment. It occurred more frequently with carotid angioplasty alone, which can be associated with dissection and thrombosis.

Table 4 Emboli Protection Devices

Occlusive devices	
Distal occlusion balloon:	PercuSurge® GuardWire™ (Medtronic, Minneapolis, Minnesota)
Proximal occlusion balloon:	Parodi Anti-Emboli System™ (ArteriA, San Francisco, California)
	MO.MA (INVAtec, Roncadelle, Italy)
Non-occlusive devices	
Supported filters:	AngioGuard™ Emboli Capture Guidewire (Cordis, Warren, New Jersey)
	NeuroShield™ (Mednova Inc., Galway, Ireland)
	AccuNet® (Guidant, Indianapolis, Indiana)
	Trap™ (Microvena, White Bear Lake, Minnesota)
Unsupported filters:	FilterWire EX® (Boston Scientific, Natick, Massachusetts)
	E-Trap™ (Metamorphic Surgical Devices, Pittsburgh, Pennsylvania)

Modern routine stenting with self-expanding elgiloy or nitinol stents reduces and treats dissections created by balloon dilatation. Contemporary antiplatelet and anticoagulant therapies also decrease procedural thrombotic complications. Ideally, patients should have been pretreated with dual antiplatelet therapy consisting of aspirin and clopidogrel. Clopidogrel pretreatment orally with 75 mg/d for five days is necessary to achieve adequate steady-state platelet inhibition. Otherwise, a loading dose of >375 mg at least five hours prior to procedure is required to achieve >80% platelet inhibition (22). Post-procedure, aspirin should be administered indefinitely, while clopidogrel should be given for at least one month. Anticoagulation with intravenous (IV) heparin should be administered to achieve an activated clotting time (ACT) of 275–300 seconds during the procedure. The use of low molecular weight heparins and direct thrombin inhibitors (such as bivalirudin or hirudin) have not been studied in the setting of CAS. With availability of EPDs, the routine use of IV GP llb/llla antagonists is not recommended given the potential risk of intracranial hemorrhage; but if they are administered, the heparin dose should be reduced to target the ACT around 250 seconds (20). In a non-randomized CAS prospective study, the 128/151 patients who received abciximab (0.25 mg/kg bolus IV, and 0.125 jag/kg/min infusion for 12 hours) had lower procedural stroke, intracranial hemorrhage or neurologic death when compared to controls (1.6% versus 8.0%, $p = 0.05$) (23). However, in a small randomized CAS study of 74 patients, the periprocedural ischemic events were not different in those randomized to abciximab (0.25 mg/kg IV bolus without infusion) (19%) compared with controls (8%) (24). These studies are of different designs, addressed different drug duration, and are too small for conclusive recommendations.

Reflex Bradycardia and Hypotension

Angioplasty of the carotid artery often stimulates the carotid baroreceptors via the afferent glossopharyngeal nerve, which is then relayed to the efferent vagal nerve decreasing cardiac chronotropy and inotropy (Fig. 5) (20). The efferent reflex arc is also relayed to the spinal cord sympathetic nervous system causing vasodilatation.

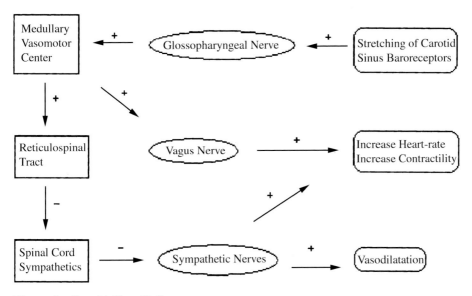

Figure 5   Carotid Sinus Reflex.

These reflex-mediated bradycardia and hypotension occur relatively frequently during CAS, 27.5% and 22.4%, respectively, in a study by Qureshi et al. (25). These are
more commonly observed during balloon inflation at the carotid bifurcation or the
proximal internal carotid artery, and usually during post-dilatation of the stent.
In a study by Yadav et al., 71% of patients developed significant bradycardia during
balloon inflation of the carotid sinus (8). These bradycardic episodes are generally
self-limited, resolving with balloon deflation, lasting only a few minutes, and do not
cause permanent high-grade atrioventricular block (8). More severe cases require IV
atropine and almost never require temporary transvenous pacemakers. The vasodila-
tory component may be more persistent, with a small proportion of patients experiencing prolonged hypotension lasting several hours that may necessitate volume
expansion and temporary vasoconstrictor therapy (e.g., pseudoephedrine, norepine-
phrine, dopamine) (20). Our protocol for post-CAS management at the Cleveland
Clinic ensures close monitoring for neurologic symptoms (i.e., headaches, altered
sensorium, focal neurologic deficits) and tight systolic blood pressure control
between 90 mmHg and 140 mmHg.

EARLY POST-PROCEDURAL COMPLICATIONS

Cerebral Hyperperfusion Syndrome

The relief of a significant high-grade carotid stenosis by CAS or CEA is accompanied by a dramatic and instantaneous increase in ipsilateral cerebral blood
flow, often in the setting of impaired cerebrovascular autoregulation due to chronic
cerebral ischemia. This cerebral hyperperfusion is transient, but may provoke severe
symptoms including ipsilateral headache, vomiting, altered sensorium, stupor,
hypertension, seizures, focal neurologic deficits, and intracranial hemorrhage. In a
series from the Cleveland Clinic, 3/323 (1%) patients suffered intracranial hemorrhage (26). Patients with high-grade stenosis (>90%), contralateral occlusion, and

severe underlying hypertension have increased risk (26). Management of this syndrome includes early recognition, with careful blood pressure (beta-blockers and diuretics) and seizure control. Prompt imaging should be performed (computed tomography or magnetic resonance imaging) to diagnose cerebral edema or hemorrhage. Transcranial Doppler may also be helpful to demonstrate increased ipsilateral flow velocity and pulsatility index (27).

Stent Thrombosis

Carotid artery stent thrombosis is relatively infrequent, occurring in ∼0.8% of cases (8). The development and utilization of self-expanding stents, and the use of dual antiplatelet therapy have lowered the risks of stent thrombosis in the current era. The use of balloon-expandable stents for the carotid bifurcation has been abandoned given the risk of stent deformation due to external compression (28). The self-expanding stents have superior apposition and conform better to vessel walls, although the precision of stent deployment is inferior to balloon-expandable stents.

Several elgiloy (e.g., Wallstent® by Boston Scientific) and nitinol (e.g., PRE-CISE™ by Cordis, SMART™ by Cordis, ACCULINK™ by Guidant, Memotherm® by Bard) self-expanding stents are now being evaluated for CAS. The Wallstent tends to foreshorten substantially and has reduced radial strength; thus operators should oversize both the diameter and length of such stents. In contrast, the nitinol stents have high radial strength, foreshorten only minimally, and have a tendency to expand after deployment. Consequently, substantial oversizing is not needed with these stents. The use of dual antiplatelet therapy (aspirin and clopidogrel) is another major contributor of reducing stent thrombosis. Aspirin is recommended life-long, and clopidogrel for at least four weeks post-CAS. Even though longer clopidogrel therapy has been shown to be beneficial for percutaneous coronary interventions (29,30), similar data for CAS is lacking.

Late Distal Embolization

Although the majority of embolization occurs during the procedure, embolic events can happen for several hours after stent deployment. These very rare late events probably arise from detachment of atherosclerotic fragments protruding through stent struts. These are typically TIAs that do not require intervention. Major deficits require CT scanning and cerebral angiography, followed by specific therapy as in distal embolization.

LATE POST-PROCEDURAL COMPLICATIONS

Stent Deformation

The use of balloon-expandable stents in the superficial carotid artery is not optimal given the possibility of external compression. Stent collapse, defined as the loss of apposition of the stent to the vessel wall (28), can occur in 0–16% of cases upon follow-up with the Palmaz balloon-expandable stents.

Bergeron et al. reported no stent compression in 96 patients treated with Palmaz stents at 13-month follow-up (31). Wholey et al. reported a stent deformation (>50% compression of stent) incidence of 2.5% in Palmaz stents at six-month follow-up (7). Yadav et al. reported 6% incidences of Palmaz stent deformation at six-month follow-up (8). Patients usually remain asymptomatic, but some may require repeat angioplasty or placement of self-expanding stents (28). Stent deformation has been eliminated with the use of self-expanding stents.

In-Stent Restenosis

Unlike stenting of other arterial beds (peripheral extremities or coronary arteries), the in-stent restenosis rates involving carotid arteries are very low. In the largest global CAS series to date, Wholey et al. reported a restenosis rate of 2.3% at six months in 4502 patients, and 3.4% at one year in 3924 patients (7). The majority of restenosis can be successfully treated with balloon angioplasty. We have successfully performed Brachytherapy for refractory carotid stent restenosis (32). The large carotid luminal diameter necessitates the use of gamma radiation, which penetrates deeper than beta radiation. CEA is not indicated for carotid stent restenosis.

CONCLUSIONS

Percutaneous carotid intervention is a rapidly evolving field with novel equipments (catheters, stents, and emboli protection devices) that have effectively reduced periprocedural complications. CAS is currently reserved for patients requiring carotid revascularization who are poor candidates for surgical endarterectomy. Upcoming studies are expected to expand its indications to lower-risk patients. Although periprocedural complications are lower with carotid stenting compared with endarterectomy in high-risk patients, operators need to be aware of potential complications that are unique to carotid stenting. Meticulous techniques, prompt recognition and management of complications are essential for the continued success of this endovascular carotid treatment.

REFERENCES

1. American Heart Association, Heart Disease and Stroke Statistics—2003 Update. Dallas, Texas: American Heart Association, 2002.
2. NASCET Investigators. Beneficial effect of carotid endarterectomy in symptomatic patients with high-grade carotid stenosis. North American Symptomatic Carotid Endarterectomy Trial Collaborators. N Engl J Med 1991; 325:445–453.
3. ECST Investigators. Randomized trial of endarterectomy for recently symptomatic carotid stenosis: final results of the MRC European Cartid Surgery Trial (ECST). Lancet 1998; 351:1379–1387.
4. ACAS Investigators. Endarterectomy for asymptomatic carotid artery stenosis. Executive Committee for the Asymptomatic Carotid Atherosclerosis Study. J Am Med Assoc 1995; 273:1421–1428.
5. Yadav J, and The SAPPHIRE Study Investigators. Stenting and Angioplasty with Protection in Patients at High Risk for Endarterectomy. Chicago, IL: The American Heart Association Scientific Sessions, 2002.
6. Kastrup A, Groschei K, Kraph H, Brehm B, Dichgans J, Schulz J. Early outcome of carotid angioplasty and stenting with and without cerebral protection devices. A systematic review of the literature. Stroke 2003; 34:813–819.
7. Wholey MH, Wholey M, Mathias K, Roubin GS, Diethrich EB, Henry M, Bailey S, Bergeron P, Dorros G, Eles G. Global experience in cervical carotid artery stent placement. Catheter Cardiovasc Interv 2000; 50:160–167.

8. Yadav JS, Roubin GS, Iyer S, Vitck J, King P, Jordan WD, Fisher WS. Elective stenting of the extracranial carotid arteries. Circulation 1997; 95:376–381.

9. Mathur A, Roubin GS, Iyer SS, Piamsonboon C, Liu MW, Gomez CR, Yadav JS, Chastain HD, Fox LM, Dean LS, Vitek JJ. Predictors of stroke complicating carotid artery stenting. Circulation 1998; 97:1239–1245.

10. Reimers B, Corvaja N, Moshiri S, Sacca S, Albiero R, Di Mario C, Pascotto P, Colombo A. Cerebral protection with filter devices during carotid artery stenting. Circulation 2001; 104:12–15.

11. Wholey MH, Jarmoiowski CR, Eles G, Levy D, Buecthel J. Endovascular stents for carotid artery occlusive disease. J Endovasc Surg 1997; 4:326–338.

12. Wholey M, Jarmoiowski C, Wholey M, Eles G. Carotid artery stent placement—ready for prime time? J Vasc Interv Radiol 2003; 14:1–10.

13. Markus HS, Clifton A, Buckenham T, Brown MM. Carotid angioplasty. Detection of embolic signals during and after the procedure. Stroke 1994; 25:2403–2406.

14. Jordan WJ, Voeliinger C, Doblar D, Piyushcheva N, Fisher W, McDowell H. Microemboli detected by transcranial Doppler monitoring in patients during carotid angioplasty versus carotid endarterectomy. Cardiol Surg 1999; 7:33–38.

15. Rapp JH, Pan XM, Sharp FR, Shah DM, Wille GA, Velez PM, Troyer A, Higashida RT, Saloner D. Atheroemboli to the brain: size threshold for causing acute neuronal cell death. J Vasc Surg 2000; 32:68–76.

16. Al-Mubarak N, Roubin G, Vitek J, Iyer S, New G, Leon M. Effect of the distal-balloon protection system on microembolization during carotid stenting. Circulation 2001; 104: 1999–2002.

17. Ackerstaff RG, Jansen C, Moll FL, Vermeulen FE, Hamerlijnck RP, Mauser HW. The significance of microemboli detection by means of transcranial Doppler ultrasonography monitoring in carotid endarterectomy. J Vasc Surg 1995; 21:963–969.

18. Jansen C, Ramos LM, van Heesewijk JP, Moll FL, van Gijn J, Ackerstaff RG. Impact of microembolism and hemodynamic changes in the brain during carotid endarterectomy. Stroke 1994; 25:992–997.

19. Tubler T, Schluter M, Dirsch O, Sievert H, Bosenberg I, Grube E, Waigand J, Schofer J. Balloon-protected carotid artery stenting: relationship of periprocedural neurological complications with the size of participate debris. Circulation 2001; 104:2791–2796.

20. Yadav JS. Technical Aspects of Carotid Stenting. EuroPCR. Version 3rd ed. Paris, 2003: 1–18.

21. Qureshi AI, Saad M, Zaidat OO, Suarez JI, Alexander MJ, Farood M, Suri K, Ali Z, Hopkins LN. Intracerebral hemorrhages associated with neurointerventional procedures using a combination of antithrombotic agents including abciximab. Stroke 2002; 33:1916–1919.

22. Savcic M, Hauert J, Bachmann F, Wyld P, Geudelin B, Cariou R. Clopidogrel loading dose regimens: kinetic profile of pharmacodynamic response in healthy subjects. Semin Thromb Haemost 1999; 25:15–19.

23. Kapadia SR, Bajzer CT, Ziada KM, Bhatt DL, Wazni OM, Silver MJ, Beven EG, Ouriel K, Yadav JS. Initial experience of platelet glycoprotein IIb/IIIa inhibition with abciximab during carotid stenting: a safe and effective adjunctive therapy. Stroke 2001; 32: 2328–2332.

24. Hofmann R, Kerschner K, Steinwender C, Kypta A, Bibl D, Leisch F. Abciximab bolus injection does not reduce cerebral ischemic complications of elective carotid artery stenting: a randomized study. Stroke 2002; 33:725–727.

25. Qureshi AI, Luft AR, Sharma M, Janardhan V, Lopes DK, Khan J, Guterman LR, Hopkins LN. Frequency and determinants of postprocedural hemodynamic instability after carotid angioplasty and stenting. Stroke 1999; 30:2086–2093.

26. Abou-Chebl A, Reginelli J, Mukherjee D, Bhatt D, Bajzer C, Yadav J. Cerebral hyperperfusion and intracranial hemorrhage following internal carotid artery stenting. J Am Coll Cardiol 2002; 39:68A.

27. Meyers PM, Higashida RT, Phatouros CC, Malek AM, Lempert TE, Dowd CF, Halbach VV. Cerebral hyperperfusion syndrome after percutaneous transiuminal stenting of the craniocervical arteries. Neurosurg 2000; 47:335–345.
28. Mathur A, Dorros G, Iyer SS, Vitek JJ, Yadav SS, Roubin GS. Palmaz stent compression in patients following carotid artery stenting. Catheteriz Cardiovasc Diagn 1997; 41:137–140.
29. Steinhubl SR, Berger PB, Mann JT III, Fry ET, DeLago A, Wilmer C, Topol EJ, CREDO Investigators. Clopidogrel for the reduction of events during observation. Early and sustained dual oral antiplatelet therapy following percutaneous coronary intervention. J Am Med Assoc 2002; 288:2411–2420.
30. Mehta Sr, Yusuf S, Peters RJ, Bertrand ME, Lewis BS, Natarajan MK, Malmberg K, Rupprecht H, Zhao F, Chrolavicius S, Copland I, Fox KA, Clopidogrel in Unstable Angina to Prevent Recurrent Events Trial (CURE) Investigators. Effects of pretreatment with clopidogrel and aspirin followed by long-term therapy in patients undergoing percutaneous coronary intervention: the PCI-CURE study. Lancet 2001; 358:527–533.
31. Bergeron P, Becquemin JP, Jausseran JM, Biasi G, Cardon JM, Castellani L, Martinez R, Fiorani P, Kniemeyer P. Percutaneous stenting of the internal carotid artery: the European CAST 1 Study–Carotid Artery Stent Trial. J Endovasc Surg 1999; 6:155–159.
32. Chan AW, Roffi M, Mukherjee D, Bajzer CT, Abou-Chebl A, Ciezki J, Bhatt DL, Ghaffari S, Yadav JS. Carotid brachytherapy for in-stent restenosis. Catheteriz Cardiovasc Interv 2003; 58:86–92.
33. Mukherjee D, Yadav J. Percutaneous treatment for carotid stenosis. Cardiol Clin 2002; 20:589–597.

10

Complications in Endovascular Therapy: Subclavian and Extracranial Vertebral Artery Occlusive Disease

Piotr S. Sobieszczyk and Andrew C. Eisenhauer
Interventional Cardiovascular Medicine, Cardiovascular Division, Brigham and Women's Hospital and Harvard Medical School, Boston, Massachusetts, U.S.A.

INTRODUCTION

The burden of peripheral arterial disease will continue to increase as a consequence of aging population and increasing prevalence of diabetes. By the 1960s, atherosclerosis of the subclavian and brachiocephalic arteries was responsible for 17% of symptomatic extracranial cerebrovascular disease (1). In patients with symptoms of cerebrovascular ischemia, vertebral arteries had greater than 50% stenosis in 22%, and 18% of patients on the left and right side, respectively (2). Subclavian artery stenosis has been noted in 3.5% of all patients referred for coronary catheterization and in 41% of patients referred for coronary catheterization who had stigmata of peripheral arterial disease (3,4). Continual improvements in non-invasive diagnostic imaging modalities, such as magnetic resonance angiography and CT-angiography allow rapid and accurate diagnosis of occlusive lesions in the subclavian and vertebral arteries (5). These developments, combined with technical innovations in endovascular therapy and growing awareness of peripheral arterial disease, will continue to foster a growth in the number of endovascular procedures. As the threshold for interventions in the subclavian, brachiocephalic and extracranial vertebral arteries becomes lower, the number of complications encountered will likely rise.

Although there are no formal guidelines for endovascular interventions in the subclavian and vertebral arteries, the most common indications include occlusive lesions causing symptoms of posterior circulation ischemia and subclavian steal, upper extremity claudication or embolization. In addition, the preservation or restoration of subclavian patency to protect an internal mammary to coronary graft is a common scenario. Atherosclerosis is the most common etiology followed by Takayasu's arteritis and giant cell arteritis (6). Radiation-induced strictures, fibromuscular dysplasia, Behçet's disease and other vasculitidies are quite rare causes of arterial stenosis in these vessels. Endovascular techniques have also been used in treatment of aneurysmal disease and traumatic injury of these arteries (7–13). The use of internal mammary arteries in coronary bypass surgery has implicated subclavian or innominate artery stenosis as a cause of angina and coronary-subclavian steal. Percutaneous intervention has been successful in reversing such symptoms (14–16).

The exact number and nature of complications resulting from endovascular procedures in the subclavian and vertebral arteries is obscured by lack of large-scale randomized trials or even large retrospective series. The frequency of these complications has changed with growing experience and transition from balloon angioplasty to direct stenting. However, based on available reports, arterial wall dissection, embolization, and perforation are the most commonly encountered vascular injuries. Stent migration, thrombosis, and restenosis are potential complications of stent implantation. Available data suggest that in the era of stenting, such complications are rare in subclavian and vertebral interventions (17–30).

MISDIAGNOSIS

Perhaps the most simple and most avoidable complication of subclavian and vertebral intervention is misdiagnosis based on inadequate diagnostic or angiographic technique.

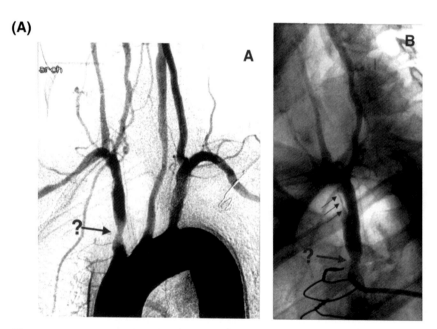

Figure 1 (**A**) The importance of appropriate angiographic views is demonstrated here. The patient had differential arm blood pressures, symptoms of right hemisphere ischemia, and an MR angiogram that suggested intrinsic brachiocephalic and right common carotid stenoses. An arch angiogram was reportedly unremarkable, yet the patient continued to have symptoms. The aortic arch angiogram in Panel A was obtained and shows what appears to be modest stenosis near the origin of the brachiocephalic. A selective view (*Panel B*), also appears to show moderate disease in the brachiocephalic but there is a subtle "string" of contrast near the main vessel (*small arrows*). (**B**) An additional angiogram of the patient in A in the orthogonal obliquity clarifies the situation (*Panel A*). It demonstrates a severe slit-like lesion of the origin of the brachiocephalic (*lower arrow*), and a near total occlusion of the common carotid (*upper arrow*). These lesions were treated with stents (*Panel B*) with resolution of the patient's symptoms.

(B)

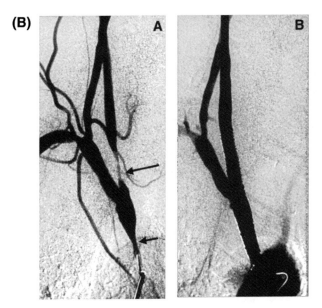

Figure 1   (*Continued*)

This can range from failure even to consider the possibility of subclavian obstruction to failure to appreciation of the importance of differential arm blood pressures (31). Angiographically, the failure to adhere to the principle of displaying all important bifurcations and imaging in orthogonal views has led to inappropriate angiographic conclusions and misdiagnosis (Fig. 1A and B).

ARTERIAL RUPTURE

This rare complication has been described during subclavian artery stenting. It is marked by extravasation of contrast, hemothorax, and precipitous hemodynamic collapse. Fortunately, it can be treated rapidly with a balloon tamponade and covered stents (32). Urgent surgery is required if hemorrhage cannot be securely controlled using interventional techniques (Fig. 2).

PSEUDOANEURYSM

Subclavian artery pseudoaneurysm has been reported as a consequence of stenting (32). This can be treated by surgical reconstruction or exclusion with a stent graft.

STENT MIGRATION AND THROMBOSIS

Intraprocedural stent dislodgement is a rare but reported complication. Hadjipetrou et al. published a series of 18 patients with symptomatic subclavian or brachiocephalic artery disease who underwent stenting (17). Stent embolization occurred in one patient and required retrieval to the femoral artery and surgical removal. Schillinger et al. also reported one case of stent embolization to the iliac artery during subclavian

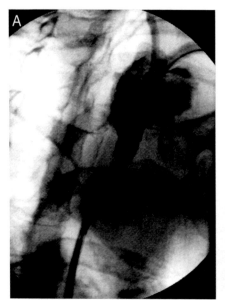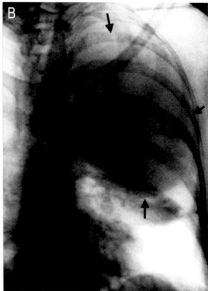

Figure 2 Perforation of the subclavian is a dreaded but rare complication. This angiogram shows extravasation of contrast into the mediastinum following balloon dilatation (*Panel A*). After prolonged balloon tamponade and stenting, there remains a large hemothorax (*Panel B*). Emergency surgical repair is required if balloon tamponade fails and a covered stent(s) cannot be delivered. *Source*: Images courtesy of Drs. M. Shotwell and G. Elkin.

intervention (33). In another series of 70 patients who underwent stenting of symptomatic subclavian artery stenosis or occlusion, stent migration distal to the lesion occurred in two cases and required deployment in the distal subclavian and brachial artery (18). In the same series, axillary artery thrombosis was noted in 3 of 69 patients (4.2%) while 5.7% had thrombosis of the brachial artery puncture site. Delayed stent occlusion occurred in 2 of 69 patients in that series. Martinez et al. published a series of 17 patients who underwent primary stenting for subclavian artery occlusion and had developed no complications of cerebral embolization except axillary artery thrombosis (34). Stent migration and misplacement can occur with self-expanding stents particularly those placed in an ostial location (Fig. 3).

Stent breakage has been reported, mostly in distal segments of the subclavian artery where the stent may be subjected to mechanical compression between the clavicle and the first rib, especially during arm abduction (35–37).

Stent infection leading to subclavian artery psudoaneurysm formation and septic embolization has also been described (38).

DISSECTION AND SIDE BRANCH OCCLUSION

Arterial wall dissection is an uncommon complication of vascular angiography and intervention. Cloft et al. estimated prevalence of iatrogenic cerebrovascular dissections to be 0.4% (39). In 69 patients undergoing subclavian artery stenting, only one had a distal subclavian artery dissection (18). Dissection of the subclavian artery can occur during routine coronary angiography while engaging left internal mammary artery (LIMA) (40). Dissection complicating subclavian angioplasty is especially worrisome

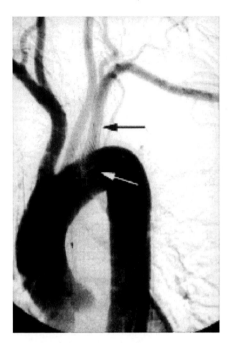

Figure 3 Stent misplacement. A self-expanding stent has been placed covering the origin of the left subclavian it extends from the proximal subclavian (*black arrow*), out of the ostium of the subclavian and nearly completely across the aorta (*white arrow*). Self-expanding stents are more difficult to place in this ostial location and may tend to "extrude" out into the lumen of the parent vessel with the passage of time. Generally, balloon expandable stents are preferable in this location while self-expanding stents may be used where the vessel is subject to movement or external compression such as between the clavicle and first rib. *Source*: From the Society of Interventional Radiology© 2003.

in patients with internal mammary grafts to the coronary circulation or isolated vertebral supply. Reported cases have been successfully treated with stenting (41,42) (Fig. 4A–C). The risk of subintimal dissection is increased when crossing total occlusions (43). Dissection with subsequent vessel occlusion has also been described (20). Dissection has been reported in stenting of subclavian and vertebral arteries: Malek et al. encountered seven such complications in 24 patients (26). Fessler placed six vertebral stents and had one dissection (28) (Figs. 5 and 6A, B).

EMBOLIZATION

Embolization of the vertebral artery has long been the primary concern in subclavian artery angioplasty. In patients with subclavian steal, reduction of culprit stenosis does not immediately restore an antegrade vertebral flow (44). This delay can range from 20 seconds to over 30 minutes, and protects the posterior circulation from periprocedural embolization (45). Nevertheless, embolization of the vertebral artery can occur, especially when antegrade vertebral flow is preserved. In a series of seven patients treated for subclavian and innominate artery stenosis, two patients who suffered periprocedural cerebral embolization had antegrade vertebral flow (46). Transient balloon occlusion of the ipsilateral vertebral artery or simultaneous inflation and deflation of the angioplasty balloon and ipsilateral arm blood pressure

(A)

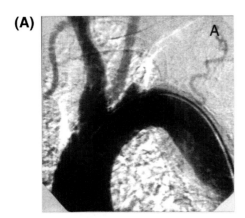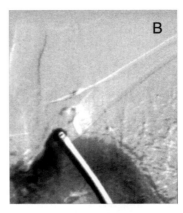

Figure 4 (**A**) Panel A shows an arch aortogram illustrating total occlusion of the proximal subclavian at its origin. Panel B is a selective injection of the occluded vessel. (**B**) (*Panel A*): Following crossing with a hydrophilic guidewire and gentle balloon dilatation at the site of prior total occlusion (*thin arrow*), there is an irregular residual stenosis but the left vertebral artery (*arrow Vert.*) and the other branch vessels are patent and fill antegrade. Following stenting (*Panel B*), the vertebral is totally occluded by the stent placement. (**C**) In Panel A, a coronary guidewire has been used to cross the stent struts into the vertebral and the origin is dilated. Following this, Panel B shows reconstitution of antegrade flow. Generally, transient mechanical occlusion is well tolerated because of patency of the Circle of Willis and the posterior communicating arteries. However, in situations with an absent or occluded contralateral vertebral or "inadequate" Circle of Willis, such occlusion can have adverse consequences.

cuff have been advocated to lower the incidence of posterior circulation stroke. In the era of balloon angioplasty, the rate of distal embolization or occlusion of the upper extremity was 2.1%, and was more likely in cases of chronic occlusion (47,48). central nervous system (CNS) complications occurred in about 1% (20,49).

(B)

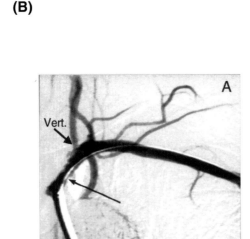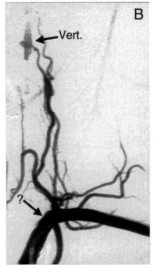

Figure 4 (*continued*)

(C)

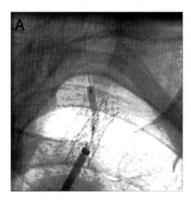

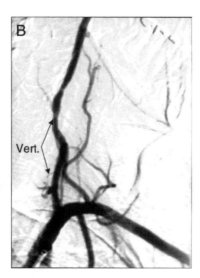

Figure 4 (*continued*)

Embolization may be less of a concern in the era of stenting. Rodriquez–Lopez et al. reported one episode of periprocedural TIA among 69 patients undergoing subclavian stenting (18). Schillinger et al. described 115 cases of subclavian angioplasty and stenting (33). One patient had a vertebral TIA and two patients had embolization to the mesenteric and renal arteries (33). Fessler et al. described a case of brief TIA in a series of six patients who underwent vertebral artery stenting (28), while Jenkins treated 32 patients with vertebral stenosis and had only one periprocedural

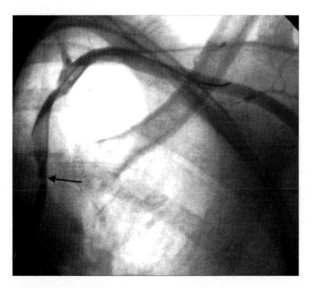

Figure 5 Spiral dissection of the subclavian from its origin and progressing antegrade past the origins of the thyrocervical trunk, internal mammary, and vertebral arteries. Unless wire position is lost, the flow to the subclavian territory can usually be salvaged by stenting. However, preservation of the branch vessels may be more difficult. The consequences of dissection and side branch occlusion should be considered when assessing procedural risk.

(A)

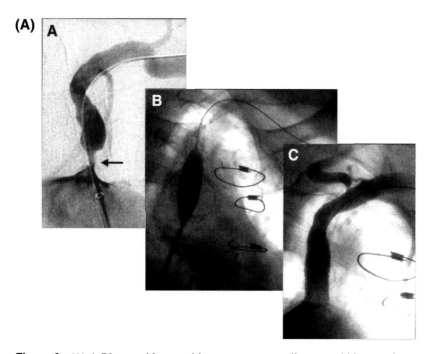

Figure 6 (**A**) A 76-year old man with coronary artery disease and history of coronary bypass surgery that included a LIMA to LAD graft underwent diagnostic angiography to evaluate angina. Panel A shows a severe stenosis at the origin of the left subclavian artery (*arrow*) compromising flow in the LIMA graft to LAD. The lesion was dilated, stented with a 10×5 mm Express stent and the aortic origin post-dilated (*Panel B*). This gave an excellent result (*Panel C*). (**B**) However, selective angiography of the IMA was performed and catheter manipulation raised a flap near the origin of the IMA that propagated distally (*small white arrows*) and proximally. Fortunately there was no flow compromise to the IMA or axillary arteries. Blood pressure was equal in both arms and the dissection was managed conservatively. Anticoagulants were continued empirically for several months and follow-up ultrasound study confirmed resolution of the dissection flap. *Abbreviations*: LIMA, left internal mammary; LAD, left anterior descending coronary.

TIA (50). Chastain et al. stented vertebral arteries in 50 patients with no periprocedural CVA or TIA (30). In another series of 83 patients who underwent primary stenting of the subclavian, innominate, and common carotid arteries, there was one case of embolization of an internal mammary graft and one case of brachial artery embolization (51). Vertebral artery occlusion has occurred because of stenting across its ostium (51). Interestingly, because of the usual dual vertebral supply to constitute the basilar artery, vertebral occlusion initially often produces no symptoms. Should the vessel remain occluded, however, stump embolization is a concern. The advent of distal protection devices will likely decrease further the risk of vertebral artery embolization during vertebral or subclavian artery stenting (Fig. 7).

RESTENOSIS

Elastic recoil and restenosis have been a problem in angioplasty of the proximal vertebral artery due to size mismatch between a large subclavian artery and a small vertebral artery.

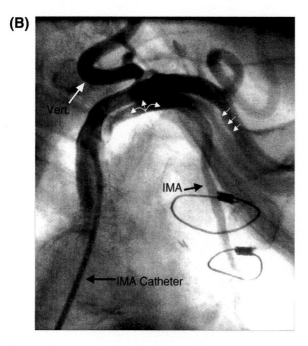

(B)

Vert.

IMA →

←IMA Catheter

Figure 6 (*continued*)

Becker et al. summarized 10 series (423 procedures) of subclavian and innominate artery angioplasties and found a recurrence rate of 19% (49). Another series reported restenosis after angioplasty of the subclavian artery to occur in 9% of cases at five months (24). Phatouros' review of literature found this to occur in 0–14% of cases at two years (52). In the early stenting procedures, the rate of asymptomatic restenosis was 7%, while symptomatic restenosis rate was 3% at 13 months (18). Schillinger analyzed 115 patients who underwent PTA or stenting of the subclavian artery. Long lesion and residual stenosis after PTA were independent predictors of restenosis as was stent placement (33). PTA had a 14% eight-year restenosis rate, while stenting yielded a 23% eight-year restenosis rate. Al-Mubarak stented 38 subclavian arteries and observed a 6% restenosis rate at 20 months (27). In another series of 50 patients with vertebral artery stenting, restenosis rate at six months was 10% (30).

HYPERPERFUSION SYNDROME

Hyperperfusion syndrome and hyperemia have been described in arterial bypass surgery and in percutaneous interventions in the carotid and iliac vessels. Full-blown hyperperfusion syndrome of the upper extremity after restoration of flow in the subclavian artery is a reported but very rare event (53). Increased blood flow can result in swelling, pain, and hyperemia of the hand and forearm. Treatment consists of analgesia and observation. Cooling of the affected areas has been reported to provide symptomatic relief. In many cases, however, a mild form of reperfusion syndrome occurs with transient erythema, mild edema, and vague tenderness. This usually responds to reassurance, elevation, and the passage of time.

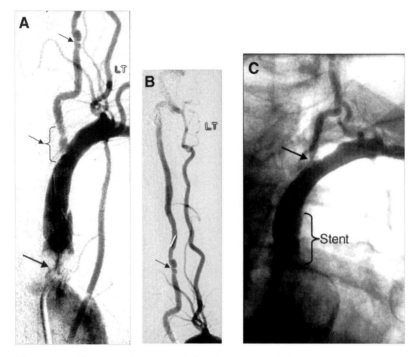

Figure 7 This patient had severe ischemic symptoms with near occlusion of the left subclavian origin. She had an occluded brachiocephalic trunk and the only supply to her posterior cerebral circulation was via the left vertebral. However, in addition to the heavily calcified, irregular stenosis (*Panel A*, *larger arrow*), the origin of the left vertebral was intrinsically compromised (*middle arrow*) and the body of the vessel had severe stenosis (*upper arrow Panel A*; *arrow Panel B*) as well. Because of this intrinsic disease distal protection was not used and the origin of the subclavian dilated and stented directly with a good result (*Panel C*) and continued patency of the vertebral (*arrow*). The patient tolerated the procedure but had a small posterior circulation infarct likely related to distal embolization of calcified atheroma. Lesions involving the origin of a single remaining or dominant vertebral vessel increase the risk of cerebrovascular complications associated with subclavian artery interventions. Generally, embolization carries more severe consequences than occlusion.

CONCLUSION

Subclavian and brachiocephalic interventions are generally safe and have replaced surgery as a first-line treatment for atherosclerotic disease in this location (17). However, complications occasionally do arise and are most often due to branch vessel compromise or embolization. Though they are uncommon, the recognition of these complications and knowledge of their appropriate treatment is extremely important in achieving optimal results.

REFERENCES

1. Fields WS, Lemak NA. Joint study of extracranial arterial occlusion. Subclavian Steal-A review of 168 cases. J Am Med Asssoc 1972; 222:1139–1143.
2. Hass WK, Fields WS, North RR, Kircheff II, Chase NE, Bauer RB. Joint study of extracranial arterial occlusion. II. Arteriography, techniques, sites, and complications. J Am Med Assoc 1968; 203:961–968.

3. English J, Donovan D, Guidera S, Carell ES. Angiographic prevalence and clinical pre-dictors of left subclavian stenosis in patients undergoing diagnostic cardiac catheteriza-tion. J Am Coll Cardiol (Abstracts for the 1999 Annual Scientific Session, abstr 1193–72).
4. Guiterrez GR, Mahrer P, Aharonian V, Mansukhani P, Bruss J. Prevalence of subclavian artery stenosis in patients with peripheral vascular disease. Angiology 2001; 52:189–194.
5. Cosottini M, Zampa V, Petruzzi P, Ortori S, Cioni R, Bartolozzi C. Contrast enhanced three-dimensional MR angiography in the assessment of subclavian artery diseases. Eur Radiol 2000; 10:1737–1744.
6. Sakaida H, Sakai N, Nagata I, Sakai H, Lihara K, Higashi T, Kogure S, Takahashi J, Ohta H, Nagamine T, Anei R, Soeda A, Taniguchi A, ShindoA, Kikuchi H. Stenting for the occlusive carotid and subclavian arteries in Takayasu's arteritis. No Shinkei Geka 2001; 29:1033–1041.
7. Lownie SP, Pelz DM, Fox AJ. Endovascular therapy of a large vertebral artery aneurysm using stent and coils. Can J Neurol Sci 2000; 27:162–165.
8. Hilfiker PR, Razavi MK, Kee ST, Sze DY, Semba CP, Dake MD. Stent-graft therapy for subclavian artery aneurysms and fistulas: a single-center mid-term results. J Vasc Interv Radiol 2000; 11:578–584.
9. Hernandez JA, Pershad A, Laufer N. Subclavian artery pseudoaneurysm successful exclusion with a covered self-expanding stent. J Invasive Cardiol 2002; 14:278–279.
10. Strauss DC, du Toit DF, Warren BL. Endovascular repair of occluded subclavian arteries following penetrating trauma. J Endovasc Ther 2001; 9:529–533.
11. Amar AP, Teitelbaum GP, Giannotta SL, Larsen DW. Covered stent-graft repair of the brachiocephalic arteries; technical note. Neurosurgery 2002; 51:247–252.
12. Redekop G, Marotta T, Weill A. Treatment of traumatic aneurysms and arteriovenous fistulas of the skull base by using endovascular stents. J Neurosurg 2001; 95:412–419.
13. Albuquerque FC, Javedan SP, McDougall CG. Endovascular management of penetrat-ing vertebral artery injuries. J Trauma 2002; 53:574–580.
14. Demir I, Yilmaz H, Sancaktar O. Coronary subclavian steal syndrome; treatment by stenting of the left subclavian artery. Japan Heart J 2002; 43:79–84.
15. Fusman B, Jolly N, Kin A, Feldman T. Endoluminal stenting of the subclavian artery to treat a surgically created left main equivalent lesion. Catheteriz Cardiovasc Interv 2002; 56:361–364.
16. Wright-Smith GR, Watson P, Svensson LG, Eisenhauer AC. Coronary subclavian steal associated with severe aortic stenosis treated with combined percutaneous stenting and minimally invasive aortic valve replacement. J Invasive Cardiol 1999; 11:676–678.
17. Hadjipetrou P, Cox S, Piemonte T, Eisenhauer A. Percutaneous revascularization of atherosclerotic obstruction of aortic arch vessels. J Am Coll Cardiol 1999; 33:1238.
18. Rodriguez-Lopez J, Werner A, Martinez R, Torruella L, Torruella LJ, Ray LI, Diethrich EB. Stenting for atherosclerotic occlusive disease of the subclavian artery. Technical aspects and follow-up results. Ann Vasc Surg 1999; 13:254–260.
19. Kumar K, Dorros G, Bates MC, Palmer L, Mathiak L, Dufek C. Primary stent deploy-ment in occlusive subclavian artery disease. Catheter Cardiovasc Diagn 1995; 34: 281–285.
20. Bogey WM, Demasi RJ, Tripp MD. Percutaneous transluminal angioplasty for sub-clavian artery stenosis. Am Surgeon 1994; 60:103–106.
21. Vitek JJ. Subclavian artery angioplasty and origin of the vertebral artery. Radiology 1989; 170:420–429.
22. Bruckmann H, Ringelstein EB, Buchner H, Zeumer H. Percutaneous transluminal angio-plasty of the vertebral artery. A therapeutic alternative to operative reconstruction of proximal vertebral artery stenoses. J Neurol 1998; 233:336–339.
23. Courtheoux P, Tournade A, Theron J, Henriet JP, Maiza D, Derlon JM, Pelouze G, Evrard C. Transcutaneous angioplasty of vertebral artery atheromatous ostial stricture. Neuroradiology 1985; 27:259–264.

24. Higashida RT, Hieshima GB, Tsai FY, Bentson JR, Halbach VV. Percutaneous trans-luminal angioplasty of the subclavian and vertebral arteries. Acta Radiol Suppl 1986; 369:124–126.

25. Kachel R, Endert G, Basche S, Grossmann K, Glaser FH. Percutaneous transluminal angioplasty (dilatation) of carotid, vertebral, and innominate artery stenoses. Cardiovasc Interv Radiol 1987; 10:142–146.

26. Malek AM, Higashida RT, Phatouros CC, Lempert TE, Meyers PM, Gress DR, Dowd CF, Halbach VV. Treatment of posterior circulation ischemia with extracranial percutaneous balloon angioplasty and stent placement. Stroke 1999; 30:2073–2085.

27. Al-Mubarak N, Liu MW, Dean LS, Al-Shaibi K, Chastain HD 2nd, Lyer SS, Roubin GS. Immediate and late outcomes of subclavian artery stenting. Catheteriz Cardiovasc Interv 1999; 46:169–172.

28. Fessler RD, Wakhloo AK, Lanzino G, Qureshi AI, Lee R, Guterman LR, Hopkins LN. Stent placement for vertebral artery occlusive disease: preliminary clinical experience. Neurosurg Focus 1998; 5:Article 15. Available at www.neurosurgery.org/focus/ october98/5-4–15.html.

29. Mukherjee D, Roffi M, Kapadia SR, Bhatt DL, Bajzer C, Ziada KM, Kalahasti V, Hughes K, Yadav JS. Percutaneous interventions for symptomatic vertebral artery steno-sis using coronary stents. J Invasive Cardiol 2001; 13:363–366.

30. Chastain HD 2nd, Campbell MS, Iyer S, Roubin Gs, Vitek J, Mathur A, Al-Mubarak NA, Terry JB, Yates V, Kretzer K, Alred D, Gomez CR. Extracranial vertebral artery stent placement: in hospital and follow up results. J Neurosurg 1999; 91:547–552.

31. Eisenhauer AC. Subclavian and innominate revascularization: surgical therapy versus catheter-based intervention. Curr Interv Cardiol Rep 2000; 2:101–110.

32. Lin PH, Bush RL, Weiss VJ, Dodson TF, Chaikof EL, Lumsden AB. Subclavian artery disruption resulting from endovascular intervention: treatment options. J Vasc Surg 2000; 32:607–611.

33. Schillinger M, Haumer M, Schillinger S, Ahmadi R, Minar E. Risk stratification for sub-clavian artery angioplasty: is there an increased rate of restenosis after stent implanta-tion. J Endovasc Ther 2001; 8:550–557.

34. Martinez R, Rodriguez-Lopez J, Torruella L, Ray L, Lopez-Galarza L, Diethrich EB. Stenting for occlusion of the subclavian arteries. Technical aspects and follow-up results. Texas Heart Inst J 1997; 24:23–27.

35. Patel AV, Marin ML, Veith FJ, Kerr A, Sanchez LA. Endovascular graft repair of pene-trating subclavian artery injuries. J Endovasc Surg 1996; 3:382–388.

36. Phipp LH, Scott DJ, Kessel D, Robertson I. Subclavian stents and stent-grafts: a cause of concern? J Endovasc Surg 1999; 6:223–226.

37. Sitsen ME, Ho GH, Blankensteijn JD. Deformation of self-expandable stent-grafts com-plicating endovascular peripheral aneurysm repair. J Endovasc Surg 1999; 6:288–292.

38. Malek AM, Higashida RT, Reilly LM, Smith WS, Kang SM, Gress DR, Mayers PM, Phatouros CC, Halbach VV, Dowd CF. Subclavian arteritis and pseudoaneurysm forma-tion secondary to stent infection. Cardiovasc Interv Radiol 2000; 23:57–60.

39. Cloft HJ, Jensen ME, Kallmes DF, Dion JE. Arterial dissections complicating cerebral angiography and cerebrovascular interventions. Am J Neuroradiol 2000; 21:541–545.

40. Frohwein S, Ververis JJ, Marshall JJ. Subclavian artery dissection during diagnostic car-diac catheterization: the role of conservative management. Catheteriz Cardiovasc Diagn 1995; 34:313–317.

41. Schmitter SP, Marx M, Bernstein R, Wack J, Semba CP, Dake MD. Angioplasty-induced subclavian artery dissection in a patient with internal mammary artery graft: treatment with endovascular atents and stent-graft. Am J Roentgenol 1995; 165:449–451.

42. Galli M, Goldberg SL, Zerboni S, Almagor Y. Balloon expandable stent implantation after iatrogenic arterial dissection of the left subclavian artery. Catheteriz Cardiovasc Diagn 1995; 34:355–357.

43. Sakaida H, Sakai N, Nagata I, Sakai H, Iihara K, Higashi T, Kogure S, Takahashi J, Ohta H, Nagamine T, Anei R, Soeda A, Taniguchi A, Shindo A, Kikuchi H. Stenting for proximal subclavian and brachiocephalic artery occlusion-preliminary results. No Shinkei Geka–Neurol Surg 2001; 29:717–725.

44. Bachman DM, Kim RM. Transluminal dilatation for subclavian steal syndrome. Am J Roentgenol 1980; 35:995–996.

45. Ringelstein EB, Zeumer H. Delayed reversal of vertebral artery blood flow following percutaneous transluminal angioplasty for subclavian steal syndrome. Neuroradiology 1984; 26:189–198.

46. Sharma S, Kaui U, Rajani M. Identifying high-risk patients for percutaneous transluminal angioplasty of subclavian and innominate arteries. Acta Radiol 1991; 32: 381–385.

47. Nastur A, Sayers RD, Bell PRF, Bolia A. Protection against vertebral artery embolization during proximal subclavian artery angioplasty. Eur J Vasc Surg 1994; 8:362–363.

48. Memis A, Oran I, Ozbek A. A simple method to avoid vertebral artery embolism during subclavian percutaneous transluminal angioplasty; provocative maneuver. Am J Roentgenol 1997; 168:569–570.

49. Becker GJ, Katzen BT, Dake MD. Noncoronary angioplasty. Radiology 1989; 170:921–940.

50. Jenkins JS, White CJ, Ramee SR. Vertebral artery stenting. Catheteriz Cardiovasc Interv 2001; 54:1–5.

51. Sullivan TM, Gray BH, Bacharach JM, Perl J 2nd, Childs MB, Modzelewski L, Beven EG. Angioplasty and primary stenting of the subclavian, innominate and common carotid arteries in 83 patients. J Vasc Surg 1998; 28:1059–1065.

52. Phatouros CC, Higashida RT, Malek AM, Meyers PM, Lefler JE, Dowd CF, Halbach VV. Endovascular treatment of noncarotid extracranial cerebrovascular disease. Neurosurg Clin N Am 2000; 11:331–350.

53. Chemelli AP, Bodner G, Perkmann R, Hourmont K, Waldenberger P, Jaschke W. Hyperperfusion syndrome of the left hand after percutaneous transluminal angioplasty and stent placement in a subclavian artery stenosis. J Vasc Interv Radiol 2001; 12:388–390.

11

Complications Associated with Endovascular Therapy for Intracranial Aneurysms and Stenotic Lesions

Jay U. Howington and L. Nelson Hopkins
Department of Neurosurgery and Toshiba Stroke Research Center (JUH, LNH),
School of Medicine and Biomedical Sciences, University at Buffalo,
State University of New York, Buffalo, New York, U.S.A.

INTRODUCTION

Endovascular therapy for the treatment of intracranial lesions represents a challenge to the interventionist for several reasons, not the least of which is the fact that the organ involved, the brain, is fundamental to life and the way we live it. Any complication resulting in a cerebrovascular accident, whether hemorrhagic or ischemic, can be devastating, and every effort should be made to prevent its occurrence. Adverse sequelae or consequences of endovascular therapy can occur immediately as with intracranial vessel and/or aneurysm perforation or vessel thrombosis, or in a delayed fashion as with recurrent vessel stenosis or aneurysm regrowth. It is crucial for the neurointerventionist to understand these complications and take the necessary steps to prevent them. Equally important is the ability to recognize the occurrence of these adverse events and then manage them appropriately. The avoidance and management of hemorrhagic and ischemic cerebral infarctions as complications of endovascular therapy for intracranial aneurysms and stenotic lesions will be the focus of this chapter.

PREDISPOSING FACTORS

Technical errors account for most complications associated with intracranial endovascular procedures and will be discussed below, but for now we will focus on those anatomic and histopathologic factors present in the intracranial circulation that must be understood to minimize such complications. Intracranial angioplasty and stenting is a technique that has evolved from one that was associated with an unacceptable high rate of morbidity and mortality to one that is relatively safe (1–6). The reason for this progression lies in the growth in understanding of the structure of intracranial vessels and their response to injury as well as improvements in endovascular devices. The endothelial lining of blood vessels inhibits platelet aggregation and the coagulation of blood and thereby preserves the fluid state required for circulation. The subendothelial elements of the vessel wall stimulate platelet adhesion and activation when an endothelial injury exposes them to blood. Platelet aggregation soon follows, as does activation of the coagulation cascade, and the degree of intimal injury and amount of subendothelial exposure govern the level of this thrombotic response (7,8). Tissue factor, a component of the subendothelium as well as atherosclerotic plaque, acts to initiate the coagulation cascade and confines procoagulant activity to the injury site in the vessel wall (9). Occurring simultaneously with platelet aggregation and the coagulation cascade is fibrinolysis, which is a natural process, directed at maintaining the patency of blood vessels by lysis of fibrin deposits. In this process, the inactive proenzyme, plasminogen, is converted to the active protease plasmin, which then breaks up clot by degrading the fibrin component of the clot (10). A checks and balances type of interaction occurs between platelet aggregation and the coagulation cascade, in conjunction with clot fibrinolysis. Although the body's response to arterial injury provides a highly effective defense mechanism against exsanguination, such an active reaction presents a formidable challenge during intracranial endovascular procedures.

Platelet aggregation and the coagulation cascade are also stimulated by the presence of foreign bodies such as the devices used in intracranial endovascular procedures. Several groups have studied the thrombogenic potential of catheter composition, and found that catheters constructed with polyurethane exhibited a lower tendency for thrombogenesis than those constructed with polyethylene, woven Dacron, or polyvinyl chloride (11–14). The microcatheters and guidewires currently used for intracranial endovascular procedures are coated with a hydrophilic membrane, which has been shown to reduce the thrombogenicity of these devices (14,15). Despite these advances in catheter and guidewire design, they are foreign bodies and do serve as potential nidi for thrombosis. Both coils and stents are thrombogenic when exposed to circulating blood, and although thrombosis is desirable within an aneurysm, it is most undesirable within an atherosclerotic vessel. In the absence of antiplatelet agents, platelets adhere to the struts of a stent soon after placement (16). Fibrinogen adherence follows, and thrombosis can occur soon after. Investigators have found that the thrombogenicity is due in part to the stainless steel used in stents as well as the geometric configuration of the stent (17,18). An increase in the number of intersections between stent struts and the amount of plaque around the stent, and a small surface area of the stent are all associated with a higher risk of thrombosis. Nitinol, a nickel–titanium alloy used in some newer-generation stents, has been shown to have a lower risk of platelet adhesion than stainless steel, but this characteristic has only been demonstrated in vitro (19).

Intracranial vessels differ from peripheral and coronary vessels in that they lack the same amount of adventitia found in these other vessels, are nearly devoid of an external elastic lamina, and have no vasa vasorum (20). The layers present in intracranial vessels are much thinner compared with those in other vascular beds. The buffering environment provided by the skull and cerebrospinal fluid replaces these supportive elements. In addition, the percentage of smooth muscle present in the wall of an intracranial vessel is 85% compared with the 60% found in the walls of peripheral vessels. Smooth muscle cells are well known to be the primary culprits responsible for restenosis following angioplasty (21–24). The vessels of the intracranial circulation are smaller and, on the basis of Poiseuille's law, are more affected by smaller changes in luminal diameters than are their counterparts in other parts of the body. Because of the decreased caliber of the intracranial vessels, an atherosclerotic lesion of 50% in the middle cerebral artery, for example, results in a greater decrease in flow when compared with a similar lesion in a vessel with a larger lumen such as the extracranial internal carotid artery. Thus, plaque-related complications may have a significantly greater effect on flow in a small-lumen vessel. As in the extracranial carotid artery, the degree of atherosclerotic stenosis in the intracranial circulation is directly correlated with the risk of neurologic events (25). However, it should be remembered that intracranial stenosis affects the brain primarily in a hemodynamic fashion, whereas extracranial carotid stenosis is mostly an embolic disease.

In their retrospective review of angiographic studies of intracranial atherosclerotic lesions in symptomatic patients treated with angioplasty alone, Mori et al. found that certain lesion morphology characteristics are predictive of both procedure-related morbidity and restenosis (25,26). Three separate groups were identified on the basis of length and location of the lesion, degree of stenosis, and eccentricity, and level of calcification present. Type A lesions (<5 mm in length, proximally located, <90% stenosis, concentric, and very little calcification) were associated with a 92% success rate according to the standard for coronary lesions (defined as a reduction of stenosis by a 20% relative improvement in luminal diameter, with less than a 50% residual stenosis) and a 0.0% rate of restenosis at one year (27). A higher rate of procedure-related complications as well as restenosis was associated with more distally located lesions that were eccentric in nature. Type B lesions (5–10 mm, eccentric or totally occluded lesions <3-months-old on the basis of symptom onset) were associated with a success rate of 86% and a restenosis rate at one year of 33%. Type C lesions (diffuse, >10 mm, extremely angulated or totally occluded for longer than three months) were associated with a 33% success rate and a restenosis rate of 56% at one year. Patients with type C lesions, however, had a cumulative occurrence of ipsilateral stroke or required ipsilateral bypass surgery or repeat angioplasty of 100% at one year. Because of the increased risk of adverse events associated with the endovascular treatment of these latter types of lesions, Mori et al. recommend not treating them with endovascular approaches.

Other anatomical peculiarities of the intracranial vessels deserve mention as they can create significant hurdles during endovascular procedures if they are not anticipated. The fragility of the vessels increases the risk of injury during the passage of wires and devices, but these risks are increased further by the tortuosities and bony confines of the internal carotid artery as it enters the cranium. The pressures exerted on endovascular devices as they are navigated through these twists and turns inevitably result in minor intimal injuries (28–31). These injuries can range from dissections that are multiple and minute to those that are large and result in arterial occlusion. After it passes through the rigidity of the carotid canal and siphon, the carotid artery gives off small branches before it bifurcates into the anterior and middle cerebral arteries. These branch vessels are fragile and can be perforated if the interventionist is not careful to maintain the position of the wires and subsequent devices within the carotid artery lumen. Also, unique to the anatomy of the intracranial circulation are the perforating vessels that arise from the main cerebral vessels. These small arteries, like other branch vessels, can be injured by the passage of devices or may even become occluded during angioplasty (28–30,32). Injury to these vessels in the posterior circulation can lead to a brainstem stroke and in the anterior circulation to a dense thalamic or internal capsule stroke.

When treating aneurysms with an endovascular technique, the anatomic and histopathologic factors mentioned above that increase the risks of intracranial angioplasty are also present, but the two most important factors influencing the decision to proceed with aneurysm embolization are the morphology of the aneurysm and the relationship of the aneurysm neck to associated branch vessels. Ideally, the neck of the aneurysm should be sufficiently smaller than its dome so that coils deployed within the aneurysm sac will not herniate into the parent vessel. In a retrospective analysis of 329 patients with a total of 339 aneurysms, Debrun et al. found that aneurysms with a dome-to-neck ratio of at least two had higher rates of complete angiographic occlusion than did those with a dome-to-neck ratio of less than 2 (33). They and others found that the absolute neck diameter also affected the morphological occlusion outcome (34–37). A neck diameter of greater than 5 mm was associated with a greater tendency for coil prolapse into the parent artery, which not only decreases the chance for complete occlusion but also can serve as a nidus for thromboemboli (38,39). Coils are made of platinum, which is three to four times more thrombogenic than stainless steel (8). Thrombogenicity is a coil property that is important for aneurysm obliteration but can be dangerous if a loop of the coil herniates into the parent vessel. The protruding loops of the coil serve as a site for potential platelet aggregation, leading to local thrombosis or distal thromboembolism.

Aneurysms with a mean diameter greater than 15 mm are associated with an increased incidence of thromboembolic events (35,38–41). The reason for this association has not been clearly demonstrated, but two possible mechanisms exist. First, larger aneurysms are more likely to have residual flow within the coil mass at the completion of the procedure. This residual flow is usually slow and prone to thrombosis, and the thrombus that forms within the coil mass may be likely to fragment and travel distally and embolize. The other mechanism to explain the association between larger aneurysms and thromboembolic complications is the fact that larger aneurysms can harbor thrombus. During an embolization, this thrombus can be dislodged, resulting in distal embolization. Another aspect of larger aneurysms that increases the risk of adverse events is the difficulty in obtaining angiographic images that delineate the interface between the neck of the aneurysm and the parent vessel, despite multiple projections. Inadequate visualization of this interface can lead to uncertainty in positioning coils and possible underfilling of the aneurysm with coils at its base. Also, larger aneurysms require longer procedure times to obtain complete embolization, and this increased time amplifies the risk of the procedure. On the other hand, smaller aneurysms (< 2 mm) are not necessarily ideal for coil embolization. Aneurysms in this category are often little more than blisters and as such are more prone to intraprocedural ruptures. Their diminished size decreases the margin for error when attempting to access the aneurysm with either a guidewire or microcatheter. As a result, the risk of aneurysm perforation is higher. Packing these aneurysms effectively with coils becomes technically difficult, as they are often too small to hold a coil without herniation into the parent vessel. Aneurysms in certain locations in the intracranial circulation, like the middle cerebral artery bifurcation, are often problematic for the interventionist because branch vessels cannot be separated radiographically from the aneurysm (33). It is often impossible to predict whether the embolization of the aneurysm will be accompanied by occlusion of one of the branch vessels. A decision to proceed with an embolization even though a branch vessel has not been cleared could result in either incomplete occlusion of the aneurysm because of fear of occluding the vessel or complete occlusion of both the aneurysm and the vessel.

Finally, it should be remembered that diagnostic cerebral angiography is not without risk. The overall risk of thromboembolic complications occurring as a result of cerebral angiography ranges from 1.0% to 2.6%; the risk of permanent neurological deficits is 0.1% to 0.5% (42–44). Although the risk is relatively low that a patient will suffer a thromboembolic complication with cerebral angiography, several factors serve to increase the risk significantly. Age greater than 60, the presence of cerebrovascular disease, longer procedure time, increased number of catheter exchanges, and higher volumes of contrast material used all serve to increase the risk associated with diagnostic cerebral angiography (42–46). With respect to cerebrovascular disease, Theodotou et al. observed a 4.5% risk for patients with transient ischemic attacks, and this risk was increased to 7.7% for those patients with evolving strokes (46). These same authors found that patients with a history of a previous but not an evolving stroke were not at an increased risk. As every patient who undergoes endovascular treatment for either intracranial stenosis or an aneurysm must also have a diagnostic cerebral angiogram, these same risk factors apply.

SHORT-TERM AND LONG-TERM CONSEQUENCES OR SEQUELAE

Because of the small caliber of intracranial vessels and their delicate histologic makeup, the risk of injury is high as is the chance for untoward sequelae that can be associated with such injury. These sequelae can occur immediately as with vessel and/or aneurysm perforation or vessel thrombosis or in a delayed fashion as with vessel restenosis or aneurysm regrowth. Both short- and long-term sequelae are usually the result of anatomic factors peculiar to the patient in conjunction with technical errors on the part of the interventionist. These complications, when they occur, may be silent or have neurologic manifestations. When a patient suffers a neurologic deficit as a result of a procedure-related complication, regardless of whether the deficit is transient or permanent, the interventionist must be able to objectively review the events and conditions that lead to the untoward result. One must be aware of the predisposing factors listed above as well as the risks associated with each of them.

Endovascular therapies for intracranial aneurysms have evolved from balloon occlusion described by Serbinenko in 1974, and detachable coil embolization described by Guglielmi et al. in 1991 (47–49) to stent and balloon-assisted coiling and liquid agent embolization, but the complications have remained the same. With respect to the treatment of intracranial aneurysms by endovascular approaches, two basic immediate complications and one long-term complication deserve mention. The two complications that have an immediate effect are aneurysm rupture and thromboembolism of the parent vessel and its distal branches. We discuss vessel perforation along with aneurysm rupture here because the consequences can be essentially the same. Perforation of a vessel or an aneurysm during an endovascular procedure is uncommon, but it is usually related to guidewire manipulation (50–52). When a normal vessel is inadvertently perforated by a guidewire, the resulting hole is small (29–30 gauge) and is usually self-sealing if the vessel is non-diseased. In such a situation, the hemorrhage that ensues is usually minor and causes only a mild headache. Unfortunately, most patients undergoing endovascular aneurysm treatment have received anticoagulation therapy with an intravenous bolus of heparin. This disruption of the coagulation cascade increases the length of time that bleeding occurs, which in turn increases the deleterious effect the perforation will have on the patient's neurologic status. If the patient is in a state of general anesthesia and is unable to report the sudden onset of a headache, the perforation may go unnoticed, and further manipulation of the wire can transform the small hole into a tear with disastrous consequences. If the perforation occurs in the dome of a recently ruptured aneurysm, the clot that initially sealed off the aneurysm could be dislodged and the resulting hemorrhage catastrophic. Because the dome of the aneurysm lacks the structure of a normal arterial wall, a small perforation can quickly expand into a sizable hole. The bleeding will eventually stop, either because of a platelet plug or because the intracranial pressure has equilibrated with the mean arterial pressure, in which case no further blood flow to the brain occurs. Brain death then rapidly ensues. Although microwires are the most common culprits of aneurysm or vessel perforation, microcatheters and coils can also penetrate or tear the dome of an aneurysm. The opening in the aneurysm is usually larger than that seen with a guidewire perforation, therefore, the hemorrhage is significantly greater and is often fatal for the reasons previously mentioned. The endovascular treatment of intracranial aneurysms may be complicated by thromboembolic events (35,37–40,44,48,53,54). Immediate or delayed thromboembolic complications associated with endovascular aneurysm treatment are the result of thrombus being dislodged during the procedure or thrombus that develops in the aneurysm as a result of the procedure and then embolizes afterward. The catheters used in the procedure may also be a source of thromboemboli.

Aneurysm size is likely the strongest risk factor for thromboembolic complications (37,39,54). Thromboemboli cause either transient ischemic attacks or strokes depending on the amount of clot burden and the vascular territory that is affected. An embolus to a non-dominant branch vessel might result in only transient weakness or sensory disturbance, whereas a small embolic event in the dominant angular artery could lead to aphasia. Pre-existing thrombus that is dislodged from the aneurysm is likely to manifest itself during the procedure. As most patients receive treatment after the induction of general anesthesia, serial angiography with an angiogram following each coil deployment provides the only means to detect thromboembolism. Microemboli will usually cause a delayed filling in the territory affected during the arterial phase of the study, rather than an obvious vessel dropout. Larger emboli will appear as a vessel occlusion and a filling void. Increasing the amount of contrast material administered during the capillary phase may demonstrate both micro- and macroemboli in the affected area. If aneurysm embolization is performed in an awake patient after the administration of sedative and analgesic agents (conscious sedation), serial neurologic exams can be used to supplement any radiographic findings. If residual filling exists within the coil mass at the completion of the procedure, thrombosis can occur after the induced coagulopathy corrects itself. The goal of treatment is to induce thrombosis within the aneurysm, but some days may pass before the thrombus becomes organized. The findings of a histopathological study performed by Bavinzski et al. (55) suggest that thrombus organization does not occur in humans until seven days after coil placement, and the works of others have supported these results. During this interim, the thrombus might actually fragment and cause distal embolization (38,39,56). The greater the residual flow in the aneurysm, the greater the tendency will be for any thrombus to remain unorganized and fragment. Any delayed ischemic event following coil embolization of an aneurysm that is not attributable to vasospasm must be assumed to be the result of thromboemboli from the aneurysm. Delayed thromboembolic events usually take place within 24 hours of the procedure, but can occur up to two months later (38,39,44).

When a balloon or stent is used to facilitate the embolization of the aneurysm, the risk of thromboembolic complications rises. Both of these techniques are used for the treatment of large-necked aneurysms, and each is associated with the occurrence of thromboembolic phenomena for different reasons. Moret et al. were the first to describe the use of a technique in which a small balloon is used to protect the vessel lumen during the deployment of coils into an aneurysm (57). They and others have reported thromboembolic events associated with this technique (58,59). With balloon-assisted coil embolization, occlusion of the parent vessel produces stasis of distal flow, which can lead to intraluminal thrombosis. Other complications attend the balloon-assistance technique and deserve mention. With each inflation of the balloon against the intimal wall, the risk of vessel dissection or rupture increases, as does the potential for thromboembolic complications. Endothelial damage can also lead to delayed stenosis. Patients with inadequate collateral reserve can suffer from hemodynamic ischemia with each successive balloon inflation. Lesions involving the basilar artery and distal internal carotid arteries are more susceptible to this treatment complication than those that occur proximally. Also, inflation of a balloon in proximity to an aneurysm is known to be associated with an increased risk of aneurysm rupture (60,61). In such cases, the balloon can cause the rupture of the aneurysm directly or indirectly by pushing a microcatheter or coils through the thin wall of an aneurysm. The technique of stent-assisted coil embolization of intracranial aneurysms was initially described by Higashida in 1997, and in that report, a coronary stent was used to buttress the neck of a fusiform vertebrobasilar aneurysm (62). Although others have reported the safe use of coronary stents as an adjunct to coiling in other vessels, using this technique to treat lesions beyond the carotid siphon or basilar artery invites complications. Coronary stents are mounted on balloons, and the combination of stent and balloon lacks the flexibility to successfully navigate the tortuosities of the siphon or vertebral arteries without a high degree of risk. An arterial dissection that results in a thromboembolic event or, worse yet, an occlusion, is possible when one attempts to maneuver the stent around a tight bend. As mentioned above, platelets adhere to the struts of a stent soon after deployment, and if an antiplatelet regimen is not in effect, thrombosis can occur with striking rapidity.

Recent advances have led to the development of stents designed for the intracranial circulation. The Neuroform™ stent (Boston Scientific, Target, Fremont, California) is a stent constructed of nitinol and possesses an open-cell design with ultra-thin struts that make it extremely pliable (63). Instead of being mounted on a balloon, the stent is self-expanding with a relatively low radial force (by comparison with coronary stents) and is delivered through a 3-French microcatheter system that can be positioned in any of the major intracranial vessels. As a result, the stent can be delivered into the distal circulation with minimal risk of intimal injury. Although the Neuroform stent represents a significant advance in the endovascular treatment of wide-neck cerebral aneurysms, it is not a panacea. Like other stents, it is thrombogenic, and this characteristic proves to be problematic when treating acutely ruptured aneurysms, because the antiplatelet regimen necessary when using a stent takes at least five hours to become partially (80%) effective (64). Patients treated on an emergency basis with a Neuroform stent are at a greater risk of thromboembolic complications than those treated electively. The relatively low radial force of the stent facilitates its passage beyond the carotid siphon, but it also makes the stent susceptible to inadvertent dislocation after deployment. A microcatheter that is being directed to an aneurysm might get caught on the struts of the stent. If this situation goes unrecognized, further manipulation of the microcatheter could dislodge the stent and move it so that it no longer spans the neck of the aneurysm. Another complication seen with the use of the Neuroform stent is poor coverage of the aneurysm neck. Unlike some stents used in the extracranial circulation that can be resheathed before full deployment if the position is undesirable, the open-cell design of this stent does not allow the operator to re-sheath, re-position, and re-deploy. Once the deployment is initiated, the only repositioning that can be accomplished is that of pulling the stent proximally before completing the deployment. The stent should span at least 4 mm of the parent vessel on either side of the aneurysm neck to ensure adequate coverage.

The main long-term complication of aneurysm coil embolization is aneurysm regrowth (33,35,36,40,48,53,65–70). This occurs as a consequence of growth of a remnant, compaction of the coil mass, or a combination of the two (35,53,68,70). The strongest factor influencing aneurysm recurrence following coil embolization is the percentage of occlusion observed angiographically at the completion of the procedure (33,35,53,69,70). Other factors that have been found to be significant predictors of recurrence include treatment during the acute phase after rupture, size of the aneurysm, and width of the aneurysm neck, but each of these increases the risk of recurrence by affecting the operator's ability to obtain a 100% occlusion. An aneurysm that is 100% occluded is much less likely to exhibit recurrence or refilling of the neck than an aneurysm with residual filling. Also, angiographic recurrences are seen more frequently in conjunction with a longer duration of follow-up evaluation (70).

Coil compaction usually occurs in larger aneurysms and is felt to be the result of the decreased packing density of the coils that is inherent in the embolization of larger lesions as well as the relationship of the coil mass to the inflow zone of the aneurysm (71–73). For example, a large basilar apex aneurysm treated with coil embolization has an inflow zone that is relatively straight as the lesion rests at the end of the basilar artery. The coil mass will therefore receive the full brunt of the pressure head generated by the column of blood flowing up the basilar artery. The repeated water-hammer effect of such a configuration increases the risk of the coil mass undergoing compaction and the aneurysm recurring over time if the packing density is less than optimal. On the other hand, in those aneurysms that have a tangential inflow zone (i.e., a posterior communicating artery aneurysm), the distal neck and wall of the aneurysm represent the inflow zone and accordingly receive the greatest amount of shear stress with each cardiac cycle. If a neck remnant involves this inflow zone, an increased risk exists for aneurysm regrowth at that particular site. As the aneurysm grows, so does the chance for hemorrhage (34–36,40,41,53,73).

The short-term complications associated with intracranial angioplasty and stenting mainly involve injury to the vessels, but thromboembolic complications can also occur. When passing a wire, catheter, balloon, or stent across an atherosclerotic lesion, the risk of intimal dissection is much higher than that encountered with normal vessels (2–6,28,74). The rate of major complications (stroke or death) associated with intracranial angioplasty ranges from 4% to 40%, and most of these complications occur during the procedure (5,28,29,74–77). Injuries can occur when any of the devices are passed through a diseased segment of an artery. Microwires and microcatheters can usually be safely passed beyond an atherosclerotic lesion if the lumen of the vessel is large enough. However, the irregular surface of such a lesion provides a possible area on which wires can snag and cause a dissection. Angioplasty balloons, with their increased size in comparison with microwires and microcatheters, carry a higher risk of intimal damage when passed through an atherosclerotic lesion. The greatest incidence of intimal injury, however, occurs with the actual process of angioplasty (3,5,6,74). Rapid inflation of a balloon during angioplasty tears the intima and creates fissures, flaps, and dissections. When an intimal injury occurs in a normal intracranial vessel, the combination of platelets and the coagulation cascade can quickly lead to vessel thrombosis, as mentioned previously. Should such an injury occur in a portion of the vessel already riddled with atherosclerosis, the response to that injury is amplified by the exposure of extracellular lipids, proteoglycans, macrophage foam cells, and smooth muscle cells to the circulation (78). Like intimal injuries associated with the endovascular treatment of aneurysms, vessel injuries occurring in the course of the treatment of intracranial atherosclerotic lesions will manifest as a filling defect on angiography. This defect may be subtle or may rapidly progress to an occlusion. Angioplasty in vessels that are associated with perforating arteries represents a unique situation because the angioplasty may "snowplow" the plaque into or over the orifice of such perforating vessels. Even though these are small vessels, they are end arteries that have minimal collateral support, and the loss of patency can be devastating.

Restenosis, the main long-term complication associated with intracranial angioplasty and stenting (3–6,28,74), is related to the intimal hyperplasia and vascular remodeling that follows the stretch injury induced by angioplasty (79,80). The remodeling occurs over four to six weeks, and there are three definite stages in that period, each dependent on the preceding stage: first is the initiating phase in which platelets, thrombin, and leukocytes release active mediators; an intermediate phase soon follows in which activated smooth muscle cells proliferate and migrate to the subintima, and finally, extracellular matrix production leads to remodeling in the chronic phase (80). Stenosis recurs in 0–33% of arteries after intracranial angioplasty with or without stenting (3,5,26,28,74,81). As mentioned previously, the rates of restenosis for lesions that are long and eccentric are statistically higher than those seen with shorter, more concentric lesions (25,26). These longer lesions tend to be irregular, complicated, and associated with breaks in the intimal surface that expose the underlying lipid core and increase the risk of thrombus formation and subsequent restenosis.

COMPLICATION AVOIDANCE AND MANAGEMENT

Complications, both immediate and delayed, are most often the result of technical errors in combination with the difficulties encountered with individual anatomic variants. Therefore, any discussion of complication avoidance and management must focus on improving the interventionist's awareness of these variants and the techniques needed for their negotiation. Armed with such an appreciation, the interventionist can anticipate different points of increased risk during a procedure and take the necessary steps to avoid a complication. However, complications are inevitable, and one should be prepared to manage them when they are encountered. Many of the complications mentioned above can be largely avoided if appropriate steps are taken. The remainder of this chapter will focus on these steps as well as the management of these complications should they occur.

Thrombi can form at the outer surface of a guidewire or microcatheter, between the inner wall of the guiding catheter and the outer wall of the microcatheter, or within the microcatheter if appropriate precautions are not taken. Essential to any intracranial endovascular procedure is the continuous irrigation of catheters with a heparinized saline solution. The authors prefer to add 5000 U of heparin to each liter of flush that is used, and the irrigation rate is titrated from 25 mL to 75 mL per hour depending on which catheter is used. Before a guide catheter is placed in either the internal carotid or vertebral artery, a bolus dose (0–70 U/kg) is given intravenously to achieve an activated clotting time (ACT) between 250 seconds and 300 seconds. As the procedure progresses, ACTs are checked and further doses of heparin are administered accordingly to maintain the ACT within this range. At the completion of the procedure, the effect of the heparin is allowed to wear off without the administration of a reversing agent. If possible, a percutaneous closure device is used to secure the access site. If not, the sheath is left in place and removed after the ACT has returned to within a normal range. For any procedure requiring angioplasty or stenting, patients are pretreated with aspirin 325 mg and clopidogrel 75 mg for at least three days. In emergent cases requiring antiplatelet therapy, aspirin (325 mg) and a loading dose (450 mg) of clopidogrel are given as soon as possible.

The intraprocedural perforation of an aneurysm manifests with a headache and can be disastrous if not recognized. Unfortunately, patients with aneurysmal subarachnoid hemorrhage often have a decreased mental status and are unable to cooperate enough to aid in the interventionist's recognition of a perforation. To make matters worse, such uncooperative patients are usually treated under general anesthesia, which further hinders the ability to recognize the signs and symptoms associated with aneurysmal rupture. The authors prefer to use local anesthesia with minimal sedation whenever possible to preserve the patient's clinical status as a sensitive indicator of aneurysmal rupture (82). The avoidance of general anesthesia is much easier in those patients who are treated electively and have been prepared for what to expect during the procedure. Movement by the patient during the procedure can be minimized with a Velcro strap or tapes across the forehead to serve as a reminder to the patient should the sedative make them drowsy. Patients who cannot cooperate because of high anxiety or decreased mental status usually require general anesthesia to keep them still enough to perform the procedure safely. When the patient is still, adequate digital subtraction angiographic roadmapping enables the interventionist to access the aneurysm safely. Should there be any question of shift in the roadmap, it should be repeated. Bladder catheterization should always be done before the procedure to provide patient comfort as well as monitor volume status.

During intracranial procedures, the interventionist must maneuver the micro-wire, microcatheter, and coils with extreme care, being ever mindful of a lack of one-to-one correlation of the movement between the devices on the screen and their manipulation. If the interventionist advances a device several centimeters and does not observe a direct response by fluoroscopy, the procedure should be stopped and not resumed until the reason for the lack of response has been discovered. An unrecognized increase in forward energy can result in a sudden release of the micro-wire and/or catheter that causes aneurysmal rupture or arterial injury. Adequate guide catheter placement can help by eliminating tortuosities that decrease the maneuverability of the devices. For aneurysms located in the anterior circulation, placing the guide catheter in the distal cervical internal carotid artery provides greater stability than leaving it in the common carotid artery. With lesions in the posterior circulation, one should make every attempt to place the guide catheter as distal as safely possible in the vertebral artery. In most instances, a 6-French angled guide catheter can be positioned so that the bend of the catheter rests in a bend in the vessel. This maneuver helps to anchor the guide catheter and increase the stability needed for the passage of the microwire and microcatheter. When accessing an aneurysm, the interventionist should always be cognizant of the location of the tip of the microwire and microcatheter.

The distal end of the microwire should be shaped according to the particular anatomy of the aneurysm and its relationship to the parent vessel. Shaping the appropriate curve increases the chance of accessing the aneurysm on the first pass, thereby decreasing the risks associated with the repeated passage of the microwire. When approaching the neck of the aneurysm, the length of wire extending beyond the end of the microcatheter should be long enough to allow full use of the shape of the wire but short enough to facilitate advancement of the microcatheter over the wire once the aneurysm is accessed. If the microcatheter has to be advanced a great distance once the tip of the wire is within the aneurysm, the risk of perforation increases. For smaller ruptured aneurysms, the authors prefer to engage the neck of the aneurysm just enough to maintain a stable purchase. As mentioned previously, these lesions tend to be little more than blisters on the artery, and their walls are extremely fragile. Keeping the microcatheter tip away from the dome of these aneurysms decreases the risk of coil perforation as a curve of the coil, rather than the tip, will make the initial contact with the aneurysm wall. The force will be spread out over the curve of the coil instead of focused at the tip. Also, with the microcatheter tip barely in the aneurysm, there is a greater tendency for a coil to back the catheter out rather than rupture the aneurysm should there be no more room for the coil. In larger aneurysms, the catheter tip should be placed well within the lesion to ensure that an adequate embolization can be performed before access to the aneurysm is lost. Attempting to reaccess an aneurysm after several coils have been deposited increases the risk of both arterial injury and aneurysm rupture.

Should an aneurysm rupture during either an attempt to access the aneurysm with a microwire and microcatheter or deployment of a coil, the effect of the anticoagulation should be reversed with protamine (1 mg/100 U heparin in the last dose; half the dose for every half-an-hour hour since the last heparin dose). The authors prefer to have 35 mg of this solution prepared and set aside on the back table so that it can be given as quickly as possible. If the rupture occurs in conjunction with microwire manipulation, the wire should be left in place until the protamine has taken effect. With normal coagulation parameters, the tiny hole created by the wire will quickly seal in some cases once the wire is withdrawn. To advance a microcatheter through the perforation and then attempt to coil the perforation can prove disastrous as it only serves to transform the 0.014-inch hole into one that is almost five times larger. However, should the perforation occur during the deployment of a coil, the heparinization is reversed and every effort is made to occlude the aneurysm as quickly as possible. The coil involved in the perforation should be deployed, then further coils deployed in rapid succession. Some authors have advocated the use of fibered coils in these situations; however, a larger microcatheter is often required to deliver these coils, and there is no time for the exchange of microcatheters (50). Time is also the major hurdle in deploying a balloon to arrest flow proximal to the aneurysm. In the time that it takes to place an occlusion balloon or exchange a larger catheter, the intracranial pressure is likely to rise to the point at which normal cerebral perfusion ceases. The authors prefer to use a 7-French guiding catheter so that a balloon can be passed easily and quickly without having to exchange to a larger catheter.

Thromboembolic complications that occur during coil embolization of intracranial aneurysms are usually the result of pre-existing intra-aneurysmal thrombus being dislodged or new thrombus forming on the coils and then embolizing (as previously mentioned). During stent- or balloon-assisted coiling, the stent or balloon can serve as a nidus for platelet aggregation and thrombus formation if the patient is not treated appropriately with antiplatelet agents and heparin anticoagulation. An appreciation of the potential for pre-existing thrombus by obtaining a magnetic resonance imaging study before the procedure, along with the use of digital subtraction roadmapping, will aid in sizing of the coils so that they do not disturb the intra-aneurysmal thrombus. Should thromboembolic events occur during the procedure despite antiplatelet and anticoagulation therapy, intra-arterial thrombolysis should be used with the understanding that the risk of intraprocedural hemorrhage will rise substantially. For those events felt to be the result of dislodged intra-aneurysmal thrombus, the authors prefer to use the third-generation recombinant tissue plasminogen activator (r-tPA) reteplase in the treatment of these thromboembolic complications. The administration of 2–8 units (U) of reteplase soon after an event will usually dissolve a fresh thrombus. This agent has an effective half-life of 13–16 min, thus endovascular treatment of the aneurysm does not have to be aborted because of fear of hemorrhagic complications if enough time is allowed to pass before resuming the embolization procedure. Other authors have reported the use of both r-tPA and urokinase in the treatment of intraprocedural thromboembolic events with mixed results (83–85). The coiling microcatheter should be removed from the aneurysm prior to attempting thrombolysis, and the microcatheter used for the intra-arterial infusion should be advanced as close to the blocked vessel as possible. Although no standard intra-arterial dose of r-tPA or urokinase has been established, the authors have found that reteplase can be given safely in 1-unit increments (1 U/5 min) up to a maximum dose of 8 units via superselective catheterization (86).

The success rate of intra-arterial thrombolysis depends on several factors such as age of thrombus, duration of occlusion, presence of collateral circulation, and degree of recanalization (84,87,88). Thrombus arising from within an aneurysm is likely to be old and devoid of intrinsically bound plasminogen, thus making it resistant to chemical thrombolysis (88). Because the brain cannot tolerate ischemia for very long, prolonged occlusion in the absence of collateral flow invariably results in an infarction. Therefore, the interventionist must act quickly as soon as a thromboembolic event is suspected. An angiogram should be performed after each unit of the thrombolytic agent has been infused, and if the blockage persists, further mechanical attempts may be used to lyse the thrombus. We refer the reader to one of several articles dealing with intra-arterial thrombolysis for specific information regarding such treatment (83–88). If the blocked vessel once again becomes patent, attention should be refocused on obliteration of the aneurysm.

Should the embolic source be platelet aggregate microemboli, which results in delayed filling of several vessels without any definite vessel dropout, intra-arterial thrombolysis might not be warranted. In these cases, the authors prefer to use an antiplatelet agent such as eptifibatide, which prevents platelet aggregation by binding to platelet glycoprotein IIb-IIIa receptors. With a half-life of 1.1 hr, eptifibatide is cleared at a relatively rapid rate (89); however, we do not advise proceeding with the coil embolization while such a strong antiplatelet agent is active in the patient's circulation. If the delay in filling improves, postponing further treatment for several hours or a day might prove to be a prudent decision. Whether the blockage is microscopic or grossly apparent within a specific vessel, the interventionist must be able to recognize such radiographic changes. Serial angiography during the procedure aids in assessing these changes. Also, by treating the patient with conscious sedation rather than general anesthesia, the interventionist has the benefit of performing serial neurologic assessments to aid in recognizing periods of cerebral ischemia.

Thromboembolic complications that occur after the procedure are most likely the result of thrombus that has formed within or on the coil mass and then broken free. The coils are thrombogenic, and platelets will immediately adhere to their surface and aggregate if appropriate antiplatelet therapy is not initiated. For ruptured aneurysms, the authors prefer to allow the systemic heparinization to wear off gradually, rather than reversing it with protamine. Aspirin (325 mg daily) is prescribed for patients for the remainder of their life, whether the aneurysm has ruptured or not. The aspirin decreases the aggregation of platelets on the coils during the process of endothelialization. For those patients treated electively, the authors prefer pretreatment with aspirin along with clopidogrel, if a stent or balloon is to be used, for at least three days before the procedure. Deactivated platelets may still adhere to the endovascular devices, but their vigorous activation and aggregation are suppressed.

When using a stent to supplement coil embolization, one must make every effort to ensure that the stent adequately spans the neck of the aneurysm. This means obtaining the appropriate views demonstrating the relationship of the aneurysm to the parent vessel and choosing a stent that is slightly larger than the diameter of the parent vessel. By oversizing the stent slightly, the stent opposes the wall more tightly, and the risk of stent migration is lessened. Should the stent not span the neck of the aneurysm, no attempt should be made to manipulate or retrieve the stent because this increases the risk of aneurysmal rupture and arterial injury.

The long-term rate of aneurysmal recurrence following coil embolization can be reduced by appropriate preparation on the front end. The decision to embolize should be made with the collaboration of both an interventionist and a neuro-surgeon. There should be a relative degree of certainty that the aneurysm can be completely coiled in one procedure. If the geometry of the aneurysm and its relation-ship to the parent vessel are not ideal, the use of adjunctive techniques (balloon or stent-assistance) should be considered or the patient referred for surgical ligation. Once the decision to coil has been made, the authors prefer to initiate the emboliza-tion with a basket-type coil that frames the aneurysm and spans the neck with several loops, and follow the deployment of this coil with the placement of progressively smaller diameter coils until no further embolization can be accomplished. If on follow-up angiography the aneurysm has recurred, one must determine the cause of the recurrence and decide whether the recurrence should be treated. With coil compaction, the resulting dome-to-neck ratio often precludes coil embolization without the use of a stent or balloon. If the recurrence is due to actual regrowth at the neck, coiling without an adjunctive device is often possible. The same precau-tions described for the original procedure should be followed for each subsequent one.

The management of thromboembolic complications associated with intracra-nial angioplasty and stenting is similar to that seen with coil embolization. However, with intracranial angioplasty, the risk of dissection is high, and the interventionist should be ready to manage this complication. If angioplasty results in a dissection, the exchange wire over which the balloon has been passed should be left in place to minimize the number of devices that must pass through the area of dissection. The intimal flap can be tacked down with a stent; however, the stent, in combination with the intimal injury, increases the risk for thrombus formation and restenosis. The authors prefer to perform the angioplasty and stenting in a staged fashion with the initial angioplasty being suboptimal. A less-aggressive angioplasty decreases the amount of arterial injury normally seen with angioplasty and results in a less vigorous cellular response within the vessel wall, allowing neoendothelialization to occur (3). An interval of four to six weeks is allowed to pass before a second angio-gram is done. If further angioplasty or stenting is warranted, the new layer of endothelium provides a smooth, uniform intimal surface.

Restenosis will invariably occur after intracranial angioplasty with or without stenting, but it may not be hemodynamically significant. Connors and Wojak have demonstrated that slow inflations produce less severe intimal disruptions and lead

to a decreased rate of significant stenosis (5). The authors have found that performing the angioplasty and stenting in separate procedures provides additional benefits
of decreased rates of thromboembolic complications and recurrent stenosis (6).
When restenosis does occur, the culprit is usually a hypercellular response as
opposed to de novo atherosclerosis. As a result, the area immediately underneath
the intima is less thrombogenic than atherosclerotic plaque. Although no large series
of the management of recurrent intracranial stenosis have been published, it would
theoretically seem that the risks of endovascular treatment would be lower than
those associated with the initial angioplasty. The periprocedural risks of intracranial
angioplasty are directly related to the irregularity of the plaque (25,26), and a plaque
that is well organized and healed over should be less likely to cause thromboembolic
complications.

CONCLUSIONS

Intracranial endovascular interventions can be associated with a high rate of both
hemorrhagic and ischemic complications, but many of these complications can be
avoided with a proper understanding of where the most common errors are made.
An old adage in surgical education is that the three most important things to
consider when performing a procedure are anatomy, anatomy, and anatomy, and
the same is true for intracranial endovascular work. The interventionist must know
both normal and aberrant cerebrovascular anatomy and be able to visualize it in
three dimensions to successfully navigate devices and minimize technical errors.
Anticipation also plays a key role in complication avoidance and management.
Being able to anticipate at which points complications are more likely to occur aids
the interventionist in taking the appropriate steps in a timely and effective manner.

REFERENCES

1. Phatouros CC, Higashida RT, Malek AM, Smith WS, Mully TW, DeArmond SJ, Dowd CF,
    Halbach VV. Endovascular stenting of an acutely thrombosed basilar artery: technical case
    report and review of the literature. Neurosurgery 1999; 44:667–673.
2. Gomez CR, Orr SC. Angioplasty and stenting for primary treatment of intracranial
    arterial stenoses. Arch Neurol 2001; 58:1687–1690.
3. Levy EI, Hanel RA, Bendok BR, Boulos AS, Hartney ML, Guterman LR, Qureshi AI,
    Hopkins LN. Staged stent-assisted angioplasty for symptomatic intracranial vertebroba-
    silar artery stenosis. J Neurosurg 2002; 97:1294–1301.
4. Chimowitz MI. Angioplasty or stenting is not appropriate as first-line treatment of intra-
    cranial stenosis. Arch Neurol 2001; 58:1690–1692.
5. Connors JJ 3rd, Wojak JC. Percutaneous transluminal angioplasty for intracranial athero-
    sclerotic lesions: evolution of technique and short-term results. J Neurosurg 1999; 91:
    415–423.
6. Levy EI, Boulos AS, Guterman LR. Stent-assisted endoluminal revascularization for the
    treatment of intracranial atherosclerotic disease. Neurol Res 2002; 24:337–346.
7. Parsons TJ, Haycraft DL, Hoak JC, Sage H. Interaction of platelets and purified
    collagens in a laminar flow model. Thromb Res 1986; 43:435–443.
8. Qureshi AI, Luft AR, Sharma M, Guterman LR, Hopkins LN. Prevention and treatment
    of thromboembolic and ischemic complications associated with endovascular procedures:
    part I—pathophysiological and pharmacological features. Neurosurgery 2000; 46:1344–1359.

9. Barry WL, Sarembock IJ. Antiplatelet and anticoagulant therapy in patients undergoing percutaneous transluminal coronary angioplasty. Cardiol Clin 1994; 12:517–535.

10. Ghigliotti G, Waissbluth AR, Speidel C, Abendschein DR, Eisenberg PR. Prolonged activation of prothrombin on the vascular wall after arterial injury. Arterioscler Thromb Vasc Biol 1998; 18:250–257.

11. Bourassa MG, Cantin M, Sandborn EB, Pederson E. Scanning electron microscopy of surface irregularities and thrombogenesis of polyurethane and polyethylene coronary catheters. Circulation 1976; 53:992–996.

12. Nachnani GH, Lessin LS, Motomiya T, Jensen WN. Scanning electron microscopy of thrombogenesis on vascular catheter surfaces. N Engl J Med 1972; 286:139–140.

13. Wilner GD, Casarella WJ, Baier R, Fenoglio CM. Thrombogenicity of angiographic catheters. Circ Res 1978; 43:424–428.

14. Kallmes DF, McGraw JK, Evans AJ, Mathis JM, Hergenrother RW, Jensen ME, Cloft HJ, Lopes M, Dion JE. Thrombogenicity of hydrophilic and nonhydrophilic microcatheters and guiding catheters. AJNR Am J Neuroradiol 1997; 18:1243–1251.

15. Leach KR, Kurisu Y, Carlson JE, Repa I, Epstein DH, Urness M, Sahatjian R, Hunter DW, Castenada-Zuniga WR, Amplatz K. Thrombogenicity of hydrophilically coated guide wires and catheters. Radiology 1990; 175:675–677.

16. Krpski WC, Bass A, Kelly AB, Marzec UM, Hanson SR, Harker LA. Heparin-resistant thrombus formation by endovascular stents in baboons. Interruption by a synthetic antithrombin. Circulation 1990; 82:570–577.

17. Rogers C, Edelman ER. Endovascular stent design dictates experimental restenosis and thrombosis. Circulation 1995; 91:2995–3001.

18. Werner GS, Gastmann O, Ferrari M, Schuenemann S, Knies A, Diedrich J, Kreuzer H. Risk factors for acute and subacute stent thrombosis after high-pressure stent implantation: a study by intracoronary ultrasound. Am Heart J 1998; 135:300–309.

19. Post MJ, de Graaf-Bos AN, van Zanten HG, de Groot PG, Sixma JJ, Borst C. Thrombogenicity of the human arterial wall after interventional thermal injury. J Vasc Res 1996; 33:156–163.

20. Lang J, Kageyama I. Clinical anatomy of the blood spaces and blood vessels surrounding the siphon of the internal carotid artery. Acta Anat (Basel) 1990; 139:320–325.

21. Andres V. Control of vascular smooth muscle cell growth and its implication in atherosclerosis and restenosis [review]. Int J Mol Med 1998; 2:81–89.

22. Pauletto P, Sartore S, Pessina AC. Smooth-muscle-cell proliferation and differentiation in neointima formation and vascular restenosis. Clin Sci (Lond) 1994; 87:467–479.

23. Carter AJ, Laird JR, Farb A, Kufs W, Wortham DC, Virmani R. Morphologic characteristics of lesion formation and time course of smooth muscle cell proliferation in a porcine proliferative restenosis model. J Am Coll Cardiol 1994; 24:1398–1405.

24. Schwartz SM, deBlois D, O'Brien ER. The intima. Soil for atherosclerosis and restenosis. Circ Res 1995; 77:445–465.

25. Mori T, Mori K, Fukuoka M, Arisawa M, Honda S. Percutaneous transluminal cerebral angioplasty: serial angiographic follow-up after successful dilatation. Neuroradiology 1997; 39:111–116.

26. Mori T, Fukuoka M, Kazita K, Mori K. Follow-up study after intracranial percutaneous transluminal cerebral balloon angioplasty. AJNR Am J Neuroradiol 1998; 19:1525–1533.

27. Ryan TJ, Bauman WB, Kennedy JW, Kereiakes DJ, King SB 3rd, McCallister BD, Smith SC Jr, Ullyot DJ. Guidelines for percutaneous transluminal coronary angio-plasty. A report of the American Heart Association/American College of Cardiology Task Force on Assessment of Diagnostic and Therapeutic Cardiovascular Procedures (Committee on Percutaneous Transluminal Coronary Angioplasty). Circulation 1993; 88:2987–3007.

28. Clark WM, Barnwell SL, Nesbit G, O'Neill OR, Wynn ML, Coull BM. Safety and efficacy of percutaneous transluminal angioplasty for intracranial atherosclerotic stenosis. Stroke 1995; 26:1200–1204.

29. Takis C, Kwan ES, Pessin MS, Jacobs DH, Caplan LR. Intracranial angioplasty: experience and complications. AJNR Am J Neuroradiol 1997; 18:1661–1668.

30. Terada T, Tsuura M, Matsumoto H, Masuo O, Tsumoto T, Yamaga H, Itakura T. Endovascular therapy for stenosis of the petrous or cavernous portion of the internal carotid artery: percutaneous transluminal angioplasty compared with stent placement. J Neurosurg 2003; 98:491–497.

31. Rasmussen PA, Perl J 2nd, Barr JD, Markarian GZ, Katzan I, Sila C, Krieger D, Furlan AJ, Masaryk TJ. Stent-assisted angioplasty of intracranial vertebrobasilar atherosclerosis: an initial experience. J Neurosurg 2000; 92:771–778.

32. Mathur A, Roubin GS, Iyer SS, Piamsonboon C, Liu MW, Gomez CR, Yadav JS, Chastain HD, Fox LM, Dean LS, Vitek JJ. Predictors of stroke complicating carotid artery stenting. Circulation 1998; 97:1239–1245.

33. Debrun GM, Aletich VA, Kehrli P, Misra M, Ausman JI, Charbel F. Selection of cerebral aneurysms for treatment using Guglielmi detachable coils: the preliminary University of Illinois at Chicago experience. Neurosurgery 1998; 43:1281–1297.

34. Fernandez Zubillaga A, Guglielmi G, Vinuela F, Duckwiler GR. Endovascular occlusion of intracranial aneurysms with electrically detachable coils: correlation of aneurysm neck size and treatment results. AJNR Am J Neuroradiol 1994; 15:815–820.

35. Vinuela F, Duckwiler G, Mawad M. Guglielmi detachable coil embolization of acute intracranial aneurysm: perioperative anatomical and clinical outcome in 403 patients. J Neurosurg 1997; 86:475–482.

36. Hope JK, Byrne JV, Molyneux AJ. Factors influencing successful angiographic occlusion of aneurysms treated by coil embolization. AJNR Am J Neuroradiol 1999; 20:391–399.

37. Pelz DM, Lownie SP, Fox AJ. Thromboembolic events associated with the treatment of cerebral aneurysms with Guglielmi detachable coils. AJNR Am J Neuroradiol 1998; 19:1541–1547.

38. Klotzsch C, Nahser HC, Henkes H, Kuhne D, Berlit P. Detection of microemboli distal to cerebral aneurysms before and after therapeutic embolization. AJNR Am J Neuroradiol 1998; 19:1315–1318.

39. Derdeyn CP, Cross DT 3rd, Moran CJ, Brown GW, Pilgram TK, Diringer MN, Grubb RL Jr, Rich KM, Chicoine MR, Dacey RG Jr. Postprocedure ischemic events after treatment of intracranial aneurysms with Guglielmi detachable coils. J Neurosurg 2002; 96:837–843.

40. Kuether TA, Nesbit GM, Barnwell SL. Clinical and angiographic outcomes, with treatment data, for patients with cerebral aneurysms treated with Guglielmi detachable coils: a single-center experience. Neurosurgery 1998; 43:1016–1025.

41. Turjman F, Massoud TF, Sayre J, Vinuela F. Predictors of aneurysmal occlusion in the period immediately after endovascular treatment with detachable coils: a multivariate analysis. AJNR Am J Neuroradiol 1998; 19:1645–1651.

42. Dion JE, Gates PC, Fox AJ, Barnett HJ, Blom RJ. Clinical events following neuroangiography: a prospective study. Stroke 1987; 18:997–1004.

43. Earnest FT, Forbes G, Sandok BA, Piepgras DG, Faust RJ, Ilstrup DM, Arndt LJ. Complications of cerebral angiography: prospective assessment of risk. AJR Am J Roentgenol 1984; 142:247–253.

44. Qureshi AI, Luft AR, Sharma M, Guterman LR, Hopkins LN. Prevention and treatment of thromboembolic and ischemic complications associated with endovascular procedures: part II–Clinical aspects and recommendations. Neurosurgery 2000; 46:1360–1376.

45. Heiserman JE, Dean BL, Hodak JA, Flom RA, Bird CR, Drayer BP, Fram EK. Neurologic complications of cerebral angiography. AJNR Am J Neuroradiol 1994; 15:1401–1411.

46. Theodotou BC, Whaley R, Mahaley MS. Complications following transfemoral cerebral angiography for cerebral ischemia. Report of 159 angiograms and correlation with surgical risk. Surg Neurol 1987; 28:90–92.

47. Serbinenko FA. Balloon catheterization and occlusion of major cerebral vessels. J Neurosurg 1974; 41:125–145.

48. Guglielmi G, Vinuela F, Dion J, Duckwiler G. Electrothrombosis of saccular aneurysms via endovascular approach. Part 2: preliminary clinical experience. J Neurosurg 1991; 75:8–14.

49. Guglielmi G, Vinuela F, Sepetka I, Macellari V. Electrothrombosis of saccular aneurysms via endovascular approach. Part 1: electrochemical basis, technique, and experimental results. J Neurosurg 1991; 75:1–7.

50. Connors JJ 3rd, Wojak JC. Rupture of a vessel, aneurysm, or arteriovenous malformation. In: Connors JJ 3rd, Wojak JC, eds. Interventional Neuroradiology: Strategies and Practical Techniques. Philadelphia: W.B. Saunders Company, 1999:775–776.

51. Halbach VV, Higashida RT, Dowd CF, Barnwell SL, Hieshima GB. Management of vascular perforations that occur during neurointerventional procedures. AJNR Am J Neuroradiol 1991; 12:319–327.

52. Cloft HJ, Kallmes DF. Cerebral aneurysm perforations complicating therapy with Guglielmi detachable coils: a meta-analysis. AJNR Am J Neuroradiol 2002; 23:1706–1709.

53. Dovey Z, Misra M, Thornton J, Charbel FT, Debrun GM, Ausman JI. Guglielmi detachable coiling for intracranial aneurysms: the story so far. Arch Neurol 2001; 58:559–564.

54. Workman MJ, Cloft HJ, Tong FC, Dion JE, Jensen ME, Marx WF, Kallmes DF. Thrombus formation at the neck of cerebral aneurysms during treatment with Guglielmi detachable coils. AJNR Am J Neuroradiol 2002; 23:1568–1576.

55. Bavinzski G, Talazoglu V, Killer M, Richling B, Gruber A, Gross CE, Plenk H Jr. Gross and microscopic histopathological findings in aneurysms of the human brain treated with Guglielmi detachable coils. J Neurosurg 1999; 91:284–293.

56. Horowitz MB, Purdy PD, Burns D, Bellotto D. Scanning electron microscopic findings in a basilar tip aneurysm embolized with Guglielmi detachable coils. AJNR Am J Neuroradiol 1997; 18:688–690.

57. Moret J, Cognard C, Weill A, Castaings L, Rey A. The "remodeling technique" in the treatment of wide neck intracranial aneurysms. Interv Neuroradiol 1997; 3:21–35.

58. Nelson PK, Levy DI. Balloon-assisted coil embolization of wide-necked aneurysms of the internal carotid artery: medium-term angiographic and clinical follow-up in 22 patients. AJNR Am J Neuroradiol 2001; 22:19–26.

59. Lefkowitz MA, Gobin YP, Akiba Y, Duckwiler GR, Murayama Y, Guglielmi G, Martin NA, Vinuela F. Balloon-assisted Guglielmi detachable coiling of wide-necked aneurysma: part II–clinical results. Neurosurgery 1999; 45:531–538.

60. Linskey ME, Horton JA, Rao GR, Yonas H. Fatal rupture of the intracranial carotid artery during transluminal angioplasty for vasospasm induced by subarachnoid hemorrhage. Case report. J Neurosurg 1991; 74:985–990.

61. Phatouros CC, Halbach VV, Malek AM, Dowd CF, Higashida RT. Simultaneous subarachnoid hemorrhage and carotid cavernous fistula after rupture of a paraclinoid aneurysm during balloon-assisted coil embolization. AJNR Am J Neuroradiol 1999; 20:1100–1102.

62. Higashida RT, Smith W, Gress D, Urwin R, Dowd CF, Balousek PA, Halbach VV. Intravascular stent and endovascular coil placement for a ruptured fusiform aneurysm of the basilar artery. Case report and review of the literature. J Neurosurg 1997; 87:944–949.

63. Howington JU, Hanel RA, Harrigan MR, Levy EI, Guterman LR, Hopkins LN. The Neuroform stent, the first microcatheter-delivered stent for use in the intracranial circulation [Guest Editorial]. Neurosurgery. 2004; 54:2–5.

64. Moshfegh K, Redondo M, Julmy F, Wuillemin WA, Gebauer MU, Haeberli A, Meyer BJ. Antiplatelet effects of clopidogrel compared with aspirin after myocardial infarction: enhanced inhibitory effects of combination therapy. J Am Coll Cardiol 2000; 36:699–705.

65. Cognard C, Weill A, Castaings L, Rey A, Moret J. Intracranial berry aneurysms: angiographic and clinical results after endovascular treatment. Radiology 1998; 206:499–510.

66. Lot G, Houdart E, Cophignon J, Casasco A, George B. Combined management of intracranial aneurysms by surgical and endovascular treatment. Modalities and results from a series of 395 cases. Acta Neurochir (Wien) 1999; 141:557–562.

67. Raymond J, Roy D. Safety and efficacy of endovascular treatment of acutely ruptured aneurysms. Neurosurgery 1997; 41:1235–1246.

68. Boulos AS, Bendok BR, Levy EI, Kim SH, Qureshi AI, Guterman LR, Hopkins LN. Endovascular aneurysm treatment: a proven therapy. Neurol Res 2002; 24(suppl 1): S71–S79.

69. Lozier AP, Connolly ES Jr, Lavine SD, Solomon RA. Guglielmi detachable coil embolization of posterior circulation aneurysms: a systematic review of the literature. Stroke 2002; 33:2509–2518.

70. Raymond J, Guilbert F, Weill A, Georganos SA, Juravsky L, Lambert A, Lamoureux J, Chagnon M, Roy D. Long-term angiographic recurrences after selective endovascular treatment of aneurysms with detachable coils. Stroke 2003; 34:1398–1403.

71. Imbesi SG, Kerber CW. Analysis of slipstream flow in a wide-necked basilar artery aneurysm: evaluation of potential treatment regimens. AJNR Am J Neuroradiol 2001; 22:721–724.

72. Asakura F, Tenjin H, Sugawa N, Kimura S, Oki F. Evaluation of intra-aneurysmal blood flow by digital subtraction angiography: blood flow change after coil embolization. Surg Neurol 2003; 59:310–319.

73. Kawanabe Y, Sadato A, Taki W, Hashimoto N. Endovascular occlusion of intracranial aneurysms with Guglielmi detachable coils: correlation between coil packing density and coil compaction. Acta Neurochir (Wien) 2001; 143:451–455.

74. Higashida RT, Tsai FY, Halbach VV, Dowd CF, Smith T, Fraser K, Hieshima GB. Transluminal angioplasty for atherosclerotic disease of the vertebral and basilar arteries. J Neurosurg 1993; 78:192–198.

75. Alazzaz A, Thornton J, Aletich VA, Debrun GM, Ausman JI, Charbel F. Intracranial percutaneous transluminal angioplasty for arteriosclerotic stenosis. Arch Neurol 2000; 57:1625–1630.

76. Touho H. Percutaneous transluminal angioplasty in the treatment of atherosclerotic disease of the anterior cerebral circulation and hemodynamic evaluation. J Neurosurg 1995; 82:953–960.

77. Marks MP, Marcellus M, Norbash AM, Steinberg GK, Tong D, Albers GW. Outcome of angioplasty for atherosclerotic intracranial stenosis. Stroke 1999; 30:1065–1069.

78. Stary H, Chandler A, Dinsmore R. A definition of advanced types of atherosclerotic lesions and a histological classification of atherosclerosis. A report from the Committee on Vascular Lesions of the Council of Arteriosclerosis, American Heart Association. Circulation 1995; 92:1355–1374.

79. Tanaka H, Sukhova GK, Swanson SJ, Clinton SK, Ganz P, Cybulsky MI, Libby P. Sustained activation of vascular cells and leukocytes in the rabbit aorta after balloon injury. Circulation 1993; 88:1788–1803.

80. Wainwright CL, Miller AM, Wadsworth RM. Inflammation as a key event in the development of neointima following vascular balloon injury. Clin Exp Pharmacol Physiol 2001; 28:891–895.

81. Lutsep HL, Barnwell SL, Mawad M, Chiu D, Hartmann M, Hacke W, Reul J, Biniek R, Guterman LR, Yahia AM, et al. Stenting of Symptomatic Atherosclerotic Lesions in the Vertebral or Intracranial Arteries (SSYLVIA): study results [abstract P83A]. Stroke 2003; 34:253.

82. Qureshi AI, Suri MF, Khan J, Kim SH, Fessler RD, Ringer AJ, Guterman LR, Hopkins LN. Endovascular treatment of intracranial aneurysms by using Guglielmi detachable coils in awake patients: safety and feasibility. J Neurosurg 2001; 94:880–885.

83. Cronqvist M, Pierot L, Boulin A, Cognard C, Castaings L, Moret J. Local intraarterial fibrinolysis of thromboemboli occurring during endovascular treatment of intracerebral

aneurysm: a comparison of anatomic results and clinical outcome. AJNR Am J Neuroradiol 1998; 19:157–165.

84. Hahnel S, Schellinger PD, Gutschalk A, Geletneky K, Hartmann M, Knauth M, Sartor K. Local intra-arterial fibrinolysis of thromboemboli occurring during neuroendovascular procedures with recombinant tissue plasminogen activator. Stroke 2003; 34:1723–1728.

85. Berg-Dammer E, Henkes H, Nahser HC, Kuhne D. Thromboembolic occlusion of the middle cerebral artery due to angiography and endovascular procedures: safety and efficacy of local intra-arterial fibrinolysis. Cerebrovasc Dis 1996; 6:222–230.

86. Qureshi AI, Ali Z, Suri MF, Kim SH, Shatla AA, Ringer AJ, Lopes DK, Guterman LR, Hopkins LN. Intra-arterial third-generation recombinant tissue plasminogen activator (reteplase) for acute ischemic stroke. Neurosurgery 2001; 49:41–50.

87. Brandt T, von Kummer R, Muller-Kuppers M, Hacke W. Thrombolytic therapy of acute basilar artery occlusion. Variables affecting recanalization and outcome. Stroke 1996; 27:875–881.

88. Zeumer H, Freitag HJ, Zanella F, Thie A, Arning C. Local intra-arterial fibrinolytic therapy in patients with stroke: urokinase versus recombinant tissue plasminogen activator (r-tPA). Neuroradiology 1993; 35:159–162.

89. Alton KB, Kosoglou T, Baker S, Affrime MB, Cayen MN, Patrick JE. Disposition of 14C-eptifibatide after intravenous administration to healthy men. Clin Ther 1998; 20: 307–323.

12

Atherosclerotic Disease of the Renal Artery

Julie E. Adams and Vikram S. Kashyap
Department of Vascular Surgery, The Cleveland Clinic Foundation,
Cleveland, Ohio, U.S.A.

INTRODUCTION

The endovascular treatment of renal artery occlusive disease has evolved significantly over the last two decades. Significant strides have been made in the design and delivery of both angioplasty balloons and stents to allow safe, percutaneous revascularization of the renal blood flow. Many of the technical advances revolve around lower profile devices on a 0.014-inch platform as opposed to the 0.035-inch platforms used in the past, rapid exchange technology, and advances in anticoagulation and antiplatelet agents. Furthermore, the possibility of improving patency by decreasing restenosis with drug-eluting stents, and the possibility of decreasing end-organ embolization by using distal protection devices support an optimistic view of endovascular renal artery treatment, supplanting bypass surgery for most patients with renal artery occlusive disease.

Despite the marked technical advances in renal artery intervention, the selection of patients for medical therapy, endovascular therapy or surgical bypass remains hotly debated. The major indications for renal intervention remain the young patient with renovascular hypertension and the older patient with uncontrollable hypertension and/or deterioration of renal function. The goal of treatment is to relieve hypertension or renal dysfunction secondary to unilateral or bilateral renal artery stenoses. Thus, a key to success, where preservation of kidney function is crucial, is to avoid any insult to the end organ that can lead to either short-term or long-term deterioration of renal function that is greater than the natural history of patients observed with medical therapy alone. This requires careful selection of patients for renal intervention and meticulous technique in the performance of the procedure. The difficulty in patient selection is underscored by the lack of an accurate functional assay that can discern renal artery stenosis (RAS) as the causative factor in renovascular disease versus other etiologies including arteriolar thickening, tubular and glomerular atrophy, glomerulosclerosis and pre-existing primary hypertension. The mechanisms of hypertension in patients with RAS are complex because not all patients with RAS have hypertension secondary to renin-dependent renovascular hypertension. Despite the major advances in the design of catheters, balloons, and stents, both minor and major complications can still occur because of the unforgiving nature of the atherosclerotic aorta and the renal artery or the pre-existing renal dysfunction in many of these patients. This chapter will summarize the main areas of complications for renal artery intervention as follows:

1. Renal artery rupture,
2. Plaque disruption leading to dissection and/or acute thrombosis, and
3. Embolization to the kidney or the periphery.

Additional relevant areas of contrast-induced renal failure and access-related complications are discussed in the introduction of this book.

CURRENT SUCCESS RATES FOR RENAL INTERVENTION

In the literature of renal artery angioplasty and stenting, complications are generally mentioned in closing. The difficulty in summarizing the specific rates of complications lies partly in the fact that authors define these complications differently. However, any discussion regarding advances in endovascular therapy, especially when compared to traditional open surgery, is not complete without an understanding of the complications of such therapy. It allows the endovascular specialist to recommend the appropriate modality of treatment for each patient with realistic expectations of success. Currently, percutaneous transluminal angioplasty (PTA) is used for primary renal lesions secondary to fibromuscular dysplasia (FMD), and distal renal artery or branch lesions. Most authorities would recommend primary renal artery stenting for ostial lesions.

In the literature, success is generally defined in terms of a satisfactory technical result at the time of the procedure and an ability to achieve the desired end point. For renal artery disease, the end point has generally included control or relief of hypertension, improvement in renal function, or a delay in the progression of ischemic nephropathy to end-stage dialysis-dependent renal failure. Recently, renal artery procedures are being performed in conjunction with endovascular treatment of complicated aortic aneurysms involving the suprarenal aorta.

The determination of technical success is done at the completion of the procedure and is usually a subjective evaluation of selective renal arteriography after intervention. In some centers, objective data with hemodynamic monitoring, intravascular ultrasound (IVUS), and post-procedure non-invasive testing is applied routinely. The literature reveals the technical success rate to be in the range of 80–100% (1–15). However, authors define technical success differently. Most give a definition of technical success as a residual diameter stenosis of less than 20% (5–9,11,13), 30% (4,13,15), or 50% (1,3,12). Some add a category for partial success or "improvement" which allows for up to 70% stenosis to be considered a satisfactory or successful outcome (1,3,4,9,10). It seems that all agree that a residual diameter stenosis of 70% or greater to be a technical failure. Some authors, however, strictly define success in terms of clinical outcome and not the radiographic appearance of the stenosis after treatment (16).

There are differences in the rates of technical success between primary angioplasty and angioplasty and stenting. A randomized prospective clinical trial evaluating balloon angioplasty and arterial stenting for ostial atherosclerotic disease found a significant difference in primary success rates between the two groups (12). Patients randomized to the angioplasty group experienced a 57% technical success rate while those receiving stents had an increase in success rates to 88%. The difference between the groups was 31% (95% confidence interval 12–50). Most individual retrospective studies reveal a similar advantage to the placement of a stent. The results of a meta-analysis concur (17). This study reviewed the literature published in 1998 evaluating 678 patients who underwent stent placement and 644 receiving angioplasty for renal artery stenoses. The authors concluded that renal artery stent placement resulted in a superior technical result and clinical improvement. Stent placement was found to have a 98% technical success rate versus a 77% success rate for angioplasty alone (17). This has led to the widespread adoption of primary stenting rather than stenting only for poor PTA results.

The three prospective randomized trials comparing balloon angioplasty to medical therapy for renovascular hypertension served as the basis for another recent meta-analysis (20–23). Of the 104 patients allocated to intervention, 11% developed clinically important hematomas at the catheter insertion site, one patient had symptomatic hypotension during the procedure, and there were five technical failures. Despite the documentation of a relatively safe procedure, balloon angioplasty had only a modest, but significant effect on blood pressure in patients with atherosclerotic RAS and poorly controlled hypertension. There was no evidence supporting the use of intervention to improve or preserve renal function, however, none of the individual trials were designed to answer this question.

Also influencing the technical success rates are various anatomic and pathologic factors (8) such as whether the lesion is ostial or non-ostial, and if the stenosis being treated is secondary to atherosclerosis or FMD. Ostial stenoses have been defined as lesions involving the proximal 5 mm of the renal artery origin or as within 1 cm of the renal artery orifice (2,13,14). Historically, overall success rates for angioplasty have been reported to be 55% for ostial lesions and 70% for all lesions (13). Ostial lesions have been thought to be more resistant to angioplasty as the nature of the plaque is different from non-ostial stenoses, with aortic plaque "spilling over" into renal ostial stenoses and therefore being more difficult to fracture. In a study by Klow, 389 stenoses secondary to atherosclerosis underwent angioplasty (10). Sixty-three percent were ostial, 32% involved the main renal artery, and 5% were in a segmental branch. The immediate technical success rates were 95%, 93%, and 84%, respectively, not reaching statistical significance. A greater difference was seen in rates of secondary patency with main renal artery lesions having an 85% secondary patency, and ostial and segmental lesions falling to 74% and 62%, respectively. Canzanello et al. studied a group of 100 consecutive patients with 125 renal artery lesions undergoing PTA for atherosclerotic renovascular hypertension (3). No statistically significant difference was found in overall success rate, but there was a trend toward decreased technical success with ostial lesions, 62% versus 72% for non-ostial lesions. Many think the addition of stent placement to the angioplasty of a RAS has further decreased the gap in technical success and patency rates for ostial stenoses.

Lesions secondary to FMD have been evaluated separately in several studies. In a study of 100 patients by Martin et al., response to angioplasty in patients with hypertension and stenoses secondary to FMD were found to have an overall benefit of 85% compared to 65% for those patients with hypertension and ostial stenoses secondary to atherosclerosis (2). The patients in this study with non-ostial atherosclerotic stenoses had outcomes similar to those with FMD. A larger study evaluating 201 patients reported less difference in immediate technical results but a difference in the clinical improvement or cure at six months (4). Technical success was 73.9% for atherosclerotic lesions (99 patients) and 71.2% for patients with FMD (37 patients). When allowing for the consideration of improvement, defined as a 30–60% stenosis

Table 1 Technical Success Rates of PTA and PTAS

Author	Year	Definition of technical success	No. of arteries treated	Complete success (%)	Partial success (%)
Sos	1983	Success = ≤50% stenosis Improvement = 50–70% stenosis	104 PTA	56.7 unilat 9.5 bilat	3 unilat 47.4 of bilateral
Martin	1985	No definition provided	100 PTA	88	n/a
Canzanello	1989	Success = ≤50% Partial success 50–70%	125 PTA	30.9 unilat 7.4 bilat	45.2 unilat 66.7 bilat
Klinge	1989	Successful = <30% Improvement = 30–60% or >15% decrease in stenosis	213 PTA	73.2	7.5
Rees	1991	<30%		96.4	n/a
MacLeod	1995	<30%; not protruding into aortic lumen	29 PTAS	100	n/a
Taylor	1996	<30%	32 PTAS	100	n/a
Boisclair	1997	<30%	35 PTAS	100	n/a
Hoffman	1998	Success = ≤30% Partial success = 30–50%	52 PTA	58	29
Klow	1998	No significant residual stenosis	552	92	3
Bakker	1999	<20% restenosis successful; 20–50% partially successful	120 PTAS	93.3	4.2
Van de ven	1999	<50% restenosis	51 PTA 52 PTA	57 PTA 88 PTAS	n/a
Yutan	2001	<30%	88 PTAS -51%	89	n/a
Ivanovic	2003	<20% restenosis	179 PTAS	98.3	n/a
Sivamurthy	2004	<30%	183	98	n/a

Abbreviations: PTA, percutaneous transluminal angioplasty; PTAS, percutaneous transluminal angioplasty and stenting; n/a, not applicable.

or at least a 15% reduction in diameter of stenosis, this total technical success rate changed to 77.6% for atherosclerotic lesions and 90.4% for lesions secondary to FMD. Additionally, a clinical cure or improvement at six months was present for 77.5% of patients with atherosclerotic lesions and 86.3% of those with FMD. Lastly, Klow et al. reported on a cohort of 49 patients with 70 stenoses secondary to FMD treated at their institution over a 10-year period (10). Only 10% were ostial, and 77% were in the main renal artery. Their immediate success rate was 99% (94% for atherosclerotic lesions). The secondary patency rates reached statistical significance when compared to atherosclerosis, 95% versus 77%. There is widespread agreement that PTA is the procedure of choice for patients with renovascular hypertension secondary to FMD.

For most patients, it is atherosclerotic disease that results in hemodynamically significant renal artery stenoses. There is evidence that success rates vary depending on whether there are bilateral lesions versus a single renal artery with atherosclerosis. As shown in Table 1, studies by Sos and Canzanello reveal a higher complete success rate with unilateral lesions (1,3). Simple elastic recoil can be the reason for a technical failure, but other complications may also contribute, such as dissection, perforation or thrombosis.

As shown in Table 1, there has been a transition over the years from angioplasty to angioplasty and stenting, as well as a general increase in technical success rates. As stated previously, this is a result of increasing experience in renal interventions as well as improvements in balloon and stent design allowing safe passage and treatment of preocclusive lesions.

Achieving technical success is only part of an uncomplicated percutaneous procedure. Other complications have been grouped in varying ways. Some authors divide complications into major or minor, depending on the patient's clinical outcome, while others have described complications as related to access or to the specific artery being treated. An analysis of complications as being anatomic or functional has been described by Ivanovic et al. and allows for a systematic approach to their discussion (14). Additionally, peripheral emboli and mortality are included.

Reported complication rates generally range between 6% and 24% (1–18). Immediate surgical intervention is only occasionally required. Anatomic complications include renal artery rupture, renal artery or aortic dissection, and acute renal artery thrombosis or occlusion.

RENAL ARTERY RUPTURE

The clinical manifestation of arterial rupture is often not subtle with bleeding into the retroperitoneum, immediate onset of back, flank or inguinal pain, tachycardia, and hypotension. Renal artery rupture is fortunately rare, with an incidence of 0–1.7% (14). It may occur secondary to the balloon dilatation in a subintimal plane or the use of too large a balloon in a non-compliant calcified artery. Oftentimes, an eccentric plaque will pierce the adventitial plane of the diseased artery causing bleeding. Unexplained back pain and hypotension mandate careful interrogation of the PTA or stented segment. Ideally, management of renal artery rupture requires recognition of this condition prior to removal of the guidewire crossing the target lesion. Successful management may consist of only reversal of heparin and prolonged balloon inflation. The PTA balloon should be inflated just till wall apposition as determined by the absence of free-flowing contrast when injected proximally in the aorta through the guiding catheter or sheath. An initial inflation time of three to five minutes will allow stabilization of the patient, reversal of heparin with protamine and thrombosis of the arterial rupture site. In cases when rupture has occurred with PTA alone, stenting should be considered if the extravasation of contrast is minimal. On the other hand, if a large arterial tear has occurred mandating surgical correction, stenting should be avoided to allow surgical repair to proceed without a metallic stent precluding primary repair. In most cases of contrast extravasation, repeat balloon inflation will cause the bleeding to stop. If the arterial rupture is not successfully treated via endovascular means, the balloon should be left inflated to allow control of hemorrhage and expeditious transfer to the operating room for renal revascularization to proceed. One should note that prolonged warm ischemia time will preclude renal salvage and excessive delay in transfer to the operating room for repair may lead to irreversible renal ischemia.

PLAQUE DISRUPTION: DISSECTION, ACUTE THROMBOSIS

Despite advances in endovascular technology, PTA remains a controlled fracture of a well-established atherosclerotic plaque. On a microscopic level, all PTA results in plaque fracture and microdissection. However, arterial dissection that is apparent on arteriographic evaluation and leading to a significant change in clinical management is uncommon. Renal artery dissection is often classified as flow limiting or non-flow limiting. Reported rates in the literature range from 0% to 7.8% (1–4,6,11,12,14). Reports are similar for angioplasty and angioplasty with stenting, 2.5% versus 2.3% (12). Some relate to a low incidence with no subsequent need for treatment (11), while others describe an emergent situation for renal salvage. Ivanovic et al. described two cases resulting in renal artery dissections, an incidence of 1.1%; one occurred in a segmental branch and resulted in a small renal infarction, and the other involved the main renal artery and required the placement of two additional stents (14). Another report gives a 5% incidence in 100 patients, four of whom underwent successful emergency aortorenal bypass (2). In a review by Sos et al. four of 51 patients (7.8%) undergoing PTA for atherosclerotic lesion developed non-occlusive renal artery dissections (1). Surgical bypass was successful in three, and one did not undergo treatment.

Aortic dissection is a known complication with any catheter or guidewire manipulation of the aorta. In the setting of endovascular treatment of renal artery occlusive disease, the aortic dissection usually occurs at the perirenal aorta. It has occurred with a 0–2.2% incidence during renal artery procedures (9,14). In a report by Ivanovic et al., there was a 2.2% incidence and no other complications related to the dissection or treatment were required (14). Hoffman et al. described the spontaneous occlusion of a false lumen of an aortic dissection following renal artery angioplasty (9). In a frank appraisal of complications after endovascular renal artery treatment, Beek and colleagues documented three renal artery dissections in 50 patients (19). In one patient, the dissection was self-limited and not viewed in further imaging. In another untreated dissection, a six-month follow-up revealed loss of the kidney. Lastly, a patient with a dissection identified after guidewire removal suffered a renal artery rupture during attempts to regain access to the distal renal artery requiring coil embolization and loss of the kidney.

Renal artery dissections occur more commonly in heavily calcified arteries with long lesions. Recognition of renal artery dissection can be difficult even to experienced clinicians. Oftentimes, multiple oblique fluoroscopic images have to be obtained to identify the length and severity of the dissection. Previously, dissection of an ostial lesion was seen frequently with PTA alone and was a common indication for stent placement. Dissection can also occur with primary stenting, usually just distal to the stent placement. Treatment for dissection includes balloon angioplasty with prolonged inflation times at the site of dissection followed by additional stenting of the renal artery if the dissection is flow-limiting. The determination of a flow-limiting dissection can often be subjective. Both hemodynamic monitoring and intravascular ultrasound (IVUS) theoretically can be helpful in this regard, but both modalities are often cumbersome to use in the setting of dissection where avoidance of dissection extension is the key.

Acute occlusion secondary to thrombosis may result from the exposure of subintimal collagen to the blood elements after plaque fracture. It can also be the result of a flow-limiting dissection or embolus. Severe spasm can also occur but is usually ameliorated with renal artery nitroglycerine infusion. The incidence of acute occlusion in the literature varies from 0% to 4.7% (1,3–5,8–12,16–18), and as with dissection, it can be associated with significant subsequent morbidity. van de Ven et al. reported a 2.5% incidence of acute thrombosis in patients undergoing PTA, and a 4.7% incidence in those with arterial stenting (12). The in-stent thrombosis was successfully treated with thrombolysis and heparin. Bakker et al. similarly reported two patients with acute thrombosis (1.7%) with the subsequent successful treatment with local thrombolysis (11), as did Hoffman et al. (9). Both patients in the former study developed small renal infarctions. Martin et al. reported a 3% incidence of segmental renal artery occlusion (2), and one patient in a study by Klinge et al. required emergency bypass for acute occlusion and recovered uneventfully (4). Not all acute occlusions are met with successful treatment, however. In a review by Sos et al., a patient with FMD required emergency nephrectomy after an unsuccessful attempt at partial nephrectomy for the segmental occlusion secondary to a renal artery dissection (1). In another series, an emergency aortorenal bypass was unsuccessful in renal salvage in a patient who developed acute renal artery thrombosis 48 hours after technically successful placement of a stent (8). The thrombosis was attributed to a contraindication for post-procedural anticoagulation because of a recent hemorrhagic stroke. Lastly, there is the report of the successful autotransplantation of kidneys in three of five patients who developed acute renal artery occlusion following balloon angioplasty (10). One also had successful thrombolysis, and the other patient required permanent hemodialysis.

From the limited literature in this area, early recognition of renal artery thrombosis after intervention is the key to renal salvage. If acute thrombosis occurs at the time of intervention, a logical treatment sequence would include catheter-directed thrombolysis followed by emergency renal artery bypass or renal autotransplantation if thrombolysis was unsuccessful.

EMBOLIZATION

Renal infarction can be diagnosed with angiography at the time of the procedure by various imaging techniques post-procedure, or clinically. Causes include renal artery thrombus/embolus, flow-limiting dissection, and cholesterol embolization. It is reported to occur in up to 12% of patients (4,8,9,14). Ivanovic reported an occurrence of 2.8% (14). Two were diagnosed with imaging and three on clinical grounds based on evidence of peripheral emboli and an increased creatinine. A 5.3% incidence was reported by Klinge et al. (4). Segmental renal artery infarction was attributed to spasm, but emergency nephrectomy was performed in two, and an emergent bypass in another. Boisclair et al. reported a 12% incidence of renal artery embolism after stenting (4 of 33 patients) one with a significant deterioration of renal function that did not require hemodialysi. Hoffman et al. relate cholesterol embolization resulting in renal infarction and hemodialysis requirement in two patients or 4% (8,9).

Peripheral cholesterol embolization is a well-described complication of the percutaneous treatment of renal artery disease. It occurred with a 10% incidence in both the PTA and percutaneous transluminal angioplasty and stenting (PTAS) groups in the review by van de Ven et al. (12) as well as the series from Hoffman et al. (9). It has been associated with major morbidity and even mortality. Other series report a 1–3.8% occurrence (4,8,11,14).

In a series of 213 patients undergoing angioplasty, a 1.6% incidence was reported (4). One patient died of mesenteric ischemia from cholesterol embolization, and another required toe amputations.

OTHER MORBIDITY AND MORTALITY

Complications related to worsening of renal function include renal infarction, a transient or permanent rise in serum creatinine, or a progression to hemodialysis, whether temporary or permanent. Hydration remains the most important factor in the prevention of renal insufficiency after intervention.

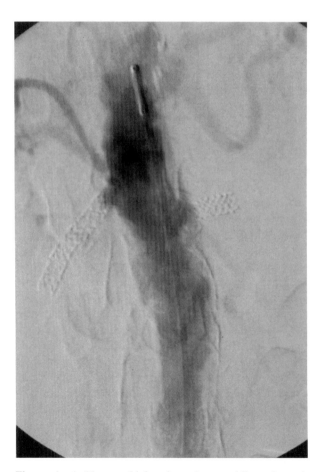

Figure 1 A 66-year-old female underwent bilateral renal artery stenting at another institution. Following the procedure, she became anuric and was transferred to The Cleveland Clinic with noninvasive evidence of stent thromboses. Aortography using gadolinium documents bilateral renal stent thromboses in the setting of a diseased aorta.

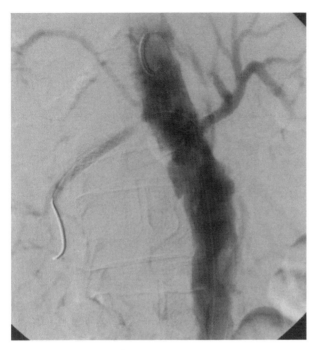

Figure 2 Both the left and right (shown in figure) renal stents are traversed and the renal artery orifices are restented after regional thrombolysis. Restoration of flow is accomplished to the kidneys with some recovery of renal function. Placement of the orginal stents into the renal arteries without correcting the orificial disease present was presumably the etiology of the stent thromboses.

Transient decreases in renal function, defined as at least a 20% increase in plasma creatinine, are often contrast related. This has been reported to occur in 24% of patients after PTA and 21% after PTAS (12). Most studies report an incidence of 2.8–8%, but definitions vary. Renal failure, defined as at least a 20% increase in plasma creatinine for one month or more is generally attributed to cholesterol embolization.

This occurred in 7.1% of patients undergoing PTAS and 4.7% of patients in PTA group in the report by van de Ven et al. (12). One of the latter had terminal renal failure. As reported by Ivanovic et al., 10 patients or 5.6% experienced a creatinine elevation lasting more than 30 days (14). Five of these 10 patients went on to hemodialysis, four within 30 days of the procedure, and four experiencing permanent hemodialysis. These patients had a mean pre-procedural creatinine of 2.3 mg/dL.

Acute renal insufficiency was reported in 26% of patients by Canzanello et al. (3). Four patients went on to require hemodialysis; their mean serum creatinine before the procedure was 4.2. Three of the four ultimately recovered renal function, but one required chronic hemodialysis. Two of 28 patients, or 7.1%, developed acute renal failure requiring hemodialysis in Rees' review (5). One died 17 days after the procedure from complications of renal failure.

The 30-day mortality following percutaneous therapy is generally low. In a meta-analysis from Leertouwer et al., mean mortality was 1% (17). Several series report a 0% mortality (1,2,12), but others report up to 4% mortality following renal artery angioplasty or stenting (3–7,9,10,13,14,16).

In the study by Klinge, a 1% mortality was reported. One patient died secondary to mesenteric ischemia from cholesterol embolization related to the intervention, and the other from a heart attack less than one month after the procedure (4). Ivanovic reported a 1.1% mortality, with the two deaths unrelated to the procedure (14). A 2% mortality rate was seen in Canzanello's study (3). One patient died of diffuse atheroembolism and the other after emergency surgery for an abdominal aortic aneurysm thought to have been perforated during the procedure. Mortality was 3.4% in MacLeod's study as one patient died of retroperitoneal hemorrhage (6). A 3.5% mortality was seen in Rees study; one of 28 patients died after developing acute renal failure requiring hemodialysis (5).

One procedure-related death was reported by Taylor, resulting in 3.4% mortality after a man who sustained a fatal myocardial infarction (MI) two days after repair of a brachial artery catheterization. Klow reported a 0.9% mortality rate (10). One patient in his study developed renal failure ultimately resulting in a cardiac death secondary to a pericardial effusion, and another died of a myocardial infarction (MI) during repair of a pseudoanuerysm at the access site. Hoffman reported a 4% one-month mortality rate with two patients dying, one of heart failure eight days after a successful angioplasty with a pre-existing infrarenal aortic occlusion, and one of hypovolemia-induced myocardial infarction attributed to a diuresis after the procedure (9).

PREVENTION OF COMPLICATIONS

The keys to success in the endovascular treatment of RAS include careful patient selection, preoperative preparation in patients with compromised renal function, and meticulous technique in the performance of the procedure. Our preferred technical steps are outlined below.

Aortography is obtained using a pigtail catheter in the visceral aortic segment. Appropriate ipsilateral oblique images (15–20°) allow delineation of the renal artery orifice and length of the main renal artery. Both gadolinium and CO_2 can be used as alternative contrast agents to low-osmolar non-ionic agents in patients with compromised renal function. Of note, most renal interventions can be performed with the use of less than 40 mL of contrast by limiting large volume aortography using a power injector. Documentation of the renal mass length is made on both sides using the late nephrogram images from aortography. Selective imaging can be obtained using a variety of end-hole 5-Fr catheters placed in the renal artery with either hand injection or power injection set at low pressure. We do not routinely obtain renal artery pressure gradients but this can be done with an end-hole catheter withdrawn through the lesion. Pressure wires are another consideration. With high-grade lesions, the downside of pressure gradient determination is that the lesion has to be re-crossed with a wire after hemodynamic monitoring and often the catheter is occlusive, falsely depressing distal pressures. We approach renal artery intervention from either transfemoral access, or a left transbrachial access in patients with a severely downsloping renal artery and ptotic kidney. A 6-Fr system is employed with either a long 6-Fr guiding sheath or 6-Fr guiding catheter. Care must be used in selection of the guiding catheter since not all stenting systems can be safely passed through the lumen of some commercially available catheters. Our preference is to cross the renal artery lesion only once with a 0.014-inch stiff wire with a floppy tip that is hand manipulated to make a gentle curve. Predilatation is rarely required with the current low-profile stenting systems. An appropriately sized pre-mounted balloon-expandable stenting system is used, usually in the 5.5–6.5 mm range. The lesion is crossed and the stent expanded with just a 3 mm overhang into the aorta. Completion images are taken with the guidewire still across the freshly treated segment. Of note, we liberally apply the use of a distal protection device in the situation of a single-functioning kidney requiring intervention. All patients are loaded with clopidogrel and continued for at least three months. Follow-up imaging is obtained using Duplex ultrasound.

Currently, the use of a distal protection device to prevent embolization to the kidney during renal artery intervention seems intuitive, but is not supported by any convincing data. A prospective randomized trial is being planned that may show the use of distal protection can reduce embolization to the kidney and further protect the organ that we are trying to revascularize with renal intervention.

REFERENCES

1. Sos TA, Pickering TG, Sniderman K, Saddekni S, et al. Percutaneous transluminal renal angioplasty in renovascular hypertension due to atheroma or fibromuscular dysplasia. NEJM 1983; 309:274–279.
2. Martin LG, Price RB, Casarella WJ, Sones PJ, et al. Percutaneous angioplasty in clinical management of renovascular hypertension: initial and long-germ results. Radiology 1985; 155:629–633.
3. Canzanello VJ, Millan VG, Spiegel JE, Ponce SP, et al. Percutaneous transluminal renal angioplasty in management of atherosclerotic renovascular hypertension: results in 100 patients. Hypertension 1989; 13:163–172.
4. Klinge J, Mali WPTM, Puijlaiert CBA, Geyskes GG, et al. Percutaneous transluminal renal angioplasty: initial and long-term results. Radiology 1989; 171:501–506.
5. Rees CR, Palmaz JC, Becker GJ, Ehrman KO, et al. Palmaz stent in atherosclerotic stenoses involving the ostia of the renal arteries: preliminary report of a multicenter study. Radiology 1991; 181:507–514.
6. MacLeod M, Taylor AD, Baxter G, Harden P, et al. Renal artery stenosis managed by Palmaz stent insertion: technical and clinical outcome. J Hypertens 1995; 13:1791–1795.
7. Taylor A, Sheppard D, MacLeod MJ, Harden P, et al. Renal artery stent placement in renal artery stenosis: technical and early clinical results. Clin Radiol 1997; 52:451–457.
8. Boisclair C, Therasse E, Oliva VL, Soulez G, et al. Treatment of renal angioplasty failure by percutaneous renal artery stenting with Palmaz stents: midterm technical and clinical results. AJR 1997; 168:245–251.
9. Hoffman O, Carreres T, Sapoval MR, August MC, et al. Ostial renal artery stenosis angioplasty: immediate and mid-term angiographic and clinical results. J Vasc Interv Radiol 1998; 9:65–73.
10. Klow NE, Paulsen D, Vatne K, Rokstad B, et al. Percutaneous transluminal renal artery angioplasty using the coaxial technique. Acta Radiol 1998; 39:594–603.
11. Bakker J, Goffette PP, Henry M, Mali WPTM, et al. The Erasme study: a multicenter study on the safety and technical results of the Palmaz stent used for the treatment of atherosclerotic ostial renal artery stenosis. Cardiovasc Interv Radiol 1999; 22:468–474.
12. van de Ven PJG, Kaatee R, Beutler JJ, Beek FJA, et al. Arterial stenting and balloon angioplasty in ostial atherosclerotic renovascular disease: a randomized trial. Lancet 1999; 353:282–286.
13. Yutan E, Glickerman DJ, Caps MT, Hatsukami T, et al. Percutaneous transluminal revascularization for renal artery stenosis: Veterans Affairs Puget Sound Health Care System experience. J Vasc Surg 2001; 34:685–693.

14. Ivanovic V, McKusick MA, Johnson CM, Sabater EA, et al. Renal artery stent placement: complications at a single tertiary care center. J Vasc Interv Radiol 2003; 14: 217–225.

15. Sivamurthy N, Surowiec S, Culakova E, Rhodes J, et al. Divergent outcomes after percutaneous therapy for symptomatic renal artery stenosis. J Vasc Surg 2004; 39:565–574.

16. Alhadad A, Ahle M, Ivancev K, Gottsater A, Lindblad B. Percutaneous transluminal angioplasty (PTRA) and surgical revascularization in renovascular disease—a retrospective comparison of results, complications, and mortality. Eur J Vasc Endovasc Surg 2004; 27:151–156.

17. Leertouwer T, Gussenhoven E, Bosch J, van Jaarsveld, B, et al. Stent placement for renal arterial stenosis: where do we stand: a meta-analysis. Radiology 2000; 216:78–85.

18. Isles CG, Robertson S, Hill D. Management of renovascular disease: a review of renal artery stenting in ten studies. QJ Med 1999; 92:159–167.

19. Beek FJ, Kaatee R, Beutler JJ, van der Ven PJ, Mali WP. Complications during renal artery stent placement for atherosclerotic ostial stenosis. Cardiovasc Intervent Radiol 1997; 20:184–190.

20. Van Jaarsveld BC, Krijnen P, Pieterman H, et al. The effect of balloon angioplasty on hypertension in atherosclerotic renal-artery stenosis. N Engl J Med 2000; 342:1007–1014.

21. Webster J, Marshall F, Abdalla M, et al. Randomized comparison of percutaneous angioplasty vs. continued medical therapy for hypertensive patients with atheromatous renal artery stenosis. J Hum Hypertens 1998; 12:32–35.

22. Plouin PF, Chatellier G, Darne B, EMMA Study Group. Blood pressure outcome of angioplasty in atherosclerotic renal artery stenosis. Hypertension 1998; 31:823–829.

23. Nordmann AJ, Woo K, Parkes R, Logan AG. Balloon angioplasty or medical therapy for hypertensive patients with atherosclerotic renal artery stenosis? A meta-analysis of randomized controlled trials. Am J Med 2003; 114:44–50.

13

Complications of Mesenteric Interventions

Timur P. Sarac
Department of Vascular Surgery, The Cleveland Clinic Foundation,
Cleveland, Ohio, U.S.A.

INTRODUCTION

Patients undergoing minimally invasive vascular procedures are susceptible to difficulties and complications that are generally applicable to all intervention cases. While minimally invasive procedures intend to treat diseases related to the mesenteric vessels with the goals of decreased risk and quicker convalescence, they are not without risks. This chapter primarily reviews complications that are unique to mesenteric interventions, in addition to a brief mention of universal complications (Table 1).

Endoluminal interventions have common risks which include access site complications such as thrombosis, embolization, and arterial dissection which can lead to arm or leg ischemia. Other difficulties related to access site complications include a wide gamut of symptoms such as a small hematoma, pseudoaneurysm formation, and massive hemorrhage. Closure devices can malfunction resulting in either thrombosis or dissection, but are also at risk for infection. The risk of hemorrhage, thrombosis, or embolization from a peripheral vascular intervention is multifactorial and may be related to size and type of introducer sheath and catheter, the physical properties of the guidewires such as stiffness and coating, the size and location of the targeted vessel, and type and degree of disease in the treatment vessel. These all can lead to unfavorable outcomes including dissection and perforation of the suspect lesion (Fig. 1). Renal insufficiency and failure are also potential complications for anyone undergoing a peripheral intervention, particularly those with underlying renal insufficiency and/or occlusive disease. In addition, anytime an intervention involves the aortic arch vessels, even if this includes using the arm for lower extremity access, there is a risk of stroke. Finally, maldeployment may lead to vessel occlusion (Fig. 2).

MESENTERIC INTERVENTION COMPLICATIONS

Early treatments of mesenteric occlusive disease by balloon angioplasty and stenting of the celiac, superior mesenteric, renal, and occasionally inferior mesenteric artery (IMA) had high recurrence and complication rates. Thus, these treatments were not

Table 1 General Complications

Complication	Incidence (%)
Arterial thrombosis	0.1–0.2
Embolization	1–2
Hematoma/hemorrhage	0.5–3
Pseudoaneurysm	1.0–1.5
Renal insufficiency	0.5–1
Rupture	0.5–1

widely accepted as a potential primary treatment modality. However, refinements in techniques and improvements in equipment such as lower profile devices, along with an increasing familiarity with visceral artery angioplasty and stenting have enabled the interventionalist to primarily treat occlusive disease of these vessels with balloon angioplasty and stents with equivalent success. Despite these improvements, there are still potential adverse sequlae.

In examining the potential deleterious effects of visceral intervention procedures (Table 2), it may be useful to categorize complications specifically related to the nature of the disease-specific intervention and target organ (Table 3). For celiac and superior mesenteric artery (SMA) procedures, distal embolization and/or acute

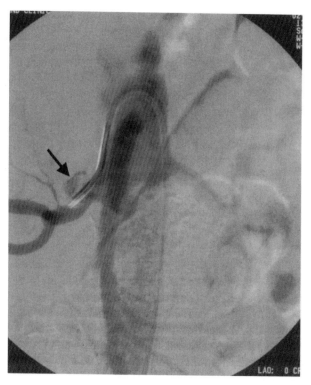

Figure 1 Extravasation of dye following balloon angioplasty of renal artery.

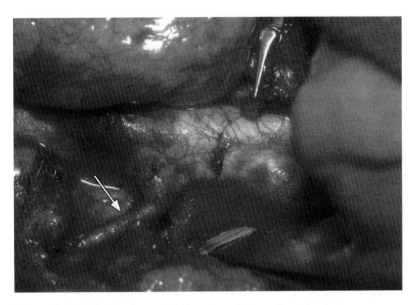

Figure 2 Maldeployed stent leading to occlusion of renal artery.

Table 2 Organ-Specific Complications by Treated Vessel

Artery	Organs at risk
Celiac	Liver, spleen, stomach, pancreas, and small and large intestine depending on status of SMA and IMA
SMA	Stomach, pancreas, small intestine, large intestine, liver and spleen, depending on status of celiac and IMA
IMA	Large intestine, small intestine, and foregut organs depending on the status of celiac and SMA
Hypogastric artery	Gluteal and lower extremity musculature
Renal arteries	Kidneys and adrenals glands

Abbreviations: SMA, superior mesenteric artery; IMA, inferior mesenteric artery.

Table 3 Complication Rates of Mesenteric Interventions for Occlusive Disease

Author	Overall rate (%)	Mortality (%)
Allen	5	5
Hallisey	6	6
Kasirajan	18	11
Maspes	9	9
Matsumoto	32	0
Sharafuddin	10	10

occlusion can lead to mesenteric ischemia resulting in stomach, small and large intestinal infarction, hepatic ischemia, ischemic pancreatitis, or ischemic colitis. While this may occur infrequently for chronic disease, in the acute setting there is as greater chance of bowel infarction and exploratory laporotomy may be indicated as a

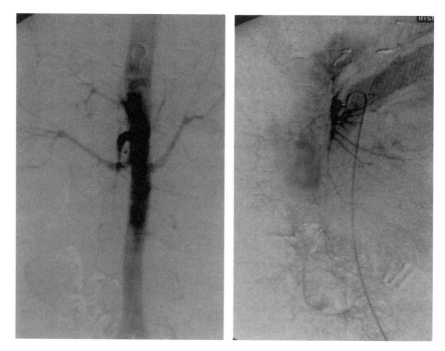

Figure 3   Manipulation of superior mesenteric artery leading to severe diffuse spasm.

oncurrent procedure. Kasirajan et al. reported the Cleveland Clinic experience of percutaneous interventions for mesenteric occlusive disease and found the incidence of
bowel infarction to be 11%, the incidence of renal insufficiency was 0%, and the mortality rate was 11% (9). The restenosis and/or occlusion rate was 27% at three years.
Recently, Sharrafudin reported his results of 26 mesenteric interventions for occlusive
disease and found the restenosis rate to be 12%, the peri-procedure mortality rate to be
3.8% and renal insufficiency also 3.8% (20). The incidence of acute thrombosis was
3.7% in both series. Additionally, compromised mesenteric perfusion may occur secondary to severe arterial spasm following endoluminal manipulation of the mesenteric
vessels (Fig. 3). Correction of the spasm may necessitate continuous intra-arterial
papaverine infusion. Coil embolization of the splenic artery and other visceral artery
aneurysms has the potential to interrupt important collaterals or lead to frank organ
infarction. While splenic infarction generally has few consequences, maldeployment of
a coil in other vessels can lead to disastrous results such as bowel or liver ischemia.

Patients requiring treatment of visceral ischemia secondary to aortic dissection
will occasionally require stenting of the celiac artery, superior mesenteric artery, or
renal artery to maintain antegrade flow through the true lumen. This most frequently
happens in acute aortic dissections, as there is insufficient time to develop collateral
flow. While the intricacies of the endoluminal management of this disease usually
involve placement of an aortic endograft, in some circumstances stenting of the true
lumen of the celiac, superior mesenteric, or renal artery may be necessary to maintain
adequate perfusion. However, in this complex scenario, distal embolization, further
dissection, and/or stenting of the false lumen can all lead to untoward consequences.
The Stanford group reported the results of 40 patients with compromised mesenteric

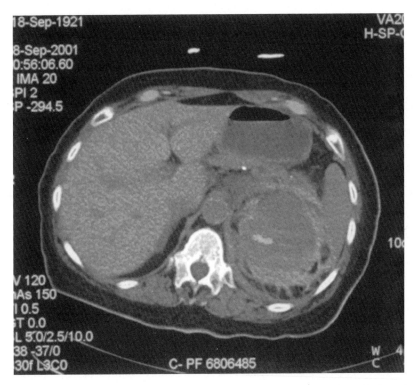

Figure 4   Perforated parenchyma of kidney from guidewire placed too far into the renal artery.

perfusion secondary to aortic dissection. These patients were treated with percutaneous visceral artery stenting, but the mortality rate was 25%, largely from sequlae of ischemia and reperfusion of severely compromised viscera.

The renal arteries are the most frequently stented visceral arteries for occlusive disease. While the procedure has minimal risk, the incidence of progression to renal insufficiency following this procedure has been reported as high as 15% for both selective angiography and percutaneous angioplasty and stenting.

This is usually attributed to pre-existing renal impairment and dosage of contrast. However, the progression to dialysis dependence is much less common and is in the range of 3%. It has yet to be seen whether embolic protection devices will prevent ischemia from microemboli following balloon angioplasty and stenting as recently reported. Although restenosis is not truly considered a complication, the group from Emory University reported restenosis rates to be as high as 16% at an average of 11 months follow-up and the acute thrombosis rate to be 1%. Additionally, rupture of the kidney capsule can occur from distal migration of the wire, which can lead to hemorrhage and organ loss (Fig. 4). Finally, severe calcification and/or device failures such as stent fractures can lead to difficulty with the procedure (Fig. 5).

While treatment of mesenteric occlusive disease has become a common intervention, internal iliac artery (hypogastric) embolization is now a widely accepted technique that extends the limitations of endovascular abdominal aortic aneurysm repair to concurrent ecstatic or aneurysmal common iliac arteries. The most commonly used method of doing this is to extend the limb of the stent graft into the external iliac artery, which is preceded by coil embolization of the internal iliac artery. In

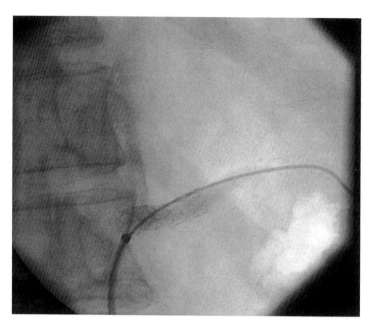

Figure 5 Fractured renal artery stent following deployment in calcified vessel.

extraordinary circumstances, both internal iliac arteries may need to be sequentially embolized. There have been many complications attributed to hypogastric embolization. Procedure-specific complications such as maldeployed coils, glue or procoagulants can lead to ischemia at an untargeted location or vessel damage with the same results. The most common complication of unilateral internal iliac artery embolization is gluteal claudication. This occurs with an incidence ranging from 28% to 50% of patients undergoing hypogastric embolization, but greater than 75% of these patient's symptoms resolve within one year. Anecdotally, claudication may be limited by placing the coils in the proximal hypogastric artery, which allows flow through uninterrupted collaterals.

Another potentially more devastating complication following hypogastric embolization is colon ischemia. Davidian et al. reported on 109 patients undergoing hypogastric embolization and found ischemic colitis to occur in 7.4% of these patients, and the mortality rate was 2.7% (5). However, Wolpert reported on a much smaller number (18 patients) and found no patient developed ischemic colitis despite seven bilateral embolizations (24). While bilateral hypogastric embolization may be done without adverse sequlae, there have been reports of catastrophic complications such as penile and scrotal sloughing and impotence. Impotence has been reported in 5% of patients undergoing unilateral embolization and 13% of patients undergoing bilateral embolization. The best chance to avoid the difficulties of bilateral hypogastric embolization is delayed sequential treatment, which allows development of collaterals.

In conclusion, complications of mesenteric ischemia are now more commonly treated with minimally invasive techniques. While these techniques have offered successful treatment options, they also have unique complications. Awareness of these can help decrease future events and provide information for quicker treatment.

REFERENCES

1. Allen RC, Martin GH, Rees CR, Rivera FJ, Talkington CM, Garrett WV, Smith BL, Pearl GJ, Diamond NG, Lee SP, and Thpmson JE. Mesenteric angioplasty in the treatment of chronic intestinal ischemia. J Vasc Surg 1996; 24:415–421.
2. Bush RL, Najibi S, MacDonald MJ, Lin PH, Chaikof EL, Martin LG, Lumsden AB. Endovascular revascularization of renal artery stenosis: technical and clinical results. Vasc Surg 2001; 33(5):1041–1049.
3. Clair DG. Aortic dissection with branch vessel occlusion: percutaneous treatment with fenestration and stenting. Sem Vasc Surg 2002; 15:116–121.
4. Cognet F, Ben Salem D, Dranssart M, Cercueil JP, Weiller M, Tatou E, Boyer L, Krause D. Chronic mesenteric ischemia: imaging and percutaneous treatment. Radiographics 2002; 22(4):863–880.
5. Powell A, Fox LA, Benenati JF, Katzen BT, Becker GJ, Zemel G. Postoperative management: buttock claudication and limb thrombosis. Tech Vasc Interv Radiol 2001; 4: 232–235.
6. Hallisey MJ, Deschaine J, Illescasas FF, Sussman SK, Vine HS, Ohki SK, Straub J. Angioplasty for the treatment of visceral ischemia. J Vasc Interv Radiol 1995; 6:785–791.
7. Holden A, Hill A. Renal angioplasty and stenting with distal protection of the main renal artery in ischemic nephropathy: early experience. J Vasc Surg 2003; 38:962–968.
8. Ivanovic V, McKusick MA, Johnson CM 3rd, Sabater EA, Andrews JC, Breen JF, Bjarnason H, Misra S, Stanson AW. Renal artery stent placement: complications at a single tertiary care center. J Vasc Interv Radiol 2003; 14(2 Pt 1):217–225.
9. Kasirajan K, O' Hara PJ, Gray BH, Hertzer NR, Clair DG, Greenberg RK, Ouriel K. Chronic mesenteric ischemia: open surgery versus percutaneous angioplasty and stenting. J Vasc Surg 2001; 33:63–71.
10. Kitchens C, Jordan W Jr, Wirthlin D, Whitley D. Vascular complications arising from maldeployed stents. Vasc Endovascular Surg 2002; 36(2):145–154.
11. Lee WA, O'Dorisio J, Wolf YG, Hill BB, Fogarty TJ, Zarins CK. Outcome after unilateral hypogastric artery occlusion during endovascular aneurysm repair. J Vasc Surg 2001; 33(5):921–926.
12. Lefkovitz Z, Cappell MS, Lookstein R, Mitty HA, Gerard PS. Radiologic diagnosis and treatment of gastrointestinal hemorrhage and ischemia. Med Clin North Am 2002; 86(6): 1357–1399.
13. Lin PH, Bush RL, Lumsden AB. Sloughing of the scrotal skin and impotence subsequent to bilateral hypogastric artery embolization for endovascular aortoiliac aneurysm repair. J Vasc Surg 2001; 34:748–750.
14. Maspes F, di Pietralata GM, Gandini R, Innocenzi L, Lupattelli L, Barzi F, Simonetti G. Percutaneous transluminal angioplasty in the treatment of chronic mesenteric ischemia: results and 3 years of follow-up in 23 patients. Abdom Imag 1998; 23:358–363.
15. Matsumoto AH, Angle JF, Spinosa DJ, Hagspiel KD, Cage DL, Leung DA, Kern JA, Tribble CG, Kron IL. Percutaneous transluminal angioplasty and stenting in the treatment of chronic mesenteric ischemia: results and long-term followup. J Am Coll Surg 2002; 194:S22–S31.
16. Matsumoto AH, Tegtmeyer CJ, Fitzcharles EK, Selby JB, Tribble CG, Angle JF, Kron IL. Percutaneous transluminal angioplasty of visceral arterial stenosis: results and long-term clinical follow-up. J Vasc Interv Radiol 1995; 6:165–174.
17. Mehta M, Veith FJ, Ohki T, Cynamon J, Goldstein K, Suggs WD, Wain RA, Chang DW, Friedman SG, Scher LA, Lipsitz EC. Unilateral and bilateral hypogastric artery interruption during aortoiliac aneurysm repair in 154 patients: a relatively innocuous procedure. J Vasc Surg 2001; 33:S27–S32.
18. Meyerson SL, Feldman T, Desai TR, Leef J, Schwartz LB, McKinsey JF. Angiographic access site complications in the era of arterial closure devices. Vasc Endovasc Surg 2002; 36(2):137–144.

19. Sabeti S, Schillinger M, Mlekusch W, Ahmadi R, Minar E. Reduction in renal function after renal arteriography and after renal artery angioplasty. Endovasc Surg 2002; 24(2): 156–160.

20. Sharafuddin MJ, Olson CH, Sun S, Kresowik TF, Corson JD. Endovascular treatment of celiac and mesenteric arterial stenosis: applications and results. J Vasc Surg 2003; 38:692–698.

21. Silber S. Hemostasis success rates and local complications with collagen after femoral access for cardiac catheterization: analysis of 6007 published patients. Am Heart J 1998; 135(1):152–156.

22. Slonim SM, Miller DC, Mitchell RS, Semba CP, Razavi MK, Dake MD. Percutaneous balloon fenestration and stenting for life threatening ischemic complications in-patient with acute aortic dissection. J Thor Cardvasc Surg 1999; 117:1118–1127.

23. Steinmetz E, Tatou E, Favier-Blavoux C, Bouchot O, Cognet F, Cercueil JP, Krause D, David M, Brenot R. Endovascular treatment as first choice in chronic intestinal ischemia. Ann Vasc Surg 2002; 16(6):693–699.

24. Wolpert LM, Dittrich KP, Hallisey MJ, Allmendinger PP, Gallagher JJ, Heydt K, Lowe R, Windels M, Drezner AD. Hypogastric artery embolization in endovascular abdominal aortic aneurysm repair. J Vasc Surg 2001; 33:1193–1198.

14

Endovascular Repair of Vascular Lesions in Solid Organ Transplantation

Wael E. A. Saad
Mallinckrodt Institute of Radiology, St. Louis, Missouri, U.S.A.

David L. Waldman
Department of Radiology, University of Rochester Medical Center, Rochester, New York, U.S.A.

LIVER TRANSPLANTATION COMPLICATIONS: ARTERIAL COMPLICATIONS

Steno-Occlusive Disease

Steno-Occlusive Disease of the transplant hepatic artery (HA) is not uncommon. It includes hepatic artery thrombosis (HAT) and hepatic artery stenosis (HAS). HAS has been speculated to progress to HAT (1–5) implicating, at least in part, that HAS and HAT are two contiguous components of the broader allograft ischemic spectrum. HAT (Fig. 1) is the most common hepatic arterial complication (1,2,6) occurring in 4–11% of adult transplants and 11–26% of pediatric transplants (1,6–10). HAS is the second most common of the arterial complications, occurring in 5–13% of transplants (1,2,11–14). As a result of the improving survival rate of hepatic transplant recipients, late vascular complications in hepatic allografts are likely to increase in prevalence (15). In addition, Doppler ultrasound (DUS) surveillance of the HA in orthotopic liver transplant (OLT) patients, which has become regularly used as of the mid-1990s, has revealed significantly more anatomic defects in the transplant HA (2,16). Prior to regular DUS surveillance, HAS and hepatic arterial kinks (HAK) represented 0–42% (weighted mean of 17%) of abnormal arterial angiograms in OLT recipients and now HAS and HAK represent 39–88% (weighted mean of 47%) of abnormal angiograms (1,7,16).

The most common site of HAS is at the HA anastomosis; it occurs in 46–75% of cases and has been described in up to 91% of HAS cases (2). However, there are numerous types of arterial anastomoses such as end to end HA anastomoses, infrarenal aortic to HA conduits, and donor celiac axis to recipient HA anastomoses. As a result, the frequency of anastomotic stenoses should be placed in the context of the type of arterial anastomosis. In case series with a high number of infrarenal aortic conduits, which have at least two to four anastomoses, the prevalence of anastomotic

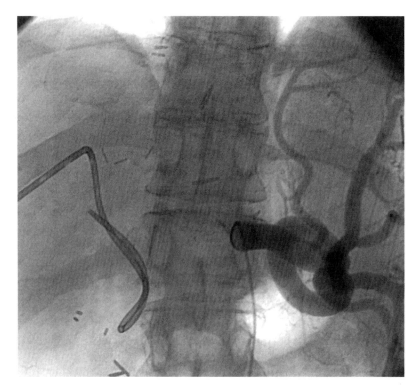

Figure 1 Celiac artery injection demonstrates complete occlusion of the hepatic artery. Without adequate collateral vessels this will lead to biliary necrosis.

stenoses is expected to be as high as it was in the case series reported by Orons et al. where 91% of their stenoses were anastomotic. In the largest case series describing end-to-end hepatic anastomoses, anastomotic stenoses and distal stenoses occurred in 46–75% (weighted mean of 65%) and 40–46% (weighted mean 41%) of HAS cases, respectively (13,14). Stenoses proximal to the anastomosis occur in 0–8% of HAS cases and may be related to pre-existing recipient inflow disease, whether atherosclerotic or compressive (2,5,13,14).

Predisposing Factors

Previous reports have outlined risk factors associated with steno-occlusive disease of the transplant HA; these are listed in Table 1 (1,6,13).

Sequelae

While asymptomatic in recipient patients before transplantation, the obliteration of collateral pathways during transplantation and the susceptibility of the biliary tract to ischemia may cause proximal stenoses to become clinically evident after transplantation.

Solely the HA perfuses the intrahepatic biliary epithelium. The arterial blood supply to the liver and biliary tree is altered following OLT whereby reciprocity of flow between the portal vein (PV) and the HA is diminished, making the integrity of the arterial flow of paramount importance (2,13,16). HAS initially causes uncomplicated, reversible, biliary ischemia. This is followed by irreversible biliary necrosis (Fig. 2), which causes allograft dysfunction incompatible with long-term

Table 1 Predisposing Factors for Steno-Occlusive Disease of the Transplant Hepatic Artery

Technical factors:
 – Clamp injury
 – Intimal tear/dissection
 – Faulty anastomotic sutures
 – Extrinsic compression
 – Excessive vessel length with arterial kinking and/or angulation
 – Differences in vessel caliber requiring oblique anastomoses
 – Complex vascular reconstructions
 – Arterial conduits
 – Arterial revisions
 – Retransplantations
 – Pediatric recipients, particularly <1 year of age
 – Recipients <15 kg
 – Arterial size <3 mm in diameter
 – Prolonged cold ischemia time
 – Microvascular preservation injury
 – Disruption of the vasa vasorum
Non-technical factors:
 – Infections
 – Rejection
 – ABO and/or HLA mismatches
 – Hypercoagulable states including polycythemia
 – Intraoperative administration of fresh frozen plasma
 – Tobacco abuse

graft survival mandating retransplantation (1,16,18,20). As a result, late detection of HAS has a high incidence of biliary complications reported to be up to 67% of OLT recipients with HAS (19). HAS can be asymptomatic, with minimal rise in the liver function tests (LFTs), in up to 20% of cases. When HAS is symptomatic, the clinical and laboratory findings are non-specific and insidious mandating a high degree of suspicion (13). DUS has become a pivotal imaging modality in the elucidation of hepatic dysfunction, for which there are many causes, and can potentially allow early diagnosis of HAS (2,19).

As a result, timely intervention can potentially be performed prior to the onset of irreversible biliary damage and even hepatic parenchymal infarction (2,13,16,19,21). It should be emphasized that the greatest morbidity associated with HAS is its potential to progress to HAT.

The majority of HAT occurs from three days to three months after OLT (1). HAT presents in three ways with equal frequency summarized in Table 2 (1,17,22,23). The current authors believe that biliary ischemia is most likely the prevalent form in the long-term due to the fulminant and dire nature of hepatic parenchymal necrosis, and those patients with relapsing bacteremia may progress to biliary ischemia. Hepatic parenchymal necrosis usually has superimposed infection with intestinal microorganisms and may rapidly progress to fulminant sepsis (23). Relapsing bacteremia most likely is due to intrahepatic microabscesses acting as occult septic foci (1). Biliary ischemia exhibits several forms, which can coexist. These include: anastomotic and extra-anastomotic biliary structures, anastomotic breakdown with biliary peritonitis, mucosal breakdown with irregular necrotic bile ducts

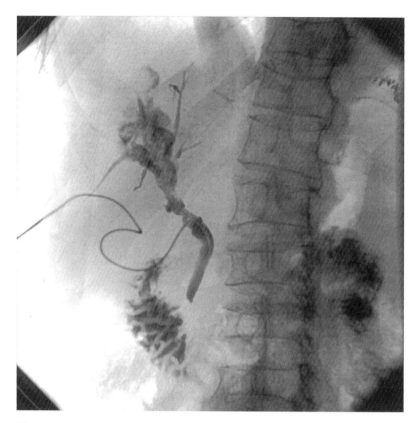

Figure 2   Filling defects seen within the confluence of the bile ducts. This is biliary necrosis most likely secondary to hepatic artery occlusion.

and intrahepatic biloma formation, as well as mucosal sloughing and formation of biliary cast syndrome (19).

Management

DUS has been reported to have a sensitivity of >80% and a negative predictive value of >0% (18,24,25). DUS findings in the setting of HAS include: a parvus-tardus wave form with a systolic acceleration time >0.1 seconds and a resistive index <0.5. In addition, if the site of stenosis is visualized it usually shows a peak systolic velocity >200 cm/sec (16). In cases of HAT, DUS shows lack of intrahepatic arterial flow. However, in the setting of HAT with collateral formation (Fig. 3) intrahepatic flow can be seen. The waveform and resistive index, however, is similar to that seen in cases of HAS. Arteriography is then used to further define the arterial abnormality.

HAT is associated with a high morbidity and mortality and is a major cause of retransplantation (1,6,13,17,22,23). The overall mortality is estimated to be 50–73% with adults having double the mortality rate of pediatric recipients estimated to be 83% and 38%, respectively (22). Pediatric recipients are thought to be more tolerant of HAT due to their ability to establish collaterals (1). Despite retransplantation being the most definitive treatment for HAT, it is associated with a high mortality estimated to be between 27% and 75% (1,22,26). In recent years revascularizing the dearterialized graft by prompt thrombectomy and revision of the arterial anastomoses has been described and may salvage up to 70% of allografts with acute throm-

Table 2 Patterns of Presentation of HAT

	Fulminant hepatic necrosis	Biliary ischemia	Intermittent/relapsing bacteremia
Onset and course	Early acute and rapid deterioration	Late, insidious. Progressive if without collaterals	Late and intermittent
Clinical picture	Rapid deterioration of liver function with septicemia and even multi-system-organ failure	Biliary peritonitis, jaundice and eventual poor liver function	Relapsing bacteremia with fevers and chills
LFTs	Rapid deterioration	Can show minimal changes initially	Can show minimal changes throughout course
Mortality	75%	57%	29%
Management	Urgent retransplantation	Percutaneous biliary and/or biloma drainage and revascularization as bridge for eventual retransplantation	Conservative treatment with antibiotics. Revascularization. Most definitive treatment is retransplantation

Abbreviations: HAT, hepatic artery thrombosis; LFT$_s$, liver function tests.
Source: From Refs. 1, 34, 46, 47.

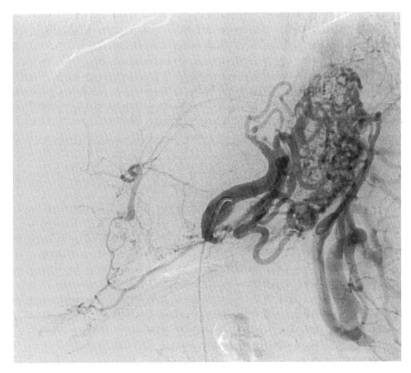

Figure 3 If a hepatic artery occlusion occurs over a long period of time adequate collaterals may form. These collateral maybe enough to maintain biliary duct integrity.

bosis when extensive parenchymal necrosis has not occurred. This in conjunction with percutaneous biloma and/or biliary tract drainage may prolong allograft survival and temporize both patient and allograft to allow retransplantation in a more favorable setting (11,27). Thrombolysis therapy has infrequently been utilized to treat acute HAT with variable results (7,11,28,29). In the early post-operative period, endoluminal thrombolytic therapy has often been avoided due to concern for bleeding complications. Successful endoluminal lytic therapy without bleeding complications has been reported as early as one week and as late as four months after transplantation (7,28,29) with some authors arguing that such attempts are warranted in order to prevent further allograft damage. Conversely, transcatheter thrombolysis has the drawback of revascularizing arteries at a slower rate than surgical thrombectomy and there is a potential for additional allograft damage until arterial flow is re-established. On re-establishing arterial flow, as in any arterial thrombolysis, the HA should be interrogated thoroughly for underlying anatomic defects. In fact, six of the seven successful and clearly described cases of HA thrombolysis in the literature had underlying anatomic defects (7,28,29). These anatomic defects should be managed definitively either endoluminally or surgically. Failure to address these lesions would most likely lead to re-thrombosis of the HA.

Traditionally, the treatment of symptomatic HAS includes anticoagulation, surgical revascularization and even retransplantation (13,15). In the past 20 years numerous case reports and case series describing endoluminal treatment of HAS (Fig. 4) have been reported (2–4,13,14,17,21,29). The largest series describing HA-PTA (2) had a technical success rate of 81%. They also had two (9.5%) complications (an arterial rupture and another patient with arterial dissection and delayed pseudoaneurysm formation). Narumi et al. also reported the development of a pseudoaneurysm following attempted angioplasty (30). In the same report by Orons et al. retransplant was required in four (24%) of those with successful PTA and in all four cases in which PTA was unsuccessful, a difference that was statistically significant (2). Furthermore, Orons et al. showed that elevated enzymes that were already established prior to HA-PTA did not significantly improve after successful PTA and that the long-term clinical success was most closely related to allograft function at the time of angioplasty, with poor function associated with the eventual need for retransplantation regardless of the success or failure of angioplasty. Similarly, Abassoglu et al. reported that the clinical outcome of patients with poor allograft function at the time of surgical revision of HAS was poorer than in cases where there was an adequately functioning allograft at the time of the surgical revision (13). These findings are contrary to the initial case reports of reversal of LFTs and even hepatic parenchymal necrosis after successful HA-PTA (3,4,20).

Denys et al. recently reported on the use of coronary stents in the management of HAS following OLT (14). In their series of 13 patients, stent deployment was technically successful in all cases. Patients were treated with heparin-anticoagulation during the procedure and long-term antiplatelet therapy (aspirin) following the procedure. The primary patency rate of the stents at six and 12 months was 62% and 53%, respectively, and the secondary patency rate of the stents at six and 12 months was 77% and 60%. One of their patients had peripheral intrahepatic HAT one day after the procedure and four (31%) other patients had restenosis of the HA within one year of their respective transplants. The authors concluded that primary stenting of transplant HAS is feasible and had an acceptable one-year patency rate. It should be noted, however, that in the setting of failure (HAT or restenosis) of stents in the treatment of HAS, the presence of a deployed stent may prolong, if not, complicate subsequent salvage attempts by surgical revascularization of the HA.

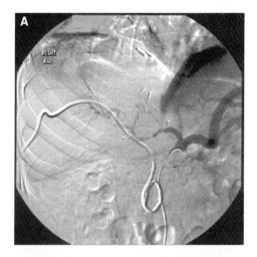

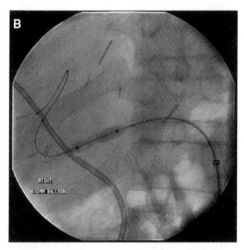

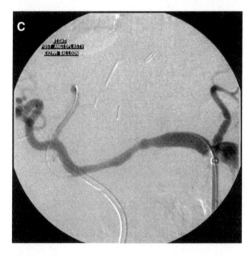

Figure 4   Initial angiogram from a celiac artery (**A**) injection shows a narrowing at the hepatic artery anastomosis. A balloon (**B**) was passed through the narrowing. Follow-up angiogram (C) demonstrates significant improvement at the anastomosis.

HEPATIC ARTERY PSEUDOANEURYSMS

Hepatic Artery Pseudoaneurysms (HA-PsAs) are relatively uncommon, occurring in 0.3–2.0% of patients after OLT (15,17,31–33). HA-PsAs are subclassified into intra- and extra-hepatic PsAs. The etiology clinical course and radiologic features differ from intra- and extra-hepatic HA-PsAs, making their location an important consideration (31). Table 3 outlines the differences between the two types based on the largest case series discussing HA-PsAs as well as numerous other case reports (11,31,32). In addition to extra-hepatic PsAs being described at the surgical anastomosis, they can also be found at the surgical stumps of ligated arterial branches such as the GDA. Additional predisposing factors for the development of extrahepatic PsAs were severe portal hypertension (Portal-HTN), adhesions from prior surgeries ("hostile abdomen") at the time of the primary OLT, and hepaticojejunostomy–biliary anastomoses (31). The latter creates the potential for colonization of the subhepatic space by enteric organisms. In fact, all nine extrahepatic PsAs reported by Marshal et al. were associated with local sepsis and subhepatic collections, with four (44%) of these PsAs being truly mycotic (fungal) pseudoaneurysms (31).

Ultrasound is better at identifying intrahepatic PsAs than extrahepatic PsAs, particularly if the extrahepatic PsA is partially thrombosed and can be mistaken for a periportal hematoma (31).

Table 3 Transplant Hepatic Artery Pseudoaneurysms: Etiology, Clinical Picture-Course and Associations

	Intrahepatic PsAs	Extrahepatic PsAs
Prevalence	31%	69%
Common site	Right hepatic lobe	Surgical anastomosis
Etiology	Percutaneous liver biopsies	Surgical-technical
	Percutaneous biliary drainage	Infection/subhepatic collections
		Complication of HA-PTA
Clinical picture	Mostly asymptomatic with a protracted subclinical course	Fever
		UGI bleeding including hemobilia (22%)
		Intraabdominal bleeding (78%)
		Mass effect – biliary obstruction
LFTs	More likely normal	Less likely normal
		Abnormalities may be due to concomitant HAT and/or sepsis
HAT	Not associated with HAT	44% associated with partial or total HAT
AVF	Can be associated with or have a component of AVF shunting either due to rupture of PsA or as a result of mutual etiology	Can lead to arterio-portal fistula formation with hyperdynamic portal hypertension if PsA ruptures into the portal vein
Mortality	50%	78%
Retransplant	Not necessary if prevented from progression	Eventually required

Abbreviations: HAT, hepatic artery thrombosis; AVF, arteriovenous fistulas.

Sequelae

HA-PsA is associated with a high morbidity and mortality. The natural history of HA-PsA is reason for this increased mortality, with it being an uncommon and often a delayed diagnosis with frequent extrahepatic rupture necessitating emergent intervention. In addition, the backdrop of sepsis adds to the morbidity and mortality associated with HA-PsA. Marshall, et al. found the overall mortality of HA-PsA to be 69% with intra- and extrahepatic PsAs having a mortality of 50% and 78%, respectively (31). Furthermore, the mortality of embolized PsA versus non-embolized PsA was 33% and 100%, respectively. The lower mortality following embolization must, at least in part, reflect a more stable group of patients who were suitable and stable enough to undergo radiologic assessment and intervention (31).

Management

Surgery has been the management of choice. Surgical management includes: excision of the HA-PsA and arterial reconstruction (using interpositioned venous graft or arterial conduit) with arterial ligation being the last resort (32). However, transcatheter coil embolization and percutaneous thrombosis of HA-PsAs have been described in recent years (11,30,31,33). In addition, HA-PsA exclusion using stents has been reported (34). However, little experience with this option has been reported and the validity of the latter option in the setting of a potential mycotic PsA is somewhat controversial. Coil embolization of the entire HA, the endoluminal equivalent of surgical ligation as a last resort, can potentially be entertained in an attempt to control hemorrhage from a ruptured PsA, thus controlling a potentially life threatening situation and temporizing the patient for an eventual elective retransplantation.

Percutaneous thrombosis of HA-PsA by direct needle administration of bovine thrombin should be reserved for intrahepatic PsA and failed transcatheter embolization of extrahepatic PsA. Features of extrahepatic PsA that are not amenable to transcatheter embolization include: inability to reach the HA-PsA due to arterial kinks and/or tortuousities and a short-wide neck of the PsA which is associated with a higher likelihood for coils to escape it and embolize distally in the peripheral HA. There is still, however, a concern for distal embolization during percutaneous thrombin administration, which has been noted in up to 2% of femoral PsA percutaneous thrombosis attempts. The key to preventing thrombin "spillage" into the native artery is a slow continuous injection of thrombin while observing flow within the pseudoaneurysm sac. Balloon inflation across the neck of the PsA during percutaneous thrombin injection or transcatheter coil embolization (in an attempt to trap the embolic material in the PsA) has the potential for in situ thrombus formation in the HA and renders this maneuver less attractive in the setting of transplant hepatic arteries. In all endoluminal management of transplant arteries, the outcome is dependent on graft function at presentation, establishing early diagnosis and the presence of comorbidities—in this particular case, sepsis (31).

ARTERIO-PORTAL FISTULAE

Arterio-Portal Fistulae (APF) in liver transplant recipients are uncommon and have been found in 0–5.6% of abnormal liver transplant angiogram series and not in liver transplants per se (1,17). Over 280 cases of APFs in native livers have been reported,

60% of which were due to percutaneous transhepatic interventions such as liver biopsies and percutaneous transhepatic cholangiograms with or without biliary drain placement. In contradistinction, few APFs have been reported in liver transplant recipients (1,17). In fact, the prevalence of APF in the transplant literature is surprisingly low in light of transplant recipients having frequent biopsies and percutaneous biliary procedures, as well as being under frequent imaging surveillance. There is no clear explanation for this, except for perhaps a result of under reporting.

Sequelae

True APFs are subclassified into intra-hepatic (75%) and extra-hepatic (25%) APFs (36). Extrahepatic APFs in transplants most likely are a result of ruptured HA-PsAs into the PV (5). Most APFs are asymptomatic and have a tendency to close spontaneously. However, when symptomatic, APFs may present with hemobilia (can be life-threatening), abdominal pain, Portal-HTN, hepatic infarcts, and when severe, congestive heart failure. DUS demonstrates reduced resistive indices of the HA, reversed flow in particular PV radicals, and even arterialization of the PV waveform. The latter is a late finding and may be due to a significantly large APF and/or concomitant hepatic disease (25). Large APFs, if neglected, may lead to graft loss and patient death as a result of Portal-HTN and/or gastrointestinal hemorrhage (35).

Management

APFs have been treated in the past by surgical ligation of the involved intrahepatic artery or by transplant segmentectomy, however, endoluminal therapy in recent years has been described to treat such lesions. Metallic coils (Fig. 5) are the frequent embolic material used (36), however, if the APF is large, a detachable balloon can potentially be used. Again, as in any intervention involving the transplant HA, concern for the development of HAT limits and complicates attempts to embolize such lesions, and thus embolization of APFs should be reserved for clinically significant cases or APFs that are progressing rapidly and/or are showing Doppler detectable portal venous changes.

VENOUS COMPLICATIONS

Portal Vein Stenosis

Portal vein stenosis (PVS) is a rare condition occurring in 1–2% of OLT (1,37). PVS typically presents late, months to years after the OLT (38). Patients present with signs and symptoms of Portal-HTN including ascites and/or variceal bleeding. PVS is difficult to detect and quantify by DUS or MRA since focal narrowing and/or size discrepancy at the anastomosis can be normally seen at the PV anastomosis. However, a three- to four-fold increase in the peak velocity at the stenosis relative to the nonstenotic segment by DUS is suggestive of PVS.

Predisposing Factors

The majority of cases of percutaneous treatment of PVS have been described in pediatric liver transplant recipients. In this particular age group, the recipient PV has a relatively smallcaliber, which requires plication of the relatively larger donor PV possibly predisposing to anastomotic stenosis (37,40). Furthermore, in live related split hepatic grafts, the PV anastomosis is technically challenging since the donor portal venous segment is relatively short and frequently requires interposition

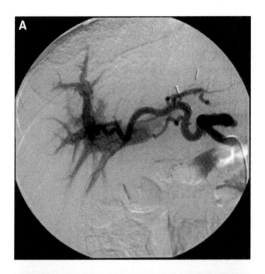

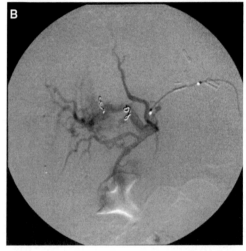

Figure 5 Initial angiogram (**A**) demonstrates prompt filling of the portal vein. Two micro coils were placed into the arteries leading to the fistula. (**B**) Follow-up angiogram showing near complete resolution of the fistula.

vascular grafts converting the portal venous connection in the transplant to two anastomoses that are more prone to delayed stenosis (41).

Management

Funaki et al. found, with approximately 30 patients, that roughly two-thirds of patients will initially respond to angioplasty and one-third will have elastic lesions exhibiting post-PTA recoil and requiring stent placement (38). In patients who initially respond well to angioplasty alone, one-half developed recurrent stenosis 1–31 months (mean 6.3 months) after the angioplasty. These patients were treated with stent placement with good long-term results. In the initial experience reported by Funaki et al. with 25 patients, two complications (8%) in the form of PV thrombosis occurred and were treated effectively with transcatheter Urokinase thrombolysis with good long-term results (39).

The percutaneous transhepatic approach is preferred over the "TIPS approach," however, any coagulopathy should be reversed prior to the former approach. Most PVs are easily assessed under ultrasound guidance. The short, direct tract through the liver provides the best mechanical advantage for negotiating severe stenoses (38). Complete hepatic allografts are generally accessed via a right intercostal approach and split (segmental) allografts are usually approached via a subxiphoid approach. Systemic heparin is administered on access of the PV and this is followed by a portal venogram and pressure gradient evaluation, with a gradient >5 mmHg considered to be significant. In the same sense a residual gradient >5 mmHg after PTA is treated with stent placement (38). Wallstents are usually utilized and should be used judiciously since malposition or "overstenting" will interfere with retransplantation should that be required. Funaki et al. concluded that percutaneous therapy is expected to be curative and that they had no delayed occlusion or stenoses with stent placement (38,39).

PORTAL VEIN THROMBOSIS

Portal vein thrombosis (PVT) is uncommon, occurring in 1–2% of liver transplants. PVT typically occurs within one month from the OLT (38,42). PVT has also been encountered during percutaneous endoluminal treatment of PVS or as a delayed complication of PV stent placement (39).

Clinical Sequelae

Patients present with hepatic dysfunction, ascites, splenomegaly, variceal bleeding, abdominal pain, and diarrhea. DUS demonstrates lack of flow or reduced flow and an echogenic thrombus may be seen within the PV. Once a diagnosis is established, immediate treatment should be performed since loss of the hepatic allograft is imminent (42).

Management

Traditionally, PVT required retransplantation or surgical thrombectomy which are associated with a high morbidity and mortality. In recent years, case reports have been published describing successful percutaneous transluminal treatment of PVT. Various combinations of pharmaceutical and mechanical thrombolysis have been described. Adjunct stent deployment has also been used to avoid thrombolysis (42). Utilizing mechanical thrombolysis and/or stent deployment has the advantage of reducing the time and overall dose of pharmaceutical thrombolytic agents and in turn reducing the risk of undesired bleeding (43). Another added advantage to stent deployment is reducing the risk of recurrence by addressing any underlying anatomic defects, namely PVS (38,43).

PORTAL HYPERTENSION (PORTAL-HTN)

Portal-HTN in liver transplant recipients may be due to arterioportal fistulas, PVS/thrombosis, hepatic venous stenoses, supra-hepatic IVC stenosis or recurrence of liver disease, particularly hepatitis C. Portal-HTN presents as recurrent-refractory ascites and gastrointestinal bleeding. Post-transplant gastrointestinal bleeding occurs in 8.9% of patients with 20% of these bleeds (1.8% of patients) attributed to portal-HTN (45).

Addressing the underlying causes should treat portal-HTN due to extrahepatic causes, however, portal-HTN due to intrahepatic pathology should be treated conservatively and the transplant recipients should be replaced on the transplant list. However, due to the limited donor pool, TIPS procedures can be used to temporize such patients until an appropriate allograft becomes available. This is an increasing problem as a result of the improved survival rate of liver transplant recipients and in turn the increased prevalence of recurrent liver disease and subsequent development of portal-HTN after liver transplantation.

Management

The added technical difficulty that a liver transplant poses to the establishment of a TIPS shunt is somewhat controversial. Richard et al. discussed technical concerns pertaining to accessing various hepatic venous anastomoses from the jugular approach, as well as the caliber discrepancy at the portal venous anastomoses and the adequate placement of the TIPS stent, particularly with eventual retransplantation in mind (46).

TIPS in the hepatic transplant recipient has been found to have a higher incidence of encephalopathy compared with nontransplant patients with TIPS. This was attributed to the advanced stages of liver disease in their eight cases as well as the presence of heavily neurotoxic drugs such as cyclosporine and tacrolimus (44). Moreover, they showed that the post-TIPS serum cyclosporine level increased after TIPS placement in transplant recipients. This was explained by the reduction of the first pass metabolism of cyclosporine by shunting portal flow away from the liver. It was therefore recommended that both the serum levels of cyclosporine and tacrolimus be monitored carefully after TIPS placement in transplant recipients. The effects of cyclosporine were further discussed by Lerut et al. as theoretically increasing the patency rates of TIPS shunts in the transplant patient based on the effect of immunosuppressant drugs on reducing stent endothelialization in coronary stents (44).

HEPATIC VEIN STENO-OCCLUSIVE DISEASE

Hepatic vein steno-occlusive disease is rare in orthotopic-full-hepatic transplants, however it occurs in approximately 4–7% of split (segmental) graft recipients (47,48). The rarity of hepatic venous stenosis (HVS) is most likely because there is usually no surgical anastomosis involved. This leaves the theory of graft rotational-growth and/or impingement as the causal factors for HVS. Hepatic vein thrombosis usually occurs secondary to IVC/hepatic vein stenosis, sepsis and/or hypercoagulable states.

Clinical Sequlae

Hepatic vein steno-occlusive disease presents with Budd-Chiari syndrome (ascites, coagulopathy and/or elevation of liver function). DUS demonstrates decreased hepatic vein and PV velocities and reduced phasicity of the waveform normally seen in the hepatic veins (47).

Management

Endoluminal therapy is the treatment of choice (38,47,48). Primary treatment utilizes PTA (47), however, due to elastic recoil, stents can be placed (38,48). Ko et al.

reported their experience in 27 patients (largest case series reported) who underwent PTA and/or stent placement (48). Technical success was 100% and the one-year clinical follow-up had achieved 73% success. The femoral, jugular or transhepatic routes may all be used successfully. However, the transhepatic approach is preferred in cases where transcaval access is difficult. Such cases include: hepatic vein thrombosis, critical stenoses at the orifice of the hepatic vein or prior IVC stent placement (38,49). Lesions are dilated to the size of adjacent vessel diameters. In general, high-pressure balloons are required to fully dilate most stenoses (38). Significant restenoses or refractory stenoses are treated with stent placement (38,48). Most patients require post-treatment DUS surveillance with repeat PTA for recurrent lesions (47).

IVC STENOSIS

IVC stenosis occurs in 0.8–2.6% of hepatic transplants and may be more prevalent in pediatric and retransplanted recipients (11,37,49,50).

IVC thrombosis is a rare entity occurring in 0.6% of hepatic transplants (37). IVC stenosis is subclassified into suprahepatic and infrahepatic stenoses with the former being more prevalent, more likely due to it being more clinically apparent and tenuous as a result of the Budd-Chiari component that presents with it (51). IVC stenosis in transplant recipients presents with leg swelling, hepatic dysfunction, ascites, pleural effusion, hypotension (due to hypovolemia and reduced venous return) and occasionally a decline in renal function (49–51).

Predisposing Factors

IVC stenoses can present early (56%) or late (44%) after OLT (38). Early IVC stenosis (<one month from the OLT) is due to technical factors such as: a tight anastomotic suture line, caval redundancy and subsequent kinking, compression of the IVC by an oversized graft or IVC torsion (51). IVC torsion is an interesting phenomenon resulting from early post-transplant graft edema, oversized graft or as a result of growth, remodeling and subsequent rotation of an initially undersized graft (51). Late IVC stenosis (greater than one month from the OLT) results from fibrosis/scarring, intimal hyperplasia at the anastomosis, or chronic thrombus. IVC thrombosis occurs secondary to IVC stenosis or IVC compression by the allograft, particularly in the setting of hypercoagulable states.

DUS findings are non-specific and variable. They include: loss of normal hepatic vein and IVC phasicity, increased hepatic vein velocities, direct visualization of the IVC stenosis with high velocities and turbulent flow and aliasing at the stenoses, as well as occasional echogenic thrombus. In critical suprahepatic IVC stenoses, reversal of the hepatic venous flow and reduction in the PV velocities can be seen. However, the gold standard for imaging remains IV cavography and pressure gradient measurement. Besides the functional value of pressure gradient measurement, cavography demonstrates the site, length and possibly the nature of the IVC stenosis. A particular diagnosis to be aware of is caval torsion, which requires stent placement (51). Torsion presents early and appears as a "ribbon-like" twisted narrowing of the IVC, which may require multiple projections to verify the diagnosis (51). Perhaps most pathognomonic findings of IVC torsion are due to inferior migration of the narrowing after stent placement (51).

Management

In the past, IVC stenosis and thrombosis were treated surgically, which involved cavotomy or atriotomy, surgical thrombectomy, revision of the anastomosis and hepatopexy. Occasionally, retransplantation was also resorted to (37,50). In cases of IVC thrombosis, endoluminal mechanical and pharmaceutical thrombolysis was thought to have a high risk for bleeding complications and/or pulmonary emboli. Both risks have been proven to be minimal, if any, by later authors (49,50). In recent years endoluminal therapy has become the treatment of choice.

Borsa et al. reported an initial technical success for PTA alone of 29% (49). Many of the lesions that were refractory to PTA may have been lesions resulting from IVC torsion or compression and not truly anastomotic stenoses. They concluded that primary stent placement (Fig. 6) was ideal for early presenting IVC narrowing due to IVC torsion, kinking or compression since stents provide a permanent support to the lumen of the IVC which is required in such lesions (49). They reserved PTA alone for delayed IVC stenoses, which are more likely due to fibrosis or intimal hyperplasia (49). Other authors advocate stent placement for all lesions paying particular attention to the resolution of any existing hepatic vein to IVC gradient, or the development of such gradients after stent placement particularly in cases of IVC torsion, where inferior torsion migration should be cleared from

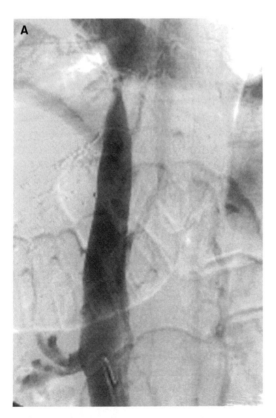
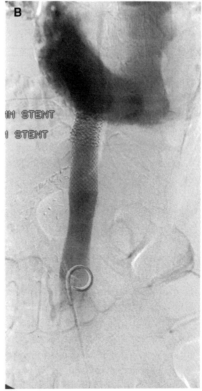

Figure 6 (**A**) Cavagram shows a narrowing of the IVC as it goes through the transplanted liver and has an anastomosis on the heart. Patient presents with recurrent ascites. Lesion would recoil with balloon dilatation. A stent (**B**) was placed with a good angiographic result. Over the next several weeks the patient's symptoms resolved.

(become inferior to) the hepatic vein region of the IVC (51). In cases where the torsion continues to involve the hepatic venous region of the IVC, further stent placement was recommended (51).

After venography and pressure measurements the lesions are crossed (heparin not necessary) and then dilated using large (12–20 mm) angioplasty balloons chosen to approximate the size of the adjacent vein (38). If the lesions resolve by PTA alone some authors do not place stents (38). However, initial angioplasty is still valued by authors who prefer primary stent placement as the balloon angioplasty aids in stent size, estimation, and assessment of the radial force required to alleviate the lesion (49,51). Wallstents are preferred by certain authors however, although Wallstents may not cause hepatic vein occlusion, any subsequent hepatic vein occlusion should be treated via a transhepatic approach (49). Gianturco Z-stents are preferred by other authors due to their increased radial force, minimal foreshortening (precise deployment feature), wide interstices (enabling transcaval hepatic vein access), as well as reduced risk of migration (38).

RENAL TRANSPLANTATION COMPLICATIONS

Arterial Stenosis

Renal transplants (RTx) are subclassified into two groups; Transplant Renal Artery Stenosis (TRAS) and proximal-TRAS. Proximal-TRAS or Pseudo-TRAS refers to pre-existing or developing atherosclerotic inflow stenosis in the native iliac arteries of the transplant recipient. TRAS is further classified into anastomotic stenoses, renal artery stenoses proper and segmental renal artery stenoses. TRAS is not uncommon, occurring in 1–16% of renal transplants and described in up to 23% of renal transplants (1–5). This wide range is due to the varying definition of significant TRAS as well as the evolving and improving surgical techniques and preoperative evaluations over the years. Proximal-TRAS is less well described and occurs in 0–2.4% of transplants and may become more prevalent with the increasing age of RTx recipients (52,54).

Predisposing Factors

The cause of TRAS is multifactorial and includes surgical techniques, allograft preservation methods, immunologic factors, CMV infection and type of allograft. Surgical techniques and practices include vascular clamp injury, intimal dissection, faulty suturing, and long transplant renal arteries. The latter predisposes to arterial kinks and torsion explaining the higher risk of such problems in right-sided renal allografts than in left-sided ones (1). The types of surgical anastomoses have been topics of numerous studies. End to side external iliac anastomoses have been hypothesized to increase the incidence of TRAS due to turbulent blood flow as a result of the hyper-acute angle between the donor Renal Artery and the recipient iliac artery (9). However, many authors believe that there is no significance in the TRAS rate between end-to-side and side-to-side anastomoses. Currel patch anastomoses performed in cadaveric RTx are considered by many to reduce the risk of anastomotic TRAS (11). Other predisposing factors for developing TRAS include vascular damage from increased cold ischemia time, Cyclosporin toxicity and allograft pulse perfusion techniques with certain perfusion liquids (1,12). Immunologic factors include acute cellular rejection, which causes an inflammatory process that can eventually lead to TRAS (13). CMV infection has been implicated in developing segmental and subsegmental TRAS (1,12). This angiographic finding can also be seen in chronic rejection (Fig. 7) and hypertensive renal allografts, two conditions which are difficult to remedy. It is important to be suspicious of CMV-related segmental stenosis since it can be treated with antiviral medication (1).

The prevalence of TRAS in different types of allografts (Cadaveric versus Liver Donor) is somewhat controversial. Certain authors believe that there is no difference between the two types of renal transplants (14). However, other authors believe that the prevalence of TRAS is less in Live Donor RTx. The latter authors' ranges of TRAS prevalence are 0.3–5.8% in Live Donor Grafts and 2.0–17.7% in Cadaveric Grafts (1,7).

Clinical Sequlae

Similar to patients with native renal artery stenosis, patients with TRAS develop renal dysfunction and hypertension or exacerbation of either pre-existing condition. In the study by Patel et al. 65% of patients presented with both hypertension and renal dysfunction and 35% had either with equal prevalence (1). The most common presentation may depend on the time of presentation. In the first week after renal transplant (RTx) patients usually present with anuria and dialysis dependence rather than severe hypertension (HTN). This is most likely because these patients are still receiving dialysis treatment and thus the intravascular volume control prevents the

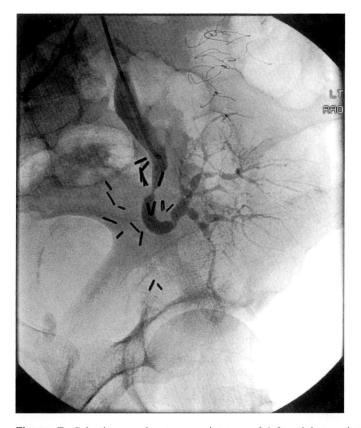

Figure 7 Selective renal artery angiogram of left pelvic renal transplant demonstrates multiple areas of severe stenosis and dilatation specifically at branch points consistent with chronic rejection.

development of severe hypertension. In contradistinction, patients with late presentation and stable baseline renal function are more likely to exhibit symptoms of renovascular HTN. Ultimately, neglected TRAS leads to allograft deterioration with patient and allograft survival rates being lower in patients with TRAS than in those without TRAS (3). Hypertension, however, may be due to many factors including: chronic rejection, steroid use, cyclosporin toxicity, recurrent glomerulo-nephritis, diseased native kidneys or TRAS (4). As a result, non-invasive imaging is warranted to evaluate for TRAS. This includes: MRA, DUS, and radionuclide renal scans. DUS is particularly valuable due to its wide availability, cost effectiveness, and reliability. DUS can produce fine morphologic details relative to the location, length, and gross appearance of a stenosis. It can depict the residual lumen of the stenotic vessel. However, it usually underestimates the degree of stenosis and thus peak systolic velocities, and Doppler waveform analysis is still required to further and more accurately evaluate the hemodynamic changes at the level of the stenosis (8). Doppler characteristics in diagnosing TRAS include: peak systolic velocity >1.8–$2.0\,m/sec$, low pulsatility index (PI of 0.9 ± 0.1), and pulses parvus et tardus wave form with a systolic acceleration time of more than or equal to $0.10\,seconds$ (8). The impact of DUS screening was shown in a study by Wong et al. where the prevalence of TRAS was 2.4% before and 12.4% after the introduction of screening DUS (10).

Management

Surgical or endoluminal management of proximal-TRAS (Fig. 8) is similar to that of iliac atherosclerotic disease and is beyond the scope of this chapter. In case of proximal-TRAS, the authors of this chapter believe that surgical treatment is preferred over endoluminal stenting if arterial stenting would potentially cover the iliac to renal anastomosis.

Surgical treatment of anastomotic and distal renal artery stenoses includes simple revisions and surgical reconstruction utilizing cadaveric ABO compatible iliac artery grafts (5,26,32). Endoluminal management includes PTA and/or, less commonly, arterial stenting. TRAS-PTA involves non-selective pelvic arteriography to exclude proximal-TRAS inflow disease. This is followed by selective iliac arteriography at multiple projections to delineate the anastomoses. A significant stenosis is considered if the diameter reduction of the renal artery is greater than 50%. If PTA is to be performed a 0.035 inch guidewire is advanced across the lesion and 3000–5000 I.U. of Heparin are administered intravenously. Balloon size is determined by direct measurement of nondiseased renal artery DSA. Post-angioplasty arteriogram is obtained with a technical success of PTA defined as a residual stenosis of less than 30% after angioplasty. The technical success rate and complication rate of TRAS-PTA is 60–94% and 0–8.3%, respectively with allograft loss rarely reported (1,12,16). Technical difficulty and complication rates increase with end-to-end anastomoses with the internal iliac artery-associated arterial kinks and elastic recoil of the stenoses.

The criteria in the literature for adequate clinical response to TRAS-PTA mostly concentrates around blood pressure control. The criterion for adequate blood pressure response to TRAS-PTA varies with the authors. Patel et al. used the following criteria for improved clinical outcome

- $>15\%$ reduction in serum creatinine
- $>15\%$ reduction in diastolic blood pressure (DBP) with no change in antihypertensive medication or $>10\%$ reduction in DBP with a reduction in anti-hypertensive medication.

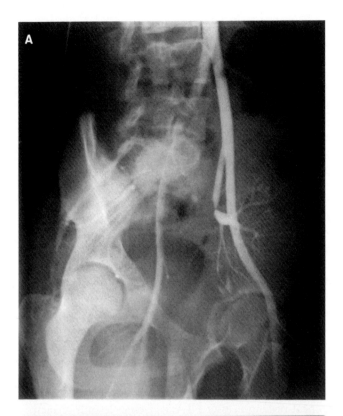

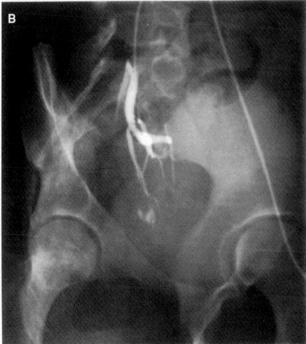

Figure 8 Stenosis is demonstrated (**A**) in the proximal renal artery in a transplant. Following balloon dilatation (**B**) no stenosis is seen.

Using the above criteria their immediate clinical success was 82% and the mean reduction in serum creatinine was from 2.6 ± 0.5 to 1.7 ± 0.3. The range of immediate and long-term clinical improvement in the literature is 69–82% and 41–67%, respectively (1,15,17). Graft survival rate following TRAS-PTA has been reported to be 95% at one year and 82% at two years (15). It appears that the degree of renal function prior to PTA is a predictor of clinical response. Greenstein et al. showed that 83% of patients with adequate renal function prior to TRAS-PTA had improved HTN after TRAS-PTA compared to the overall 76% of their patients who had improved HTN (10).

The efficiency of PTA versus surgical repair of TRAS is somewhat controversial. In one study evaluating surgical and endoluminal therapy of TRAS, surgery had an immediate and long-term success rate of 92.1% and 81.5%, respectively, and PTA had an immediate and long-term success rate of 69% and 40.5%, respectively (15). In addition TRAS-PTA carries a restenosis rate of 10–12% (6,10,12) and has been reported in up to 20% of cases (17). Almost all restenoses occur within eight to nine months of their respective PTA. The relatively high restenosis rate in transplants, not limited to RTx, may be related to accelerated atherosclerotic disease as a result of immunologic and metabolic processes associated with transplantation (18). Despite the relatively high restenoses rate after PTA and some reports of better long clinical outcome of surgical management of TRAS, almost all authors still recommend PTA as the first line of therapy (5,12,15,16,19). This is because endoluminal therapy is less invasive with a lower periprocedural morbidity and does not negate the surgical option (5,12,15,16). Surgery is reserved as a first line treatment for arterial kinks and lesions that are inaccessible or refractory to PTA (16).

Transplant renal artery stent placement for treatment of TRAS is infrequently reported and is reserved for repeat restenosis after PTA, as well as lesions refractory to primary PTA, such as lesions with elastic recoil and severe anastomotic stenoses. Stent placement should not be placed primarily since it carries an even higher rate of restenosis of 25% (19). In addition stent placement, unlike PTA, complicates future surgery adding to it morbidity.

ARTERIAL DISSECTION

Arterial dissection after RTx is rarely documented (20). It is either spontaneous or iatrogenic. Spontaneous renal artery dissection (RAD) usually presents in the early postoperative period, usually within two to seven days (20). RAD usually presents with anuria and dialysis dependence. This presentation has a wider differential diagnosis including: renal vein thrombosis (RVT), renal artery thrombosis (RAT), critical TRAS and acute rejection. DUS usually has difficulty visualizing the intimal flap but is usually capable of detecting arterial flow compromise. RAD can lead to renal artery thrombosis (RAT) and/or renal vein thrombosis. The endoluminal management of RAD, whether spontaneous or iatrogenic, is by stabilizing the intimal flap with stent placement. Adjunct thrombolysis has been described if associated graft thrombosis occurs.

Arterial Injury

Arterial injury is a collective term given by the current authors to include arteriovenous fistulas (AVF), intrarenal pseudoaneurysms (PsA) and arterio-calyceal fistulas.

They are combined as such, as their etiology, manifestations, and management are similar. In addition, these three entities, particularly AVF and PsA, may coexist in up to 30% of cases (21); they occur in 0.2–2.0% of renal allografts after percutaneous biopsy, however they have been reported in up to 15–16% of renal allografts (22). Arterial injuries are almost always caused by percutaneous transplant renal biopsies occurring from zero to 70 days (mean 10.5 days) after the biopsy. As in native renal arteries, RTx, AVFs, and PsAs can resolve spontaneously, however they can lead to dramatic symptoms prompting immediate management. Gross hematuria followed by extravasation and hypovolemia are the most common two presentations involving up to 92% of cases (21). Other manifestations include renal insufficiency, HTN, and high cardiac output failure (21). Embolization is the treatment of choice in symptomatic cases with a technical success rate of 71–100% and alleviations of symptoms in 57–88% of cases (21). Minor infarcts, representing less than 30% of the allograft, have been reported in up to 100% of cases using coil embolization only and having no long-term consequences with regards to allograft survival (21). However, major infarcts involving more than 30–50% of the allograft leading to allograft loss, have been reported in up to 28.6% of cases using combined coil embolization and PVA and/or gelfoam (23). The current authors believe that aggressive embolization with the aim of complete obliteration of the AVF/PsA at the time of the embolization is not necessary and that partial obliteration may suffice to obtain eventual occlusion of the lesion and, if not, reduction or resolution of symptoms. If symptoms persist, a "second-look" angiogram with possible repeat micro-coil embolization would be warranted.

RENAL GRAFT THROMBOSIS (RGT)

Renal Graft Thrombosis (RGT) collectively refers to both renal artery thrombosis (RAT) and renal vein thrombosis (RVT) (Fig. 9). It is difficult to clearly separate the two entities in some of the reports in the reviewed literature. The prevalence of RGT is 0.3–6.1% and has not significantly changed in the past three decades. In the two studies that clearly described and defined the two entities RAT represented 31–43% of RGT with a RAT rate of 1.7–1.9% (25,26). Moreover, both RAT and RVT coexisted in 11.5% of cases of RGT (25). In addition, a report by Robertson, et al. showed that 15% of patients with RVT had associated RAT (27). RGT usually occurs within two weeks of the RTx with 80% occurring within one month and 93% occurring within one year of the RTx. RGT usually presents with oliguria, hematuria, rising serum creatinine and occasional graft pain and tenderness (24). The RVT component of RGT has been associated with lower extremity DVT and in this setting accompanying lower extremity swelling. Accompanying hypovolemia presenting with tachycardia and hypotension has been described in cases of graft rupture with RGT. DUS in the setting of RVT demonstrates graft edema and swelling with no venous flow. Thrombus filling defects can be seen in the renal veins. The arterial Doppler signal shows a high resistive index with reversal of the diastolic arterial flow.

Predisposing Factors

Factors predisposing to RGT are listed in Table 4. Renal transplant patients receiving cyclosporin immune suppression have a higher rate of RGT than patients

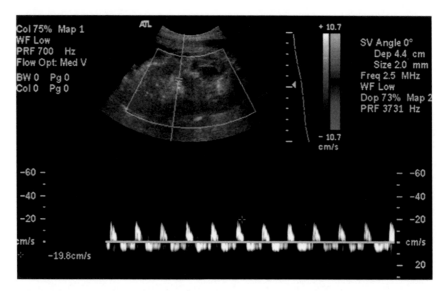

Figure 9 Ultrasound of a kidney two hours following transplant demonstrates poor resolution of the kidney parenchyma. The kidney is swollen and hypoechoic. Vascular evaluation shows reversal of the diastolic flow. Findings are non-specific although are consistent with renal vein thrombosis. This child was brought back to the operating room where the kidney had to be removed.

receiving noncyclosporin immune suppression (28). In fact, the rate of RVT in patients receiving cyclosporin was found to be 7.6% compared to 1.1% in patients receiving immunosuppressants other than cyclosporin (28). Similarly, the RAT rate for patients receiving cyclosporin is 1.8–7.0% compared to 0–1.0% for patients receiving azathioprine and prednisone (29,30). Cyclosporine contributes to vascular thrombosis by reducing blood flow, enhancing platelet aggregation and causing endothelial vascular damage. In addition, patients with endstage renal disease awaiting renal transplantation were found to have a high prevalence of hypercoagulable states (13.6%) with a 3.5-fold increase in the risk of developing RGT within the first year of RTx. The factors predisposing to RAT listed in Table 1 contribute mostly to RAT within the first month after RTx. Beyond the first month, RAT is usually due to rejection or high-grade TRAS. Similarly, delayed RVT is usually associated with lower extremity DVT that propagates to the pelvis and the renal allograft.

Clinical Sequelae

RGT is a serious complication of RTx usually leading to graft loss. In one study RGT represented 45% and 37% of renal allograft loss at three months and twelve months after RTx, respectively (25). Traditionally, and to present, RGT is mostly treated by laparotomy, evaluating graft viability and accordingly either graft nephrectomy or surgical thrombectomy. However, numerous case reports and case series have discussed endoluminal therapy for RGT.

Table 4 Factors Predisposing to Renal Graft Thrombosis (RGT)

Anatomic/technical factors:
Right donor kidney (RVT and RAT)
– Left lower quadrant transplantation (RVT)
– Surgical/technical factors (RVT and RAT – see TRAS)
– Repeat renal transplant (RVT)
– Arterial or venous kinks and/or tortuosity (RAT and RVT)
– Compression of vessels by peri-graft collections (RVT > RAT)
– Underlying atherosclerotic disease (RAT)
– Extreme donor ages (RAT and RVT)
– Pediatric recipients (RVT)
Vircow's Triad factors:
– History of DVT (RVT)
– Hypercoagulable states (RVT > RAT)
– Cyclosporine related hypercoagulable states and vascular damage (RVT and RAT)
– Hypovolemia, postoperative hypotension (RVT > RAT)
Other factors:
– Pretransplant DM (RVT and RAT)
– Pretransplant peritoneal dialysis (RVT)
– Posttransplant ATN/glomerulonephritis (RAT and RVT)
– Acute rejection (RAT)

Abbreviations: RVT, renal vein thrombosis; RAT, renal artery thrombosis.

Management

In cases of RAT, the maximum duration of normothermic ischemia compatible with complete recovery of renal function in native kidneys is estimated to be 30 to 45 minutes. Severe renal damage followed by irrecoverable renal damage can be expected at 1 to 2 hours followed by three hours, respectively. Case reports of successful renal allograft salvage by revascularization of acute arterial thrombus within 24 hours, and even 48 hours in one case, have been reported with recovery of renal function (31). This suggests that renal allograft may have the capacity to recover function even when the three-hour critical delay is exceeded. There is no clear explanation for this discrepancy. One explanation is that the clinical symptoms of RAT precede the actual renal artery occlusion. Another explanation is that the reported RAT in cases of revascularization after 24 hours are incomplete occlusions or that these allografts have collateral flow (24). Indeed, Nicholson et al. who reported graft salvage by means of surgical thrombectomy 48 hours after the start of symptoms noted minimal distal arterial perfusion by angiography despite the arterial occlusion (32). It was not clear to them the exact source of the distal perfusion although it was presumed to be due to collateral flow (32). In addition, evidence of collateral flow is suggested by the presence of renal artery back bleeding during transplant nephrectomy or surgical thrombectomy. In the largest case series discussing Renal Artery Thrombolysis by Rouviere, et al., three of their four cases were technically successful and two of those had clinical recovery (24). Renal artery flow was re-established in 10 to 22 hours (mean of 16 hours) after starting urokinase infusion. In those three cases the tip of the catheter was placed within the thrombus one centimeter distal to the surgical anastomosis. Urokinase infusion was started using an intra-thrombotic bolus of 200,000 I.U. followed by an infusion at a rate of 2500 I.U./kg/hr along with an I.V. Heparin infusion at a rate of 500 I.U./kg/d (RAT). The unsuccessful case had a heavy clot burden with the arterial thrombus propagating to the external iliac artery (24). As a result of transcatheter thrombolysis having the drawback of revascularizing arteries at a slower rate than surgical thrombectomy, evaluating clot burden during the initial diagnostic angiogram is important. Heavy clot burden, such as in the fourth case by Rouviere et al. should be deferred to surgical thrombectomy, leaving the option for transcatheter thrombolysis, for low clot burden (24). On re-establishing arterial flow the renal artery should be interrogated thoroughly for underlying anatomic defects such as TRAS and/or arterial kinks. These anatomic defects should be managed definitively either endoluminally or surgically. Failure to address these lesions would most likely lead to re-thrombosis of the renal artery. Two cases in point are the second and third cases reported by Rouviere et al. where their second case demonstrated an underlying arterial kink and the third case showed a significant anastomotic TRAS (24). The latter was treated successfully with PTA (24).

REFERENCES

1. Wozney P, Zajko AB, Bron KM, Point S, Starzl TE. Vascular complications after liver transplantation: a 5-year experience. AJR 1986; 147:657–663.
2. Orons PD, Zajko AB, Bron KM, Trecha GT, Selby RR, Fung JJ. Hepatic artery angioplasty after liver transplantation: experience in 21 allografts. J Vasc Interv Radiol 1995; 6:523–529.
3. Abad J, Hidalgo EG, Cantarero JM, Parga G, Fernandez R, Gomez M, Colina F, Moreno F. Hepatic artery anastomotic stenosis after transplantation: treatment with percutaneous transluminal angioplasty. Radiology 1989; 171:661–662.
4. Castaneda F, Samuel KS, Hunter DW, Castaneda-Zuniga WR, Amplatz K. Reversible hepatic transplant ischemia: case report and review of the literature. Cardiovasc Interv Radiol 1990; 13:88–90.
5. Nemcek AA Jr. Interventional radiology for transplantation: arterial interventions. SIR Proceedings 2003; Categorical Course: P315–P320.
6. Cheng YF, Chen YS, Huang TL, de Villa V, Chen TY, Lee TY, Wang CC, Chiang YC, Eng HL, Cheung HK, Jawan B, Wang SH, Goto S, Chen CL. Interventional radiologic procedures in liver transplantation. Transpl Int 2001; 14:223–229.
7. Bjerkuik PS, Vatne K, Mathisen O, Soreide O. Percutaneous revascularization of postoperative hepatic artery thrombosis in a liver transplant. Transplantation 1995; 59: 1746–1748.
8. Cienfuegos JA, Pardo F. Incidence and clinical manifestations of arterial complications of liver transplantation. Rev Esp Enferm Dig 1991; 80:103.
9. Wazques J, Santamaria ML, Gomez M, et al. Hepatic artery thrombosis in the pediatric liver transplant. Cir Pediatr 1991; 4:185.
10. Tan KC, Yandza T, de Hemptinne B, Clapuyt P, Claus D, Otte JB. Hepatic artery thrombosis in pediatric liver transplantation. J Pediatr Surg 1988; 23:927–930.
11. Orons PD, Zajko AB. Angiography and interventional procedures in liver transplantation. Radiol Clin North Am 1995; 33:541–558.
12. Zajko AB, Campbell WL, Logsdon GA, Bron KM, Tzakis A, Esquivel CO, Starzl TE. Cholangiographic findings in hepatic artery occlusion after liver transplantation. AJR 1987; 149:485–489.
13. Abbasoglu O, Levy MF, Vodapally MS, Goldstein RM, Husberg BS, Gonwa TA, Klintmalm GB. Hepatic artery stenosis after liver transplantation-incidence, presentation, treatment and long-term outcome. Transplantation 1997; 63:250–255.

14. Denys AL, Qanadli SD, Durand F, Vilgrain V, Farges O, Belghiti J, Lacombe P, Menu Y. Feasibility and effectiveness of using coronary stents in the treatment of hepatic artery stenosis after orthotopic liver transplantation: preliminary report. AJR 2002; 178: 1175–1179.
15. Merion RM, Burtch GD, Ham JM, Turcotte JG, Campbell DA. The hepatic artery in liver transplantation. Transplantation 1989; 48:438–443.
16. Dodd GD, Memel DS, Zajko AB, Baron RL, Santaguida LA. Hepatic artery stenosis and thrombosis in transplant recipients: Doppler diagnosis with resistive index and systolic acceleration time. Radiology 1994; 192:657–661.
17. Karatzas T, Lykaki-Karatzas E, Webb M, Nery J, Tsaroucha A, Demirbas A, Khan F, Ciancio G, Montalvo B, Reddy R, Schiff E, Miller J, Tzakis AG. Vascular complications, treatment and outcome following orthotopic liver transplantation. Transplant Proc 1997; 29:2853–2855.
18. Segel MC, Zajko AB, Bowen A, Bron KM, Skolnick ML, Penkrot RJ, Starzl TE. Hepatic artery thrombosis after liver transplantation: radiologic evaluation. AJR 1986; 146:137–141.
19. Orons PD, Sheng R, Zajko AB. Hepatic artery stenosis in liver transplant recipients: prevalence and cholangiographic appearance of associated biliary complications. AJR 1995; 165:1145–1149.
20. Raby N, Karoni J, Thomas S, O'Grady J, Williams R. Stenoses of vascular anastomoses after hepatic transplantation: treatment with balloon angioplasty. AJR 1991; 157: 167–171.
21. Stein M, Radich SM, Riegler JL, Perez RV, Link DP, McVicar JP. Dissection of an iliac artery conduit to liver allograft: treatment with an endovascular stent. Liver Transpl Surg 1999; 5:252–254.
22. Tzakis AG. The dearterialized liver graft. Semin Liver Dis 1985; 5:375–376.
23. Moderators: Busuttil RW; Discussants: Goldstein LI, Danovitch GM, Ament ME, MEMSIC LDF. Liver Transplantation today. Ann Int Med 1986; 104:377–389.
24. Richard HM, Silbersweig JE, MiHy HA, Lon WY, Ahn J, Cooper KM. Hepatic arterial complications in liver transplant recipients treated with pretransplantation chemoembolization for hepatocellular carcinoma. Radiology 2000; 214:775–779.
25. De Gaetano AM, Cotrneo AR, Maresca G, Di Stasi C, Evangelisti R, Gui B, Agnes S. Color Doppler sonography in the diagnosis and monitoring of arterial complications after liver transplantation. J Clin Ultrasound 2000; 28:373–380.
26. Tisone G, Gunson BK, Buckels JA, McMaster P. Raised hematocrit a contributing factor to hepatic artery thrombosis following liver transplantation. Transplantation 1988; 46:162–3.
27. Bhattacharjya S, Gunson BK, Mirza DF, Mayer DA, Buckels JA, McMaster P, Neuberger JM. Delayed hepatic artery thrombosis in adult orthotopic liver transplantation—l 12-year experience. Transplantation 2001; 71:1592–1596.
28. Vorwerk D, Gunther RW, Klever P, Riesner KP, Schumpelick V. Angioplasty and stent placement for treatment of hepatic artery thrombosis following liver transplantation. J Vasc Interv Radiol 1994; 5:309–311.
29. Cotroneo AR, Di Stasi C, Cina A, De Gaetano AM, Evangelisti R, Paloni F, Marano G. Stent placement in four patients with hepatic artery stenosis or thrombosis after liver transplantation. J Vasc Interv Radiol 2002; 13:619–623.
30. Narumi S, Osorio RW, Freise CE, Stock PG, Roberts JP, Ascher NL. Hepatic artery pseudoaneurysm with hemobilia following angioplasty after liver transplantation. Clin Transplant 1998; 12:508–510.
31. Marshall MM, Muiesan P, Srinivasan P, Kane PA, Rela M, Heaton ND, Karani JB, Sidhu PS. Hepatic artery pseudoaneurysms following liver transplantation. Incidence, presenting features and management. Clin Radiol 2001.

32. Lowell JA, Coopersmith CM, Shenoy S, Howard TK. Unusual presentations of nonmy-cotic hepatic artery pseudoaneurysms after liver transplantation. Liver Transpl Surg 1999; 5:200–203.

33. Madariaga J, Tzakis AG, Zajko AB, et al. Hepatic artery pseudoaneurysm ligation after orthotopic liver transplantation—a report of seven cases. Transplantation 1992; 54: 824–828.

34. Paci E, Antico E, Candelari R, Alborino S, Marmorale C, Landi E. Pseudoaneurysm of the common hepatic artery; treatment with a stent-graft. Cardiovasc Intervent Radiol 2000; 23:472–474.

35. Marizarbeitia C, Jonsson J, Rustgi V, Oyloe VK, Olson L, Hefter L, Kankam C. Man-agement of hemobilia after liver biopsy in liver transplant recipients. Transplantation 1993; 56:1545–1547.

36. Tomczak R, Helmberger T, Gorich J, Schutz A, Merkle E, Brambs HJ, Rieber A. Abdominal arterio-venous and arterio-portal fistulas: etiology, diagnosis, therapeutic possibilities. Zeitschrift fur Gastroenterologie 1997; 35:555–562.

37. Lerut J, Tzakis AG, Bron K, Gordon RD, IwatsukiS, Esquivel CO, Makowka L, Todo S, Starzl TE. Complications of venous reconstruction in human orthotopic liver transplantation. Ann Surg 1987; 205:404–414.

38. Funaki B. Interventional radiology for transplantation: venous interventions. SIR Pro-ceedings 2003; Categorical Course: P320–P323.

39. Funaki B, Rosenblum JD, Leef JA, Zaleski GX, Farrell T, Lorenz J, Brady L. Percuta-neous treatment of portal venous stenosis in children and adolescents with segmental hepatic transplants: long-term results. Radiology 2000; 215:147–151.

40. Rollins NK, Sheffield EG, Andrews WS. Portal vein stenosis complicating liver trans-plantation in children: percutaneous transhepatic angioplasty. Radiology 1992; 182: 731–734.

41. Millis JM, seaman DS, Piper JB, Alonso EM, Kelly S, Hackworth CA, Newell KA, Bruce DS, Woodle ES, Thistlethwaite JR, Whitington PF. Portal vein thrombosis and stenosis in pediatric liver transplantation. Transplantation 1996; 62:748–754.

42. Baccarani U, Gasparini D, Risaliti A, Vianello V, Adani GL, Sainz M, Sponza M, Bresadola F. Percutaneous mechanical fragmentation and stent placement for the treat-ment of early post-transplantation portal vein thrombosis. Transplantation 2001; 15: 1572–1582.

43. Gibson M, Dick R, Burroughs A, Rolles K. Incidence, risk factors, management, and outcome of portal vein abnormalities at orthotopic liver transplantation. Transplantation 1994; 57:1174.

44. Lerut JP, Goffette P, Molle G, Roggen FM, Puttemans T, Brenard R, Morelli MC, Wallemacq P, Van Beers B, Laterre PF. Transjugular intrahepatic portosystemic shunt after adult liver transplantation: experience in eight patients. Transplantation 1999; 68:379–384.

45. Tabasco-Minguillan J, Jain A, Naik M, Weber KM, Irish W, Fung JJ, Rakela J, Starzl TE. Gastrointestinal bleeding after liver transplantation. Transplantation 1997; 63: 60–67.

46. Richard JM III, Cooper JM, Ahn J, Silberzweig JE, Emre SH, Mitty HA. Transjugular intrahepatic portosystemic shunts in the management of Budd-Chiari syndrome in the liver transplant patient with intractable ascites: anastomotic considerations. J Vasc Interv Radiol 1998; 9:137–140.

47. Egawa H, Tanaka K, Uemoto S, Someda H, Moriyasu F, Sano K, Nishizawa F, Ozawa K. Relief of hepatic vein stenosis by balloon angioplasty after living-related donor liver transplantation. Clin Transplant 1993; 7:306–311.

48. Ko GY, Sung KB, Yoon HK, Kim JH, Song HY, Seo TS, Lee SG. Endovascular treatment of hepatic venous outflow obstruction after living-donor liver transplantation. J Vasc Interv Radiol 2002; 13:591–599.

49. Borsa JJ, Daly CP, Fontaine AB, Patel NH, Althaus SJ, Hoffer EK, Winter TC, Nghiem HV, McVicar JP. Treatment of inferior vena cava anastomotic stenoses with the Wallstent Endoprosthesis after orthotopic liver transplantation. J Vasc Interv Radiol 1999; 10:17–22.

50. Pfammatter T, Williams DM, Lane KL, Campbell DAJ, Cho KJ. Suprahepatic caval anastomotic stenosis complicating orthotopic liver transplantation: treatment with percutaneous transluminal angioplasty, Wallstent placement, or both. AJR 1997; 168: 477–480.

51. Weeks SM, Gerber DA, Jaques PF, Sandhu J, Johnson MW, Fair JH, Mauro MA. Primary Gianturco stent placement for inferior vena cava abnormalities following liver transplantation. J Vasc Interv Radiol 2000; 11:177–187.

52. Patel NH, Jindal RM, Wilkin T, Rose S, Johnson MS, Shah H, Namyslowski J, Moresco KP, Trerotola SO. Renal arterial stenosis in renal allografts: retrospective study of predisposing factors and outcome after percutaneous transluminal angioplasty. Radiology 2001; 219:663–667.

53. Fervenza FC, Lafayette RA, Alfrey EJ, Petersen J. Renal artery stenosis in kidney transplantation. Am J Kidney Dis 1998; 31:142–148.

54. Becker BN, Odorico JS, Becker YT, Leverson G, McDermott JC, Grist T, Sproat I, Heisey DM, Collins BH, D'Alessandro AM, Knechtle SJ, Pirsch JD, Sollinger HW. Peripheral vascular disease and renal transplant artery stenosis: a reappraisal of transplant renovascular disease. Clin Transplant 1999; 13:349–355.

55. Halimi JM, Al-Najjar A, Buchler M, Brimele B, Tranquart F, Alison D, Lebranchu Y. Transplant renal artery stenosis: potential role of ischemia/perfusion injury and longterm outcome following angioplasty. J Urol 1999; 161:28–32.

56. Rengel M, Gomes-Da-Silva G, Inchaustegui L, Lampreave JL, Robledo R, Echenagusia A, Vallejo JL, Valderrabano F. Renal artery stenosis after kidney transplantation: diagnostic and therapeutic approach. Kidney Int Suppl 1998; 68:S99–S106.

57. Wong W, Eynn SP, Higgins RM, Walters H, Evans S, Deane C, Goss D, Bewick M, Snowden SA, Scoble JE, Hendry BM. Transplant renal artery stenosis in 77 patients-does it have an immunological course?. Transplantation 1996; 61: 215–219.

58. Lacombe M. Arterial stenosis complicating renal allotransplantation in man: a study of 38 cases. Ann Surg 1997; 181:283.

59. Cloudon M, Lefevre F, Hestin D, Martin-Beitaux A, Hubert J, Kessler M. Power Doppler imaging: evaluation of vascular complications after renal transplantation. AJR 1999; 173:41–46.

60. Morris PJ, Yadav RV, Kincaid-Smith P, Anderton J, Hare WS, Johnson N, Johnson W, Marshall VC. Renal artery stenosis in renal transplantation. Med J Aust 1971; 1: 1255–1257.

61. Greenstein SM, Verstandig A, McLean GK, Dafoe DC, Burke DR, Meranze SG, Naji A, Grossman RA, Perloff LJ, Barker CF. Percutaneous transluminal angioplasty: the procedure of choice in the hypersensitive renal allograft recipient with renal artery stenosis. Transplantation 1987; 43:29–32.

62. Osman Y, Shokeir A, Ali-el-Dein B, Tantawy M, Wafa EW, el-Dein AB, Ghoneim MA. Vascular complications after live donor renal transplantation: study of risk factors and effects on graft and patient survival. J Urol 2003; 169(3):859–862.

63. Gray DW. Graft renal artery stenosis in the transplanted kidney. Transplant Rev 1994; 8:15–21.

64. Macia M, Paez A, Tornero F, DeOleo P, Hidalgo L, Barrientos A. Post-transplant renal artery stenosis: a possible immunological phenomenon. J Urol 1991; 145:251–252.

65. Fanchald P, Vatne K, Paulsen D, Brodahl U, Sodal G, Holdaas H, Berg KJ, Flatmark A. Long-term clinical results of percutaneous transluminal angioplasty in transplant renal artery stenosis. Nephrol Dial Transplant 1992; 7:256–259.

66. Benoit G, Moukarzel M, Hiesse C, Verdelli G, Charpentier B, Fries D. Transplant renal artery stenosis: experience and comparative results between surgery and angioplasty. Transplant Int 1990; 3:137–140.

67. Shames BD, Odorico JS, D'Alessandro M, Pirsch JD, Sollinger HW. Surgical repair of transplant renal artery stenosis with preserved Cadaveric iliac artery grafts. Ann Surg 2003; 237(1):116–122.

68. Raynaud A, Bedrossian J, Remy P, Birsset JM, Angel-Gaux JC. Percutaneous transluminal angioplasty of renal transplant arterial stenoses. AJR 1986; 146(4):853–857.

69. Berliner JA, Navab M, Fogelman AM, Frank JS, Demer LL, Edwards PA, Watson AD, Lusis AJ. Atherosclerosis: basic mechanisms, oxidation, inflammation, and genetics. Circulation 1995; 91:2488.

70. Nicita G, Villari D, Marzocco M, LiMarzi V, Trippitelli A, Santoro G. Endoluminal stent placement after percutaneous transluminal angioplasty in the treatment of post-transplant renal artery stenosis. J Urol 1998; 159:34–37.

71. Takadashi M, Humke U, Girndt M, Kramann B, Uder M. Early post-transplantation renal allograft perfusion failure due to dissection: diagnosis and interventional treatment. AJR 2003; 180:759–763.

72. Maleux G, Messiaen T, Stockx L, Vanrenterghem Y, Wilms G. Transcatheter embolization of biopsy-related vascular injuries in renal allografts: long-term technical, clinical and biochemical results. Acta Radiologica 2003; 44(1):13–17.

73. Martinez T, Palomares M, Bravo JA, Alvarez G, Galindo P, Entrena AG, Osuma A, Asensio C. Biopsy-induced arteriovenous fistula and venous aneurysm in a renal transplant. Nephol Dial Transplant 1998; 13:2937.

74. Dorffner R, Thurnher S, Prokesch R, et al. Embolization of iatrogenic vascular injuries of renal transplants: immediate and follow-up results. Cardiovasc Intervent Radiol 1998; 21(2): 129–134.

75. Rouviere O, Berger P, Beziat C, Garnier JL, Lefrancois N, Martin X, Lyonnet D. Acute thrombosis of renal transplant artery: graft salvage by means of intra-arterial fibrinolysis. Transplantation 2002; 73:403–409.

76. Nakir N, Sluites WJ, Ploeg RJ, vanSon WJ, Tegzess AM. Primary renal graft thrombosis. Nephrol Dial Transplant 1996; 11(1):140–147.

77. Ismail H, Kalicinski P, Drewniak T, Smirska E, Kaminski A, Prokurat A, Grenda R, Szymczak M, Chrupek M, Markiewicz M. Primary vascular thrombosis after renal transplantation in children. Pediatr Transplant 1997; 1(1):43–47.

78. Robertson AJ, Nargund V, Gray DWR, Morris PJ. Low dose aspirin as prophylaxis against renal-vein thrombosis in renal transplant recipients. Nephrol Dial Transpl 2002; 15:1865–1868.

79. Merion RM, Calne RY. Allograft renal vein thrombosis. Transpl Proc 1985; 17: 1746–1750.

80. Rigotti P, Fleschner SM, VanBuren CT, Payne WT, Kahan BD. Increased incidence of renal allograft thrombosis under cyclosporine immunosuppression. Int Surg 1986; 71:38.

81. The Canadian Multicenter Transplant Study Group. A randomized clinical trial of cyclosporine in Cadaveric renal transplantation. N Engl J Med 1983; 309:809.

82. Zajko AB, McLean GK, Grossman RA, Barker CF, Freiman DB, Ring EJ, Alvai A, Perloff LJ. Percutaneous transluminal angioplasty and fibrinolytic therapy for renal allograft arterial stenosis and thrombosis. Transplantation 1982; 33:447.

83. Nicholson JD, Burleson RL, Bredenberg CE. Survival of a renal allograft after correction of an early total acute renal artery occlusion. Transplantation 1978; 26:131.

84. Swanson DA, Sullivan MJ. Thromboendarterectomy for anuria $4\frac{1}{2}$ years post-renal transplant: a case report. J Urol 1976; 116:799.

85. Renders L, Goerig M, Schreiber M, Kasprzak P, Houser I. Successful surgical revascularization of a kidney transplant after PTA-induced arterial dissection of the allograft renal artery. Nephrol Dial Transplant 1997; 12:1264.

86. Herrera RO, Benitez AM, Abad MJH. Renal vein partial thrombosis in three recipients of kidney transplantation. Arch Esp Urol 2000; 53(1):45–48.

15

Complications in Aortoiliac Arterial Interventions

Michael Wholey
Cardiovascular and Interventional Radiology, University of Texas Health Science Center at San Antonio, San Antonio, Texas, U.S.A.

INTRODUCTION

With the rise in peripheral vascular disease in the general population, there has been an increased awareness of the severe atherosclerotic disease affecting the aortoiliac arteries and the lower extremities. The disease progression is complex and can be multifactorial including any level of disease in the aorta, iliac, or infrainguinal arteries. There are many causes of narrowing of the aortoiliac arteries but the most common has been atherosclerotic disease. Occasionally, we will encounter other causes such as fibromuscular dysplasia (FMD), radiation fibrosis, and causes of vasculitis.

The objective of this chapter is to gain a better understanding of aortoiliac anatomy, interventional options to treat the disease, and most importantly, complications that can occur from intervention.

ANATOMY

The infrarenal abdominal aorta measures approximately 12–20 mm in diameter extending from below the take off of the renal arteries to the iliac bifurcation located approximately at the L4 vertebral body. There are bilateral lumbar arteries that originate off the posterior oblique angle of the aorta in addition to the inferior mesenteric artery that originates off approximately L3 anterior-lateral border. The inferior mesenteric artery has a superior branch flowing to the descending colon and an inferior branch to the rectosigmoid colon (Fig. 1).

The wall of the aorta is similar in structure to the common iliac arteries. The common iliac arteries measure approximately 7–9 mm in diameter and take off from the aorta and extend until the bifurcation of the internal and external iliac arteries (Fig. 2). The internal iliac artery branches into the anterior and posterior divisions.The anterior internal iliac artery has many of the important branches to the organs in the pelvis including the ovary/uterus/prostate, bladder, and collaterals to

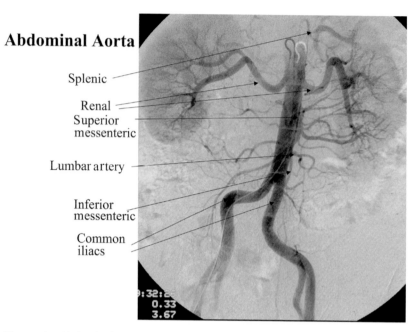

Abdominal Aorta

Splenic

Renal

Superior
messenteric

Lumbar artery

Inferior
messenteric

Common
iliacs

Figure 1   Abdominal aortagram with major branches revealed.

the colon. One of the complications of embolizing the internal iliac, is a slow decrease in the posterior branch, which can cause buttocks claudication. The external iliac artery is a muscular type, measures approximately 5–7 mm in diameter and extends to the femoral head where it becomes the common femoral artery.

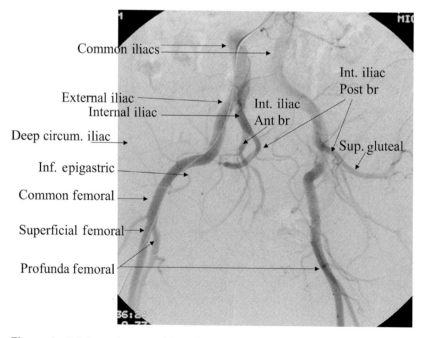

Common iliacs

External iliac
Internal iliac

Deep circum. iliac

Inf. epigastric

Common femoral

Superficial femoral

Profunda femoral

Int. iliac
Ant br

Int. iliac
Post br

Sup. gluteal

Figure 2   Pelvic angiogram with major branches revealed.

AORTOILIAC ARTERIAL INTERVENTIONS

The major types of aortoiliac interventions depend upon the type of disease and location. These include interventions of aortoiliac stenoses versus total occlusions.

Aortoiliac Stenoses

A relatively common finding in a patient with peripheral vascular disease is a focal lesion in the iliac artery and less commonly a focal aortic lesion. How you approach each of these depends on the severity of the lesion, location, and size of vessel. Some general rules that we have utilized include the following: we almost always place a stent for iliac lesions. Our choice of stent depends upon lesion location and length of lesion. Generally, we will use balloon-mounted stents for lesions in the proximal common iliac artery to precisely deploy the stent at the ostium. For lesions approaching the distal external iliac and for long lesions, we will use self-expandable stents. We will use angioplasty alone for external iliac lesions crossing the inguinal ligament, rare cases of FMD or markedly small vessels (<4 mm diameter).

For aortoiliac lesions, we will prefer to use balloon-mounted stents and place them at the bifurcation extending several millimeters into the aorta. We try to avoid the use of self-expandable stents. For pure aortic lesions, we will prefer to place either a balloon-mounted or self-expandable stent depending upon diameter of the vessel, length of lesion and characteristics of the lesion. Other interventionalists have advocated angioplasty alone and have stated equivalent results.

Aortoiliac Occlusions

There are several different techniques in treating occlusive disease of the aortoiliac arteries. An important distinction has been acute versus chronic occlusions. For chronic lesions, we have had good technical success in recanalizing short lesions with the use of a hydrophilic guidewire and a 4–5 French diagnostic catheter (1). As stated, we will use roadmap techniques to carefully cross short focal lesions and then place a small self-expanding stent.

Another approach we have used is to place an infusion catheter or guidewire at or in the occluded vessel and begin thrombolytic therapy. We will infuse Urokinase (Abbott Labs, Chicago, Illinois) at approximately 120,000 units per hour in addition to heparinzation with the goal of reopening the vessel and reducing lesion length. We will then proceed with angioplasty and possible stent placement. In a large series of 250 patients with chronic arterial occlusions of the iliac and femoro-popliteal arteries, we were able to achieve a 77% technical success rate in reopening these vessels with thrombolytic therapy (2). The development of new mechanical thrombectomy catheters such as from Bacchus may speed the usual overnight process that was required in the past.

Newer devices carried over from coronary recanalization also offer promise in treating longer lesions and possibly improving long-term results. There have been good reports from the use of laser in recanalizing long lesions; Scheinert et al. reported in a series of 212 patients with chronic iliac occlusions, a 90% technical success and 88% clinical improvement in two to three grades (3). Likewise, there have also been good reports with the use of LuMend Frontrunner catheter (Redwood City, California) and IntraLuminal catheter system (Carlsbad, California) (4).

Whichever technique, recanalization with a wire, laser or other device, maintenance of patency is imperative with good and frequent surveillance and re-interventions.

For acute occlusions of the aortoiliac arteries, we will use the traditional method of overnight thrombolysis infusion catheters to reopen the vessel followed by angioplasty and stent placement. We will accelerate the treatment with the use of mechanical thrombectomy catheters such as Trellis catheter (Bacchus Vascular, Inc., Santa Clara, California) and the AngioJet System (Possis Medical Inc., Minneapolis, Minnesota).

COMPLICATIONS IN AORTOILIAC INTERVENTIONS

Dissection

Etiology and Frequency

Dissection of the iliac arteries during iliac artery intervention is fairly common and can occur during multiple phases of the procedure. It can occur during the following:

1. It can occur during passage of the guidewire and/or diagnostic catheter through diseased and even normal segments of the iliac artery (Fig. 3A–C). In these cases, it may be caused by not watching under fluoroscopy the careful advance of the guidewire and catheter in the iliac arteries.
2. Dissection can also occur from a bad arterial stick, in which the needle is in the media and the wire creates a dissection plane (Fig. 4A–C).
3. Another cause of dissection can occur from passage of the guidewire and catheter past high-grade lesions, in which the wire will course underneath the plaque.
4. A major cause of dissection can occur during angioplasty and stent placement. Predilatation of a high-grade lesion almost always causes a small dissection, fortunately most of these are small and inconsequential. Occasionally, these will expand or spiral; hence, it is important to inject contrast after dilatation and prior to stent placement. Stent placement can also cause dissections related to the injury created by the stent edge, which is particularly related to balloon-mounted stents. Also, dissection occurs from the angioplasty balloon wings that extend past the stent edge.
5. Other less common causes of dissection include too hard a contrast injection from the sheath located distal to a recently angioplastied or stented lesion.

How to Avoid Dissections

The simplest advice is to use caution. Other important tips to avoid dissection include the following:

- As stated, always watch guidewire and catheter movement under fluoroscopy. If a guidewire is stuck, do not ever force it.
- Do not advance a catheter without a guidewire leading the way first.
- Watch the use of hydrophillic guidewires. Glidewires (Terumo, Boston Scientific, Natick, Massachusetts) are useful in crossing difficult lesions; but they have a high tendency to go through vessel walls. We avoid the use of torque devices with these wires. Also, once across a difficult lesion, we will switch to the more conventional stainless steel wires.

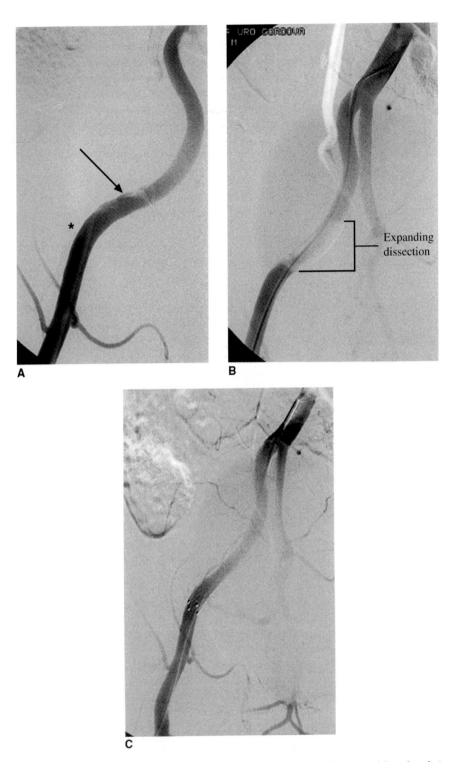

Figure 3 (**A**) Inadvertant dissection (*arrow*) caused by the guidewire exiting sheath (*asterisk*) which faces the vessel wall. (**B**) With access past the dissecting flap, contrast injected revealed dissection expansion resulting in a near occlusion. (**C**) Self expandable stent placed resulting in return of flow.

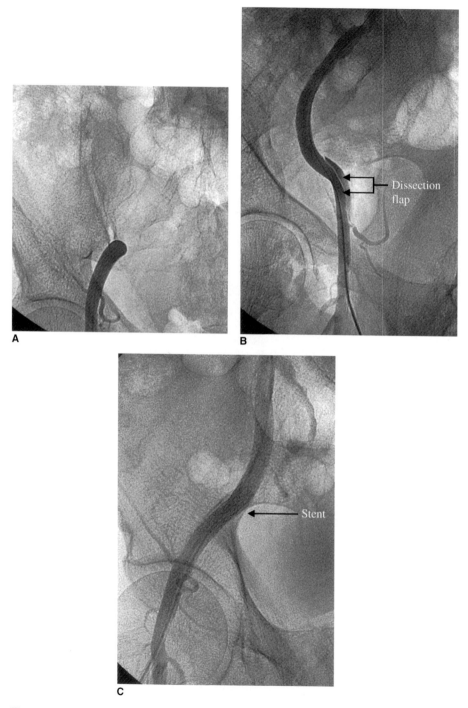

Figure 4 (**A**) Through a 19 gauge seldinger needle 0.035" wire was advanced resulting in a near complete occlusion of right external iliac. (**B**) Access was achieved past the dissection flap (*arrow*) with a torquable wire followed by the catheter. (**C**) Short stent placed at origin of flap placed with return of flow.

- Watch the sheath position and avoid injecting below lesions just angioplastied or stented.
- Use good fluoroscopy and roadmapping to cross difficult lesions.
- Use small angioplasty balloons to predilate when needed. Hence, we will use predilatation to insure that our sheath or stent will cross the lesion easily. Our choice of predilatation balloon is usually 4 mm in diameter. This minimizes the risk of dissection.
- Use balloon catheters with minimal wings extending proximally and distally from balloon-mounted stents.
- Be careful of excessive post-balloon dilatation once the vessel is stented and avoid dilating vessel segments not covered by a stent.
- Be careful of patients on hemodialysis, for these have a high tendency to dissect. Also of concern are lesions with marked amounts of calcium.

How to Manage Dissections

Once a dissection occurs, it is important to control the extent of damage. When a dissection occurs from wire or catheter interruption of the vessel wall or from angioplasty, it is important to determine the location and extent of dissection. One of the most important rules to remember is never to lose guidewire across the dissection. Another important rule is not to waste time for the dissections can spiral in length and occlude the vessel; that is why it is important to heparinize the patient well.

With the wire in place, you can advance a diagnostic catheter or your sheath (with coaxial introducer in place) and perform an angiogram from above the lesion to assess the damage. For lesions in the common and external iliac, we will conventionally stent these with a stent sized to the vessel. For lesions near the inguinal ligament, we will first try to tack up the dissection flap with an angioplasty balloon catheter, again sized to the vessel wall, inflated for one to two minutes.

If you lost wire access or never had it as in a poor arterial puncture and the vessel has shut down, then you must regain access in the true lumen. This can be obtained in two ways: carefully try to get in the true lumen from below or more easily, make a contralateral arterial access and get in from above. In both cases, we will use a 5F diagnostic catheter with a slight angle and carefully manipulate a torqueable guidewire, such as a Wholey (Mallinckrodt, St. Louis, Missouri) or a glidewire. You must be certain that you are not making the dissection worse. Good imaging including roadmapping again is crucial to utilize in these situations. Once access has been secured, we will angioplasty or stent the lesion. We prefer to stent in most situations because of the risk of recurrence. Even though dissections created from retrograde direction have less risk of spreading, they still have the potential of closing the vessel off completely. We will try to stent the entire dissection (Fig. 3C) but occasionally, we can treat the major flap of the dissection and solve the problem (Fig. 4C).

Placing an additional stent, making sure that you overlap the adjoining stent, can treat dissections that occur from stent placement. Which stent to use varies with the comfort ability of the interventionalist. Theoretically, self-expanding nitinol may provide greater support, but we have not seen much difference.

Some dissections from stent placement occur underneath the stent. Ulcerations and heavily calcified plaques can mimic a dissection. If a dissection extends fairly deep (Fig. 5A–C) below the stented lesion, these need to be treated with prolonged balloon inflation. Additionally, these patients need to have a CT-scan (non-contrast)

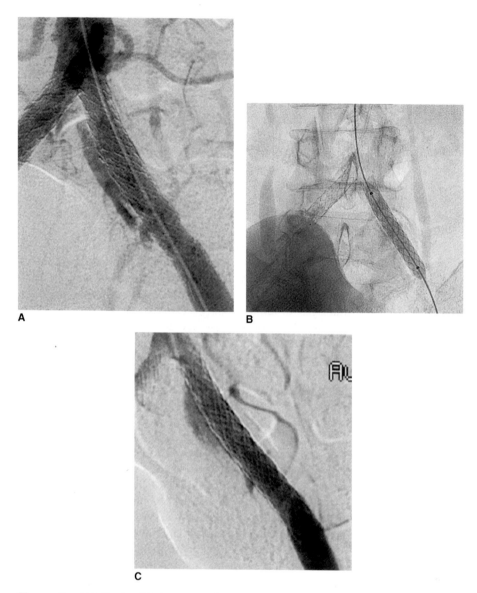

Figure 5 (**A**) During kissing stent placement, a large deep dissection has occurred. (**B**) Prolonged balloon dilatation performed over the site. (**C**) After balloon dilatation, contrast injection revealed improvement of deep dissection.

to evaluate the lesion, making sure that it does not extend out of the vessel or that a pseudoaneurysm has not been created. Also, we will admit these patients into the intensive care unit and monitor serial hematocrits.

Extravasation

This a life-threatening situation caused from a guidewire, catheter or stent causing a disruption of the three layers. Dissections if severe can lead to an extravasation. See below for more information.

Patient Follow-Up

Most dissections once treated with stent or even angioplasty alone become inconsequential. However, if left untreated or missed, these lead to vessel occlusion requiring greater intervention. It is important to regularly follow these patients in clinic with imaging modalities as needed.

Extravasation

Etiology and Frequency

Extravasation is a potentially life-threatening complication that results from a disruption of the three layers of arterial wall. It can occur from a guidewire or catheter perforation of the wall or from complication incurred during endovascular aortic aneurysm stent graft placement. We see it most frequently related to penetrating and blunt arterial injuries, unrelated to aortoiliac interventions.

How to Avoid Extravasation

Use the same keys as above in the dissection section. For extravasation related to abdominal aortic aneurysm (AAA) stent grafts, it is important not to try to advance the large sheaths and delivery systems in small, tortuous or heavily calcified iliac arteries.

How to Manage Extravasation

We will always have available a covered stent 8–10 mm in diameter for such emergencies. Covered stents are available from Wallgraft (Boston Scientific, Natick, Massachusetts), Atrium (Hudson, New Hamsphire), Bard Fluency (CR Bard, Murray Hill, NJ), and Gore Viabahn (W.L. Gore, Flagstatt, AZ) Most require large sheaths for access and are difficult to advance over the aortic bifurcation; hence, an ipsilateral approach is required.

Occasionally, an area of extravasation can be watched and not intervened. We have had a wire perforation (0.035-inch glidewire) of an internal iliac in a patient with a AAA; the perforation was monitored with CT and serial hematocrits (Fig. 6A–C). The patient did well and was later embolized and a AAA stent graft placed. This watch-and-wait method is controversial. For wire perforations of other sites, such as in the kidney, embolization of the bleeding vessel is required.

If the extravasation should occur in branches off the external iliac or in internal iliac branches, we will embolize these bleeding sites with coils. These are almost always trauma related from blunt or penetrating accidents. The key features for this management include: good diagnostic images of the bleeding vessel, selection of the vessel with a diagnostic catheter or a microcatheter, and embolization with coils to effectively stop bleeding.

Patient Follow-Up

Regular patient follow-up is needed.

Stent Migration

Etiology and Frequency

Stent migration used to be more common in the recent past prior to the advent of premounted balloon stents. Migration of the balloon-mounted stents still occurs today with the loose placement of an unmounted stent on an angioplasty balloon catheter, particularly those with hydrophilic coating. It can also occur by stripping

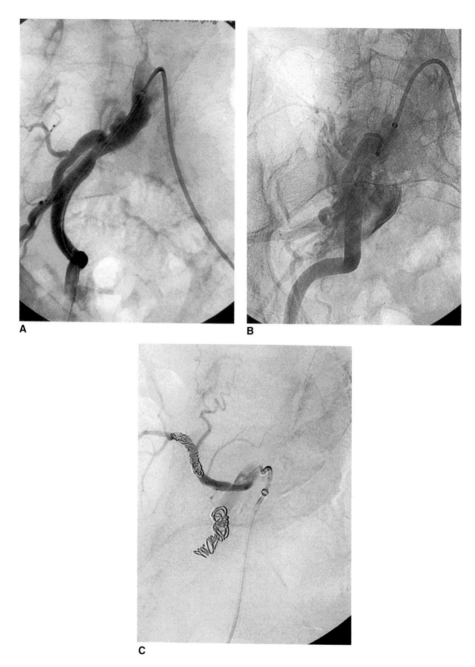

Figure 6 (**A**) During initial evaluation of right internal iliac prior to AAA stent placement, perforation of vessel occurred. (**B**) Contrast injection showed extravasation around iliac vessels. (**C**) With both anterior and posterior arteries selected, with a microcatheter, microcoils were placed to occlude these iliac branches prior to stent placement.

the balloon-mounted stent by the arterial sheath by inadvertently pulling the balloon-mounted stent back into the sheath. Also, stent migration can occur in tight, calcified lesions not effectively predilated (Fig. 7A–C). The tight lesion can strip the stent off the balloon even with premounted stents.

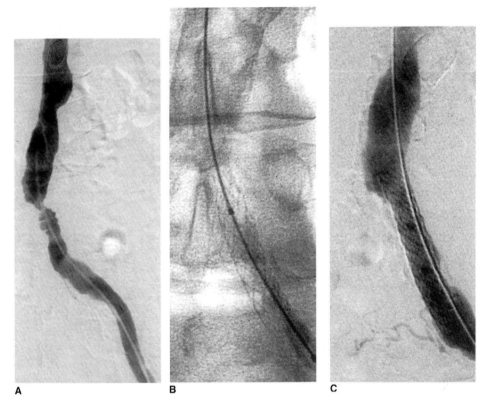

A   **B**   **C**

Figure 7A–C Initial attempt of primary stenting. Because lesion was not predilated to allow easy passage of stent, we could not advance stent past lesion. Stent became wedged and had to be deployed in the common iliac. Second stent was used to bridge into the abdominal aorta.

Another cause of migration of a stent is undersizing of the stent to the vessel. This can occur in balloon-mounted as well as self-expanding stents.

How to Avoid Stent Migration

The following tips are useful:

1. Use premounted stents mounted on low profile balloon catheters.
2. For your premounted stents on balloon catheters, do not aspirate on the balloon catheter segment prior to advancing the balloon and stent through the sheath for this could weaken the hold on the stent.
3. Dip your balloon and stent in a contrast media.
4. Use long sheaths. We will use 25 cm 6- and 7-French sheaths in order to get past the lesion. Once our balloon and stent are in position, we will pull the sheath back proximally and deploy the stent.
5. If you suspect a tight aortoiliac lesion, always predilate with a 3–4 mm balloon. We will even use an occasional 5 mm balloon catheter.
6. Do not undersize a stent to the vessel wall.

How to Manage Stent Migration

When a stent migrates, there are different strategies depending upon where the stent is located. When it is slightly off the balloon, you can either deploy the stent where it lies and when most of the stent is opposed to the wall, use the same or different balloon advanced into the remaining underexpanded stent and then dilate this segment. Or, occasionally, we can recapture the stent and apply light pressure (1 atm) to reposition it. But depending upon the slippage, most the time it is safer to deploy the stent where it is rather than take the risk of causing a dangerous dissection by moving the migrated stent.

If the stent is completely off the balloon catheter, you have more problems. Again, the first thing to remember is never lose access of your wire through the stent. Depending upon the balloon used, you will probably have to exchange for a very low profile balloon such as a 3 or 4 mm that goes over a 0.035 inch wire. If you are using a 0.014-inch or 0.018-inch wire, then you can use a small percutaneous transluminal coranary angioplasty (PTCA) balloon such as 2–3 mm with the purpose of expanding the stent to allow a larger balloon such as 5–6 mm and then finally, a balloon to have the stent apposed to the wall (Fig. 8A–C).

When the stent is off the balloon and wire, you can try an endovascular approach if it is still in the iliacs. If the stent has gone to the common femoral artery, you and the patient may be better off by going to surgery for a cutdown and removal of the stent by surgery. For endovascular techniques, you can snare the stent and try to pull it though a larger sheath (9–10F). Alternatively, you can place a new stent next to it in the iliac and expand the new stent, crushing the migrated one against the wall.

When a self-expandable stent migrates, your options are limited. Self-expandable nitinol is difficult to snare and capture into a large sheath. The Wallstent can be snared a little more easily. We had a case of a 14 mm Wallstent that migrated to the right atrium from a superior vena cava stenosis. We were able to retrieve it by gaining access above and below with two guidewires and removing it with a cutdown (Fig. 9A–C). This would probably be too dangerous to do in the aortoiliac. For a misplaced Wallstent, you may be better off by gaining access through the stent and placing a balloon-mounted stent to pin the Wallstent against the arterial wall.

Patient Follow-Up

Routine follow-up is required. If there was a risk of dissection with movement of the stent, then follow-up computerized tomography-scan may be indicated. With all stent cases, we place them on clopidogrel (Plavix) and aspiring after the procedure.

Other Problems and Accidents

Balloon Rupture During Aortic Stent Placement

Etiology and Frequency. When placing a balloon-mounted stent in treating a purely aortic lesion, rupture of the angioplasty balloon catheter during the beginning of the inflation was actually fairly common before new, stronger wall balloon catheters became available. Fortunately, now with new balloons and also with new self-expanding stents (with larger diameters), this has become less of an issue.

How to Avoid. As stated above, make sure your angioplasty balloon catheter has a strong balloon surface (Duralyn or other material) that can take a stent and dilate it safely. Also, consider a self-expanding stent if the size and length of lesion is allowable.

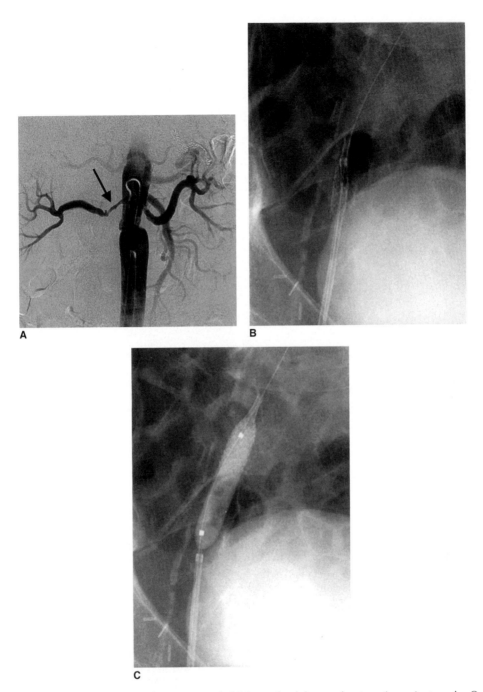

Figure 8 (**A**) Initial angiogram reveals high grade right renal artery (*arrow*) stenosis. On initial advancement stent became wedged on lesion and then stripped off balloon catheter. (**B**) Candal end of balloon mounted stent was dilated to allow it to be temporarily placed on sheath. (**C**) Serial dilationof caudal end allowed the stent to be opposed against the wall of the graft. The cephaliac end was then serially dilated.

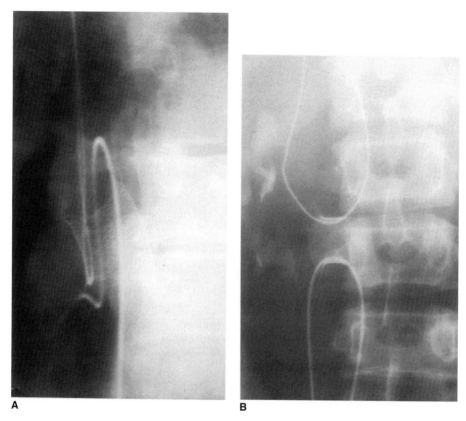

A   B

Figure 9 (A) Superior vena cava wall stent has migrated into the right arterium. Through two rim catheters wire was advanced to allow control of both stent coils. (B) With jugular and femoral venous control, migrated stent could have axis rotated and stent subsequently pulled down to femoral vein.

Before you mount the stent onto the balloon, make certain that there is no air in the balloon by careful aspiration. Then mount the stent carefully, again making sure that it cannot be moved or pulled off the balloon. Use a long enough sheath to go past the lesion, and then deploy the stent.

Management of the Complication. If the balloon should rupture, you will notice it simply by no increased pressure in the inflation syringe as you push it forward. You could also tell a rupture by aspiration of blood back into the syringe. But the key is not to wait too long, rather, quickly inflate forcefully the existing saline/ contrast mixture in the balloon to expand the stent as much as possible against the aortic wall. Then replace the balloon with a new balloon and quickly (and carefully under fluoroscopy) reinflate to expand the stent.

Wrong Location of Stent Placement

Etiology and Frequency. Misplacement of a balloon-mounted stent can occur as stated above when it should slide off the balloon. But a much more frequent cause is operator error in misjudging lesion location in which the operator places the stent in either the wrong location or the stent is deployed incorrectly. If the lesion is not predilated, heavy calficied lesions can cause a balloon-mounted stent to move

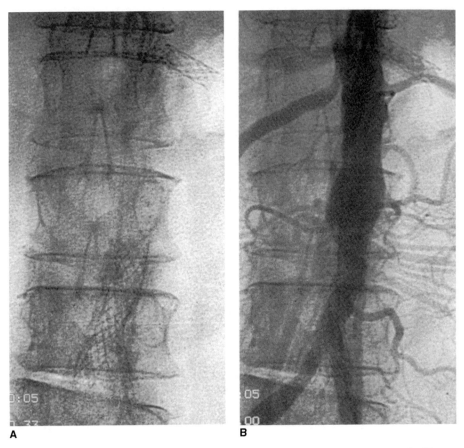

A   B

Figure 10 (**A**) Operation misjudgement resulted in inadvertent misplacement of self-expandable stent from common iliac aretry into abdominal artery. (**B**) Injection revealed good flow through stent struts.

forwards or backwards off the lesion. For self-expandable stents, occasionally, there will be much slack which causes the stent to lunge forward, and deploy past the targeted spot. That is why it is difficult to deploy nitinol stents at the iliac bifurcation for they have a tendency to jump forward into the aorta (Fig. 10A–B).

How to Avoid. The best way to avoid such mistakes is to pay attention to the lesion and surrounding vessel. If you are not sure of the vessel diameter, a quick way is to use a predilatation balloon catheter, which will allow you an idea as to the size of the vessel and length of the lesion. Other ways include measuring guidewires and catheters. Intravascular ultrasound is useful but may be a little too much expense and effort.

Management of the Complication. Place an additional stent overlapping with the misplaced stent.

CONCLUSIONS

Iliac artery intervention, namely angioplasty and stent placement, has evolved into a relatively safe procedure with good long-term results. Its use will increase in the future with greater frequency. Complications with iliac intervention will also grow, especially with more interventionalists who have not had dedicated peripheral training. Becoming aware of potential complications and how to manage these complications will be essential in all internventionalists who become dedicated in stent placement.

REFERENCES

1. Reyes R, Maynar M, Lopera J, Ferral H, Gorriz E, Carreira J, Casteneda WR. Treatment of chronic iliac artery occlusions with guide wire recanilization and primary stent placement. J Vasc Interv Radiol 1997; 8:1049–1055.
2. Wholey MH, Maynar MA, Wholey MH, Pulido-duque JM, Reyes R, Jarmolowski CR, Castenda WR. Comparison of thrombolytic therapy of lower extremity acute, subacute and chronic arterial occlusions. Catheteriz Cardiovasc Diagn 1998; 44:159–169.
3. Scheinert D, Schroder M, Ludwig J, Braunlich S, Mockel M, Flackskampf FA, Balzer JO, Biamino G. Stent supported recanalization of chronic iliac artery occlusions. Am J Med 2001; 110:708–715.
4. Biamino G, Schofer J, Schluter M. A new vascular approach to chronic total occlusions of the superficial femoral artery. Presented Feb 2000, Interventional Cardiology Aspen, CO 2000.

16

Complications of Endovascular Therapy: The Common Femoral Artery

Krishna Rocha-Singh
Vascular Medicine Program, Prairie Heart Institute, Springfield, Illinois, U.S.A.

OVERVIEW

Over a half century ago, Sven Seldinger, M.D., first described the concept of percutaneous vascular entry and thereby introduced a new era of percutaneous therapies (1). Today, with considerable evidence supporting the efficacy of a variety of percutaneous therapies of coronary and non-coronary vascular bed pathologies, diagnostic and therapeutic vascular interventional procedures performed via the common femoral artery (CFA) are increasing. Technological advances in the design of guidewires, sheaths, and guiding catheters to address carotid, brachiocephalic and infrainguinal, renal and mesenteric atherosclerosis, as well as the percutaneous deployed grafts for thoracic and infrarenal aortic pathologies are now effectively treated with percutaneous endovascular techniques. The CFA, in the majority of these interventions, is the preferred portal of entry to this revolution in endovascular therapies.

The goal of these minimally invasive endovascular therapies is compromised if the CFA cannot be closed with minimal morbidity. Still, "20–30 minutes hand-held pressure" after catheter removal followed by prolonged bedrest originally described by Seldinger, remains the primary method for management after percutaneous interventions. However, with the increasing popularity and complexity of percutaneous interventions, the aging patient population, and the concomitant use of potent antithrombotics and anticoagulants, there is increasing concern for the associated complications of percutaneous therapies. This chapter will highlight the changing landscape of CFA access, the diagnosis and management of the associated major complications, and new methodologies to minimize complications. Finally, the increasing popularity of percutaneous CFA closure devices will be discussed and the new challenges of diagnosis and management of closure device associated complications are reviewed.

CFA ACCESS COMPLICATIONS

The CFA is the access site of choice for the vast majority of percutaneous endovascular procedures, in part, due to its relatively large diameter and superficial location

269

over the femoral head of the femur and proximity to the proceduralist, which allows for manual compression after access sheath removal. Over the past four decades, manual compression to achieve hemostasis followed by four to eight hours of bed rest has been the mainstay of post-procedural CFA access management. However, the increasing adoption of non-coronary interventions of increasing complexity and duration, requiring larger size sheaths, and the use of potent anticoagulants, has drawn attention to the hemorrhagic and ischemic complications associated with CFA access management (Table 1).

HEMORRHAGE

Access site bleeding is the most frequent complication following CFA puncture and a leading cause of morbidity after percutaneous interventions (2–4). Much of the data regarding the incidence of CFA access complications is culled from interventional cardiology device trials and more recent trials of vascular closure devices (3–10). It is noteworthy that there is no standardization regarding the reporting of "minor" and/or "major" complication rates which vary significantly from 0.4% to 27% depending on the definition of the complications used (8–10). Clearly, many reports site only "major" complications which require surgery, suggesting that "minor" complications may go unreported.

Reports by Popma et al. (3) first identified major access site complications as a significant problem noting a 14% bleeding rate associated with percutaneous coronary interventions (PCI). In 2001, Dangas (8) compared manual compression to the use of vascular closure devices after PCI and reported an overall complication rate with manual compression of 12.1%, focusing attention on the high incidence of complication rates associated with the "gold standard." The relatively high complication rates associated with manual compression may reflect the increasing complexity of interventional techniques, the use of more aggressive antithrombotic and anticoagulation regimens, and changing patient demographic with percutaneous procedures performed on older, sicker, and more obese patients who are at higher risk for vascular complications.

Despite meticulous technique and adequate compression after CFA catheter removal, complications may occur. Expanding groin hematomas secondary to localized hemorrhage is the most common complication. Any complaint of groin, hip,

Table 1 CFA Access Complications and Incidences After Interventional Procedures

Complication	Range of incidence (%)
Hematoma (requiring prolonged observation, blood transfusion, surgical evacuation)	2–6
PA	0.6–9
AVF	≤0.2
Femoral neuropathy	≤0.2
Percutaneous closure devices (all complications)	
Collagen-mediated	0–12.9
Suture-mediated	0.3–7.7

Abbreviations: CFA, common femoral artery; PA, pseudoaneurysm; AVF, arterial venous fistula.

back or lower extremity discomfort, coolness, or mottling should be evaluated thoroughly. The patient may frequently complain of pain over the CFA puncture site and careful examination to exclude a pseudoaneurysm (PA), arterial venous fistula (AVF), or continued hemorrhage should be performed.

Retroperitoneal Hemorrhage

The incidence of retroperitoneal hemorrhage in hematoma formation has been reported at 0.12–0.4% in patients after interventional procedures (11). The risk of hemorrhage into the retroperitoneal space is increased by a high CFA puncture (above the inguinal ligament) and with inadvertent puncture of the posterior wall of the CFA. Therefore, knowledge of the common femoral vasculature and inguinal anatomy is important to minimize risk associated with a retrograde CFA puncture. Successful access of the CFA overlying the medial 1/3 of the femoral head has been advocated as the ideal access point (Fig. 1).

Retroperitoneal hemorrhage may present as unexplained hypotension, abdominal or flank distension, fullness, or discomfort (12). A high index of suspicion in any patient with unexplained hypotension, particularly on continued anticoagulants or antithrombotic agents should result in discontinuation/reversal of the anticoagulant or antithrombotic agent and exclusion of a hemorrhage by computed tomography or abdominal or pelvic ultrasound. Emergent assessment of the patient's hematocrit and

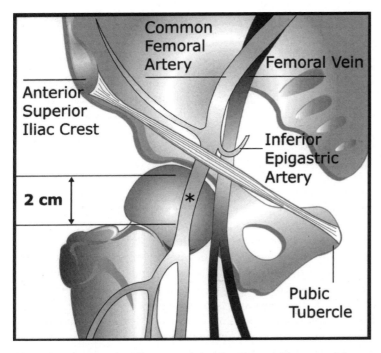

Figure 1   Use bony and fluoroscopic landmarks to guide successful percutaneous CFA access. Puncture of the CFA (below the inguinal ligament and above the SFA/PFA bifurcation) is made by first locating anterior superior iliac spine laterally and the pubic tubercle medially. Puncture the CFA approximately 1 cm lateral to the most medial cortical edge of the mid femoral head. *Abbreviations*: CFA, common femoral artery; SFA, superficial femoral artery; PFA, profunda femoris artery.

hemoglobin and consideration of typing and crossing the patient in the event of requiring blood transfusion should also be performed. Volume resuscitation with crystalloid and/ or blood products should be administered if volume depletion is evident.

If, despite cessation of antithrombotics/anticoagulants and fluid or blood product resuscitation, the patient's clinical situation continues to deteriorate, emergent angiography performed via the contralateral femoral access to localize the bleeding site or surgical exploration of the groin and evacuation of the hematoma should be considered. The use of prolonged balloon inflation and consideration of covered stent (e.g., WallGraft, Boston Scientific Corporation, Watertown, Massachusetts) deployment should be considered to seal the puncture site.

PSEUDOANEURYSMS (PA)

A PA is a well-established complication associated with vascular access and commonly involves the CFA. A PA is defined as a pulsatile mass caused by extravasation of blood outside of the artery, which is confined by the surrounding soft tissues. Available evidence suggests that PA is a rather uncommon complication following diagnostic angiography occurring at rates of 0.7–2% (13,14). However, the PA rates associated with interventional procedures have been reported to occur with increasing intervals approaching 5.5–20% (14,15). This suggests that sheath size may predict PA formation; however, increasingly complex procedures requiring longer procedure times and anticoagulation may also contribute. Specifically, the use of protracted heparinization, post-sheath removal heparinization and the use of glycoprotein IIB/ IIIA inhibitors may additionally contribute to increased incidence.

The anatomy of a PA consists of a track or "neck" between the arterial wall and the extravascular accumulation of blood. The blood is confined in a "sac" which may be painful and pulsatile. While many PAs may be small and, therefore undetected and clinically insignificant, other PAs may expand in size and result in compression of other elements of a neurovascular bundle. Therefore, a large PA may result in thrombosis of the CFA artery, femoral nerve compression or neuropathic discomfort. A more serious complication relates to possible infection of the PA, PA sac rupture and the potential for distal embolization of thrombus contained within the PA into the distal SFA or infrapopliteal circulation.

A high index of clinical suspicion should always accompany the post-procedure inspection of the access site. Painful access sites associated with a pulsatile mass and an auscultated bruit over the site are typical clinical findings. However, any one of these findings may be absent and the patient may have only an extensive area of ecchymosis. An arterial duplex ultrasound should be performed. Arterial duplex ultrasonography is ideal in the diagnosis of a CFA pseudoaneurysm. By using standard commercially available ultrasound equipment and probes, the native artery is typically easily visualized. If the access site is particularly edematous, ecchymotic and associated with significant pain, intravenous analgesics should be administered. Typically, the extravasated blood contained in the PA "sac" is anterior to the artery with a classic "to-and-fro" waveform, which is pathognomonic of a PA (15) (Fig. 2). This represents the systolic flow out of the native artery into the PA sac and the backflow from the sac into the artery during diastole. Given the accessibility of duplex ultrasonography and its use in the management of a PA (see below), angiography is rarely needed for either diagnosis or treatment. Clearly, an additional arterial access site carries the risk of additional formation of a PA.

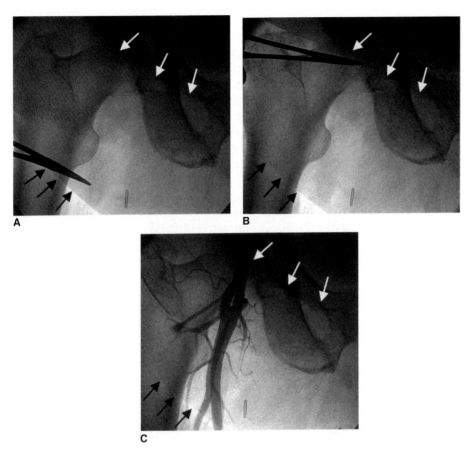

Figure 2 Do not use inguinal skin folds as a landmark to guide CFA access. (**A**) The use of the inguinal skin fold in this obese patient to guide location of the maximal pulsation would have resulted in puncture of the superficial femoral artery. (**B**) Target the CFA pulse by identifying the femoral head under fluoroscopy and placing a metallic instrument approximately 1 cm lateral to the medial edge of the femoral edge. The skin puncture should be made 1–2 cm below this point. (**C**) Note the relationship of the redundant skin fold (*white arrow*) and the inguinal skin fold (*black arrow*) to the CFA access site. *Abbreviation*: CFA, common femoral artery.

The management of PA must consider the size of the aneurysm and the associated patient symptomatology (pain, erythema, need for repeat access at a later date). Clearly, if a patient is to receive post-procedure anticoagulation or prolonged antithrombotic therapy (i.e., full dose aspirin and clopidogrel) even a small PA may be closed due to concern for subsequent expansion. In a large series of 196 PAs, 72 were observed without intervention while the remainder underwent either acute or delayed surgical intervention. Surgical intervention was prompted by a PA size ≥3 cm, expansion of the PA on follow-up duplex, limb ischemia, pain, possibility of infection, and need for long-term anticoagulation (17). Clearly, in an active or an obese patient, early intervention may be considered due to fear of further expansion. The 72 aneurysms observed in the trial which were managed conservatively, all thrombosed. There was a 3% perioperative complication rate in the patients who were managed surgically.

Surgical repair, while considered the "gold standard," carries the risk of local wound infection, requirement for discontinuation of parental anticoagulant or antithrombotic therapies (which may place patients with acute coronary syndromes at risk), wound dehiscence, and protracted discomfort. More recently, PAs have been successfully managed without surgery using a variety of compression devices in association with duplex ultrasonography. Several case series have reported the combined use of a "C-clamp" applied over the PA guided by ultrasound. After compression times approximating 30 minutes, PAs can be induced to thrombosis (16,18). However, the use of external compression devices in patients with large PAs, with a very painful edematous groin may not be ideal candidates for extrinsic compression. Other investigators used a combination of duplex ultrasonography and manual compression with improved results. In a large series of over 100 patients, ultrasound-guided manual compression was successful in 98% of the patients not receiving anticoagulation, and 86% of the patients receiving therapeutic heparinization (19).

The mean compression time was noted at 33 minutes; in PAs noted for more than 14 days, the mean compression time was prolonged to 51 minutes. Surgery still may be considered the gold standard in patients with very large PAs, those who will require follow-up anticoagulation where primary closure of the arterial site may be preferable.

More recently, a novel non-surgical intervention using arterial duplex ultrasound-guided thrombin injection has been reported (20–25). In this procedure, the PA sac is clearly defined by duplex ultrasonography and a 20-gauge 1.5-inch long needle on the end of a stop caulk is filled with agitated saline. Once the PA is identified by duplex ultrasonography and the size of the PA and distance from the center of the sac is defined, the skin overlying the PA is anesthetized. After adequate anesthesia, the 20-gauge needle is inserted into the PA sac; once the needle punctures the sac and intra-PA position documented by the injection of a small amount of agitated saline, a small amount (0.1–0.2 mL) of dilute bovine thrombin is injected repetitively into the sac under continuous imaging. After each injection, the physician should observe increasing thrombus formation within the sac (Figs. 3 and 4). Multiple aneurysm sacs should be injected individually. Once thrombosis of the sac has been demonstrated, the patient should be kept in a supine position for at least two hours, repeat duplex Doppler examination of the thrombosed aneurysm site should be completed within 24 hours to document persistent thrombosis of the PA. This procedure has been found to be relatively inexpensive as most hospitals have bovine thrombin available at a relatively nominal cost. Other instruments are disposable and reusable.

Using this methodology, several groups have reported successful series ranging from 93% to 99% (20–25). A multicenter series of 98 patients has suggested successful thrombosis in 91 patients. Importantly, this procedure may be used in complex multi-sac PAs and may be extended to the use in post-surgical PAs involving bypass grafts (20). Thrombotic complications have been reported using this methodology and include inadvertent native femoral artery thrombosis (25). However, this non-surgical, relatively inexpensive methodology is generally very safe in skilled experienced hands.

ARTERIOVENOUS FISTULA (AVF)

The incidence of iatogenic AVF is relatively infrequent with a reported incidence of 0.05–0.14% (26). However, these studies might underestimate the true incidence of AVF due to retrospective analyses of surgical data of patients referred for surgical

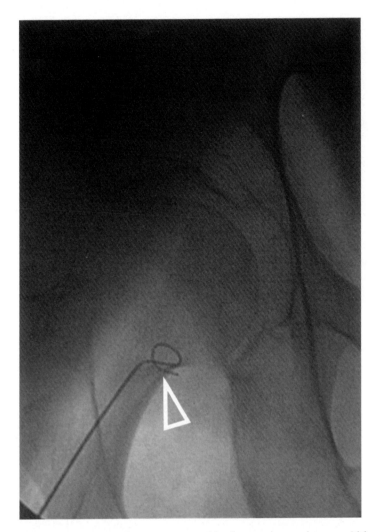

Figure 3 Do not advance access guidewires against resistance. Although the puncture site relative to fluoroscopic landmarks appears correct, the needle placement may be extravascular (posterior vessel wall) or subintimal. Forcing the guidewire may result in vessel dissection or perforation. The guidewire should be withdrawn and the access needle repositioned to follow the longitudinal axis of the artery.

intervention. A more recent prospective evaluation of over 10,000 patients after cardiac catheterization reported a 0.86% incidence of iatogenic AVF (27). This study also cited the risk factors for development of AVF to be similar for other groin complications including periprocedural heparin or coumadin therapy, hypertension, and the female gender. Interestingly, multivariate analysis identified left groin puncture as a risk factor for AVF formation; the authors hypothesized that the two-fold increase in AVF risk with the left groin puncture may be secondary to different angulation of the needle in an attempt to puncture the artery if the operator was standing on the patient's right-hand side in puncturing the left groin.

The most common sites of AVF formation are the superficial and deep femoral artery (Fig. 5). AVFs occur most readily when the artery is punctured below the

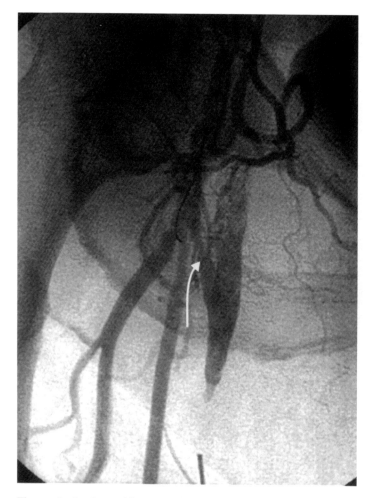

Figure 4 Angiographic appearance of a CFA-superficial femoral vein fistula. Note the direct communication between the artery and vein. This AVF was an incidental finding at the time of planned SFA intervention. *Abbreviations*: CFA, common femoral artery; AVF, arterial venous fistula.

bifurcation of the superficial femoral and profunda femoris arteries (28). Typically, at the level of the femoral head, the common femoral vein and CFA lie side-by-side; at the level of the bifurcation, the femoral vein is inferior to the artery and can be easily punctured. The force of blood from a high-pressure vessel to a lower pressure vessel causes bruit and is an important sign of both AVF formation and PA. Frequently, the AVF is asymptomatic and is incidentally identified on angiography or duplex ultrasound examination for other groin pathologies. They are easily identified by a palpable thrill or bruit; many fistula close spontaneously. However, the patient may experience pain and endovascular exclusion or surgical repair is required.

Femoral Neuropathy

Femoral neuropathy may occur after development of a large groin hematoma or PA; alternatively, femoral neuropathy may be a late complication from the chronic

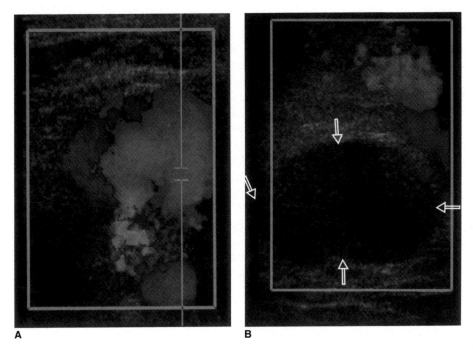

A   **B**

Figure 5 This color duplex ultrasound (shown here in gray scale) is diagnostic of a CFA PA. The classic "to-and-fro" appearance found in the PA "sac" is illustrated by the duplex color pattern (**A**). No color flow is observed in the PA "sac" confirming successful thrombosis after ultrasound-guided percutaneous thrombin injection (**B**). *Abbreviations*: CFA, common femoral artery; PA, pseudoaneurysm.

accumulation and irritation of the femoral nerve. Permanent neuropathy resulting in a foot drop, paresthesias, and chronic pain have been reported although the general incidence is low (29). The development of an iatogenic femoral artery PA may cause compression or irritation of cutaneous branches of the femoral nerve. Irritation, compression, or stretching of the anterior femoral cutaneous nerve may cause femoral neuralgia syndrome. Meralgia paresthetica, a mono-neuropathy of the lateral femoral cutaneous nerve, can lead to significant chronic discomfort, numbness, and dysesthesias involving the anterior lateral aspect of the extremity (30). Additional risk factors for the development of femoral neuropathy include excessive anticoagulation and the use of external groin compression devices (e.g., FemoStop, Bard Medical) to compress the groin after sheath removal. Most of the symptoms resolve once compressive force is relieved by treatment of the PA or resolution of the hematoma. Additionally, a more severe and potentially permanent neuropathy may occur as a consequence of a large retroperitoneal hematoma in which the femoral nerve is compressed resulting in weakness of the upper extremity and chronic pain in the thigh and calf (31).

COMPLICATIONS ASSOCIATED WITH VASCULAR CLOSURE DEVICES

The use of percutaneous vessel closure devices to manage common femoral arteriotomies continues to expand. It is estimated that 30% of all procedures requiring femoral access in the United States are closed with either a suture-mediated or collagen-based device (32). The advantage of these closure devices centers principally around patient comfort with shorter times to ambulation and early hospital discharge. Limiting the time of bed rest required may also increase angiography suite schedule flexibility, increase patient volumes, and reduce physician and ancillary staff requirements for manual compression. However, percutaneous closure devices are not without complications. The expanding use of these devices has resulted in the increased prevalence of a unique series of device-related complications which include infection, arterial thrombosis, and peripheral embolization (33–38). Therefore, the decision to use a closure device must weigh the benefits of patient comfort and staff/physician efficiency versus the small but apparent risk of a major complication.

The risks associated with manual compression persist with closure devices in elderly patients >65 years of age, female gender, diabetes, hypertension, small body size, previous catheterization within 30 days, and systemic anticoagulation (activated clotting time >300 seconds) (39). Additionally, obese diabetic patients with poor hygiene, the immuno-compromised host on chronic steroid therapy, or patients requiring long sheath dwell times warrant antibiotic prophylaxis or consideration of manual compression to avoid a potential increased risk of groin infections (36,38,40). The usual infectious organism is a Gram-positive cocci, similar to those with any arterial catheterization. The staphylococcal species may cause bacteremia, abscess formation, endocarditis, and endarteritis, which are associated with the presence of a foreign material within the arterial lumen (41,42).

Steps that angiographers/interventionalists should employ to reduce the incidence of infections include consideration of administration of prophylactic antibiotics, changing of gloves between the procedure and groin closure procedure, re-preparation of the groin site, use of a new sterile table, and irrigation of the groin with antibiotics (33). Kahn et al. (43) reported a large series using a suture-mediated device in which investigators routinely re-sterilized the access site, used new drapes and gloves and reported no infections in over 1000 closures.

The assessment of whether device design (suture closure versus collagen closure) may affect the efficacy and complication rates requires randomized head to head comparison. To date, however, there are few randomized trials amongst various devices. Furthermore, the rapid evolution of these devices with improved ease of use and reduced device complexity makes direct comparisons among the different closure devices difficult.

COMPLICATION PREVENTION

CFA Catheterizations

The CFA is the most frequent access site for angiography in part due to its proximity to the surface of the skin, its relatively large caliber and ability to accommodate angiographic tools and relative ease of compression against the femoral head. The CFA is contained within the femoral sheath and as such, periarterial bleeding is limited.

CFA percutaneous access is the essential initiating step to many diagnostic and therapeutic interventions. As the majority of complications in endovascular interventions are related to the access site, proficiency in percutaneous CFA access is essential. Access to the CFA should occur at the infrainguinal level. Higher suprainguinal punctures carry the risk of uncontrolled hemorrhage due to inability to use appropriate external compression due to the retroperitoneal location and obstruction to compression by the inguinal ligament. Likewise, lower punctures are associated with more complications as direct entry to the superficial femoral are more prone to AVF and PA formation.

The majority of CFA punctures are retrograde (against arterial blood flow) although antegrade punctures (in the direction of arterial blood flow) may be performed (Fig. 6). Ideally the CFA should be accessed over the mid- or lower 1/3 of the femoral head in order to facilitate compression at the termination of the procedure. Ideal methods for cannulation should combine manual compression to define the point of maximal impulse, presumably over the femoral head, and fluoroscopic visualization of the femoral head. Importantly, in large individuals, surface landmarks including the inguinal crease are unreliable, and therefore fluoroscopically guided localization of the CFA is ideal in these patients (Fig. 4). Using fluoroscopy, a metal instrument is placed on the skin at the anticipated point of access over the medial 1/3 of the femoral head. The entry site in the skin should be 1–1.5 cm below the intended entry site into the artery. In a difficult to palpate CFA, fluoroscopic guidance is essential; in these instances, the use of a Doppler-tipped needle (SMART Needle™) is ideal (Table 2). CFA related complications could be minimized by the use of anatomic landmarks to locate and guide CFA puncture. The CFA begins at the level of the inguinal ligament just inferior to the inferior epigastric artery and spans a line between the anterior superior iliac spine and the pubic symphysis (Fig. 6). Localization of the point of maximal pulsation of the CFA generally correlates with only

Table 2 Trouble-Shooting Difficult CFA Access

Challenge	Solution
Obese patient	– Use bony landmarks and fluoroscopy to identify the medial aspect of the femoral head. Locate the maximal arterial impulse and puncture 1–2 cm inferior to this point. – Use a Doppler-tipped needle (SMART Needle™) to locate the maximal arterial impulse.
Non-palpable artery	– Use bony and fluoroscopic landmarks and vessel wall calcification to locate the vessel at the level of the femoral head. – Use a Doppler-tipped needle (SMART Needle™, Peripheral Systems Group) to guide vessel location. – Consider direct sonographic localization with a 7.5-MHz ultrasound probe.
Inability to pass J-wire	– Inject a small amount of dilute contrast in through the puncture needle under fluoroscopy to define position. – Re-position the puncture needle to achieve pulsitile blood return and re-insert the J-wire. – Consider using a 5F micropuncture 0.018-inch wire system (Flexor™ Cook, Bloomington, Indiana) system. After access is achieved, exchange for a 0.035-inch 6F system.
Inability to insert femoral sheath	– Use a soft 4F dilator over the J-wire, then exchange for a 0.0350-inch extra-stiff J-wire – Use serial 4–6F dilators over the extra-stiff J-wire.

Abbreviations: CFA, common femoral artery.

(A)

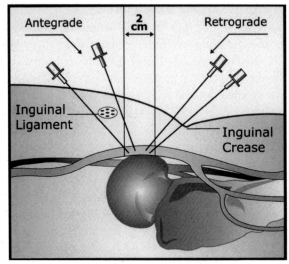

(B)

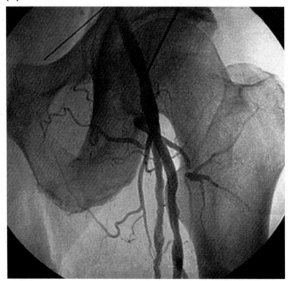

Figure 6 (**A**) The proper needle angles for retrograde and antegrade CFA punctures are illustrated. Both approaches target the CFA at the level of the femoral head. Note that proper antegrade puncture into the CFA is made below the level of the inguinal ligament and frequently requires a more acute angle of approach. (**B**) Prior to inserting the guidewire and sheath, angiographic verification of the puncture location is recommended to avoid unintended insertion into profunda femoris or superficial femoral arteries. *Abbreviations*: CFA, common femoral artery.

the CFA segment above the femoral head. However, in obese individuals and the elderly, the inguinal crease and fat creases are unreliable surface markers for the CFA.

In these instances, manual palpation to locate the common femoral segment should be confirmed under fluoroscopy. Using the inguinal crease or fat crease may result in puncture of the CFA or the deep femoral artery both of which are difficult to compress and may lead to a higher incidence of AVF and PAs.

Fluoroscopically guided identification of the femoral head in these patients is ideal. However, despite appropriate use of anatomical landmarks and fluoroscopic identification of the femoral head, improper needle angulation may place the puncture site above the inguinal ligament and into the external iliac artery (Fig. 7). In this instance, compression after sheath removal may also be problematic. Therefore, the importance of point compression with direct finger pressure must be emphasized.

The needle should be advanced slowly through the cutaneous nick at a 45° angle slowly until arterial pulsations are transmitted via the needle. The bevel of the needle should be slanted superiorly. Frequently, a slight resistance is encountered as the needle enters the vessel lumen. Ideally, blood flow should be pulsatile and vigorous. However, when blood flow through the needle does not correlate with the quality of the arterial pulsations, the needle tip may be partially transmural, encased in plaque or in the orifice of a small branch vessel. If this is encountered, the needle should be slowly withdrawn and reintroduced; alternatively, a soft J-wire may be introduced only if no resistance to the advancement of the wire is encountered. Gentle retraction of the needle and re-positioning of the tip may be required. When the guidewire will not advance freely, the needle should be fluoroscopically evaluated. Changing the alignment of the needle with the long access of the artery or slight alteration in the angle of the needle as it approaches the artery may be required.

If vigorous pulsatile flow is not achieved or a J-wire cannot be advanced, a small injection of dilute contrast using a non-lure lock syringe may be helpful in the localization of the needle tip. The use of a Doppler-tipped entry needle (SMART Needle™) to locate the point of maximal arterial flow may be helpful. Only after vigorous blood flow return should a J-wire be passed. Easy passage of the J-wire is essential; the J-wire should not be forced. The use of guidewires should be avoided during sheath placement.

Antegrade CFA puncture is frequently required in difficult situations including patients undergoing infrainguinal revascularization for long occlusive disease, patients with aortobifemoral bypass graft where a contralateral approach is ill-advised or in individuals with challenging contralateral around the "aortic bifurcation" access. In this situation, the documentation of landmarks and the fluoroscopically-visualized femoral head are essential. Antegrade puncture may be particularly difficult in obese individuals. Many of the same techniques in cannulating the CFA are similar to the retrograde approach (Fig. 6). However, particular attention should be paid to avoiding puncture of the external iliac artery, or superficial femoral, or profunda femoris. Visualization using a small amount of contrast prior to placement of an arterial sheath is important to avoid cannulazation of the SFA, PFA, or external iliac artery.

A "hostile groin" may be encountered as a result of multiple previous percutaneous or surgical procedures/scars or significant obesity. Importantly, if the distal anastomosis of an aortobifemoral bypass graft or the proximal anastomosis of a femoral-popliteal bypass graft is present, then ascertainment of the age of the graft, the graft material used, and the level of the vascular anastomosis is important. Many times, an arterial or synthetic graft can be punctured relatively soon after surgery, if necessary. Antibiotics are usually not necessary when puncturing a synthetic graft if entrance is uncomplicated and the sheath is removed promptly. In the post-surgical groin where significant scarring may be encountered, particularly when a CFA anastomosis is present, the use of extra-stiff guidewires (e.g., Amplatz™ wire) and serial vascular dilators may be required in order to place the femoral sheath.

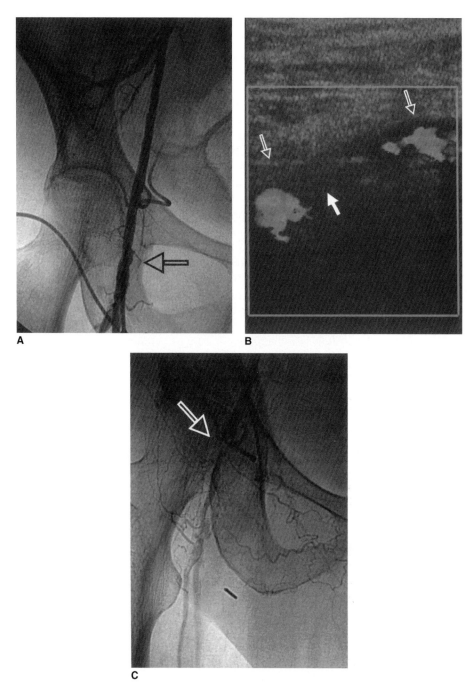

Figure 7 This patient developed lower extremity pain and numbness 18 hours after CFA access site closure with a collagen-mediated device. (**A**) Focal atherosclerotic plaguing is noted at the CFA puncture site on the screening angiogram prior to use of the closure device. (**B**) Color duplex ultrasound (shown here in gray scale) of the access site confirms sub-total CFA occlusion with flow within the arterial segment noted above and below the previous puncture site. (**C**) CFA angiography documented a high-grade eccentric lesion at the previous access site. Surgical exploration of the CFA repair confirmed a combination of atherosclerotic plaque and thrombus. Percutaneous closure devices should not be deployed in diseased arterial segments. *Abbreviation*: CFA, common femoral artery.

REFERENCES

1. Seldinger S. Catheter replacement of the needle in percutaneous arteriography. Acta Radiol 1953; 39:368–376.
2. Wiley J, White C, Uretsky B. Non-coronary complications of coronary interventions. Catheteriz Cardiovasc Interv 2002; 57:257–265.
3. Popma J, Satler L, Pichard A, et al. Vascular complications after balloon and new device angioplasty. Circulation 1993; 88:1569–1578.
4. Waksman R, King S, Douglas J, et al. Predictors of groin complications after balloon and new-device coronary interventions. Am J Cardiol 1995; 75:886–889.
5. Schomig A, Neumann F, Kastrati A, et al. A randomized comparison of antiplatelet and anticoagulant therapy after the placement of coronary-artery stents. N Engl J Med 1996; 334:1084–1089.
6. Leon M, Baim D, Popma JJ, et al. A clinical trial comparing three antithrombotic regimes after coronary-artery stenting: Stent Anticoagulation Restenosis Study Investigators. N Engl J Med 1998; 339:1665–1671.
7. EPILOG investigators. Platelet glycoprotein IIb/IIIa receptor blockade and low-dose heparin during percutaneous coronary revascularization. N Engl J Med 1997; 336: 1689–1696.
8. Dangas G, Mehran R, Koklois S, et al. Vascular complications after percutaneous coronary interventions following hemostasis with manual compression versus arteriotomy closure devices. J Am Coll Cardiol 2001; 38:638–641.
9. Sanborn T, Gibbs H, Brinker J, et al. A multicenter randomized trial comparing a percutaneous collagen hemostasis device with conventional manual compression after diagnostic angiography and angioplasty. J Am Coll Cardiol 1999; 22: 1273–1279.
10. Baim D, Knopf W, Hinohara T, et al. Suture-mediated closure of the femoral access site after cardiac catheterization: result of the suture to ambulate and discharge (STAND I and STAND II) trials. Am J Cardiol 2000; 85:864–869.
11. Kent K, Moscucci M, Mansour K, et al. Retroperitoneal hematoma after cardiac catheritezation: prevalence, risk factors, and optimal management. J Vasc Surg 1994; 20:905–911.
12. Sreeram S, Lumsden A, Miller J, et al. Retroperitoneal hematoma following femoral artery catheterization: a serious and often fatal complication. Am Surg 1993; 59:94–98.
13. Katzenschlager R, Ugurluoglu A, Ahmadi A, et al. Incidence of pseudoaneurysm after diagnostic and therapeutic angiography. Radiology 1995; 195:463–466.
14. Wyman R, Safian R, Portway V, et al. Current complications of diagnostic and therapeutic cardiac catheterization. Am Coll Cardiol 1988; 12:1400–1406.
15. Abu-Yousef M, Wiese J, Shamma R, et al. The "to-and-fro" sign: duplex Doppler evidence of femoral artery pseudoaneurysm. Am J Radiol 1988; 150:632–634.
16. Toursarkissian B, Allen B, Petrinec D, et al. Spontaneous closure of selected iatrogenic pseudoaneurysms and arteriovenous fistulas induced by arterial puncture. J Vasc Surg 1993; 17:125–133.
17. Coley B, Roberts A, Fellmeth D, et al. Postangiographic femoral artery pseudoaneurysms: further experience with US-guided compression repair. Radiology 1995; 194:307–311.
18. Agrawal S, Pinheiro L, Roubin G, et al. Nonsurgical closure of femoral pseudoaneurysms complicating cardiac catheterizations and percutaneous transluminal coronary angioplasty. J Am Coll Cardiol 1992; 20:610–615.
19. Cox G, Young J, Gray B, et al. Ultrasound-guided compression repair of postcatheterization pseudoaneurysms: results of treatment in one hundred cases. J Vasc Surg 1994; 19:683–686.

20. Mohler A, Mitchell M, Carpenter J, et al. Therapeutic thrombin injection of pseudoaneurysms: a multicenter experience. Vasc Med 2001; 6:241–244.

21. Gorge G, Kunz T. Thrombin injection for treatment of false aneurysms after failed compression therapy in patients on full-dose antiplatelet and heparin therapy. Catheteriz Cardiovasc Interv 2003; 58:505–509.

22. La Perna L, Olin J, Goines D, et al. Ultrasound-guided thrombin injection for the treatment of post-catheterization psuedoaneurysms. Circulation 2000; 102: 2391–2395.

23. Kang S, Labropoulos N, Mansour A, et al. Expanded indications for ultrasound-guided thrombin injection of pseudoaneurysms. J Vasc Surg 2000; 31:289–298.

24. Friedman S, Pellerito J, Scher L, et al. Ultrasound-guided thrombin injection is the treatment of choice for femoral pseudoaneurysms. Arch Surg 2002; 137:462–464.

25. Forbes T, Millward S. Femoral artery thrombosis after percutaneous thrombin injection of an external iliac artery pseudoaneuysm. J Vasc Surg 2001; 33:1093–1096.

26. Kim E, Orron D, Skillman J, et al. Role of superficial femoral artery puncture in the development of pseudoaneurysms and arteriovenous fistula complicating percutaneous transfemoral cardiac catheterizations. Catheteriz Cardiovasc Diagn 1992; 25: 91–100.

27. Perings S, Kelm M, Jax T, et al. A prospective study on incidence and risk factors of arteriovenous fistulae following transfemoral cardiac catheterization. Internat J Cardiol 2003; 88:223–228.

28. Sidway A, Neville R, Adib A, et al. Femoral artery arteriovenous fistula following cardiac catheterization: an anatomic explanation. Cardiovasc Surg 1993; 1:134–137.

29. Kent K, Moscucci M, Gallager S, et al. Neuropathy after cardiac catheterization: incidence, clinical patterns and long-term outcome. J Vasc Surg 1994; 19:1008–1014.

30. Bulter R, Webster M. Meralgia paresthetica: an unusual complication of cardiac catheterization via the femoral artery. Catheteriz Cardiovasc Interv 2002; 56: 69–71.

31. Hallett J, Wolk S, Cherry K, et al. The femoral neuralgia syndrome after arterial catheter trauma. J Vasc Surg 1990; 11:702–706.

32. Brown D. Current status of suture-mediated closure: what is the cost of comfort? J Vasc Interv Radiol 2003; 14:677–681.

33. Carey D, Martin J, Moore C, et al. Complications of femoral artery closure devices. Catheteriz Cardiovasc Interv 2001; 52:3–7.

34. Wagner S, Gonsalves C, Eschleman D, et al. Complications of a percutaneous suture-mediated device versus manual compression for arteriotomy closure: a case-controlled study. J Vasc Interv Radiol 2003; 14:735–741.

35. Wilson J, Johnson B, Parker J, et al. Management of vascular complications following femoral artery catheterization with and without percutaneous arterial closure device. Ann Vasc Surg 2002; 16:597–600.

36. Geary K, Landers J, Fiore W, et al. Management of infected femoral closure devices. Cardiovasc Surg 2002; 10:161–163.

37. Starnes B, O'Donnell S, Gellespie D, et al. Percutaneous arterial closure in peripheral vascular disease: a prospective randomized evaluation of the Perclose device. J Vasc Surg 2003; 38:263–271.

38. Hollis W, Rehring T. Femoral endarteritis associated with percutaneous suture closure: new technology, challenging complications. J Vasc Surg 2003; 38:83–87.

39. Hoffer E, Bloch R. Percutaneous arterial closure devices. J Vasc Interv Radiol 2003; 14: 865–885.

40. Nienaber C, Hamm C. Peripheral embolism of hemostasis collagen (Vasoseal). Z Kardiol 1992; 81:543–545.

41. Smith T, Cruz C, Mousi M, et al. Infectious complications resulting from use of hemostatic puncture closure devices. Am J Surg 2001; 182:658–662.

42. Rinder M, Tamirisa P, Taninchi M, et al. Safety and efficacy of suture-mediated closure after percutaneous coronary interventions. Catheteriz Cardiovasc Interv 2001; 54:146–151.
43. Kahn Z, Kumar M, Hollander G, et al. Safety and efficacy of the Perclose suture-mediated closure device after diagnostic and interventional catheterization in a large consecutive population. Catheteriz Cardiovasc Interv 2002; 55:8–13.

17

Complications of Infrapopliteal Endovascular Interventions

Gary M. Ansel

Peripheral Vascular Intervention, Section of Cardiology, Riverside Methodist Hospital, MidOhio Cardiology and Vascular Consultants, Columbus, Ohio and Department of Internal Medicine, Medical College of Ohio, Toledo, Ohio, U.S.A.

GENERAL

Percutaneous treatment for various manifestations of symptomatic peripheral vascular disease continues to be utilized at an escalating rate. Technological improvements and increasing operator experience are having a positive impact on patient options for the treatment of arterial occlusive disease.

The indications for endovascular treatment of the infrapopliteal arteries include limb salvage, failing bypass grafts due to compromised outflow, and rarely, claudication. As in every medical procedure, endovascular procedures carry an inherent risk of complication to the patient. This inherent risk for procedural complication is significantly elevated in patients undergoing tibial endovascular therapy due to the high prevalence of comorbidities such as diabetes, cerebrovascular disease, coronary artery disease, and renal insufficiency. Any therapeutic maneuver that is considered in this population needs to be low-risk since the five-year mortality in patients with limb-threatening ischemia approaches 50% (1). Thus, it is paramount that physician operators have the proper training, anticipation, and treatment insight as complications arise during these distal endovascular procedures.

The treatment of arterial occlusive disease present in patients with limb-threatening ischemia involving the infrapopliteal arterial bed is often complex. The atherosclerotic lesions found in patients with limb-threatening ischemia are associated with a high incidence of multilevel disease, long complex arterial occlusions, and diffuse lesion calcification. Technology directed to the successful treatment of infrapopliteal disease is usually limited to cardiac devices that were created for shorter lesions and even today, percutaneous angioplasty continues to be the mainstay of tibial artery endovascular therapy. There is, however, increasing yet undefined roles for more complex interventions such as cutting balloon angioplasty, atherectomy, laser, and stents.

There is a growing body of literature demonstrating efficacy of balloon angioplasty for the treatment of limb-threatening ischemia (2–4). However, much of this data comes from the treatment of focal tibial disease and there has been a reticence to proceed with percutaneous treatment of longer or more complex lesions (5). Some feel only 20–30% of patients with tibial disease have favorable anatomy suitable for endovascular treatment (2,6). However, since open surgical bypass carries a significant perioperative risk and increased metabolic demands to heal the surgical wound, the overall combined rates of death and amputation may be lowered with a percutaneous approach. Long-term success is dependent, however, on the development of careful surveillance with secondary interventions (7).

Complications of tibial intervention may occur both at the local intervention site as well as remote to the site of intervention. Major complications arising from tibial intervention have been reported in 2–6% of procedures (8). Limb salvage patients have shown a higher procedural complication rate compared to claudicants (9). The majority of tibial procedural complications appear to be centered around access site hematomas, dissection leading to acute vessel occlusion, and contrast nephropathy. However, as operators become more aggressive with endovascular limb salvage other types of possible complications must be anticipated and effectively managed. When endovascular complications do occur, over 86% are usually evident in the endovascular site (10). Periprocedural complications leading to amputation should be seen in <1% of procedures with major amputation usually limited to patients with pre-existing critical limb ischemia (11).

COMPLICATIONS

Contrast Nephropathy

With such a high prevalence of diabetes and hypertension in patients undergoing lower limb angiography and endovascular procedures the incidence of contrast-induced nephropathy is significantly increased. The incidence of contrast nephropathy may double when treating patients with limb-threatening ischemia (12). Patients that develop contrast-induced nephropathy are at increased risk of complications and mortality (13). Contrast nephropathy is characterized by the development of a quickly rising creatinine that often resolves within two to three weeks. This is in contrast to atheroembolic renal failure, which typically demonstrates a decline in renal function over several weeks.

When manifested, contrast-induced nephropathy is treated conservatively by keeping the patient well hydrated, blood pressure controlled, and discontinuing medication that could be nephrotoxic. The incidence of contrast nephropathy is decreased by preparing the patient with sufficient hydration and possibly by the periprocedural use of *n*-acetylcystine for those at risk (14).

Alternative imaging strategies may also be utilized to decrease the risk of contrast nephropathy by evaluating the patient's vascular anatomy as thoroughly as possible without the use of nephrotoxic dye. A thorough vascular exam, duplex scanning, and magnetic resonance imaging (MRA) may all play a role in limiting the nephrotoxic dye utilization. For example, a patient who is found on physical exam to have normal femoral and popliteal pulses, or duplex scanning showing lack of occlusive disease to the popliteal arteries may not need angiography of these vessels. Alternatively, though expensive, an MRA may be utilized for pre-procedural imaging of the arterial anatomy. Advancement of catheters through the various vascular beds while evaluating for evidence of significant hemodynamic pressure reduction can confirm the non-invasive findings. This technique often allows for

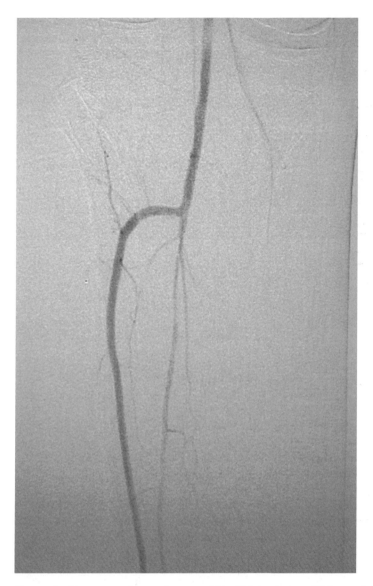

Figure 1   Representative angiogram of the tibial arteries utilizing gadolinium as the imaging agent. Injection was completed at the level of the popliteal artery through a 5-French catheter.

limited angiography of the tibial arteries. Alternatively, non-nephrotoxic imaging agents such as gadolinium may substitute for nephrotoxic dye for tibial angiography (15,16) (Fig. 1).

Access Site Complications

Access site bleeding, hematoma, psuedoaneurysm, and arteriovenous fistula may complicate tibial artery intervention. Factors that may predispose to access site complications include obesity, vessel wall calcification, advanced age, hypertension, and anticoagulation.

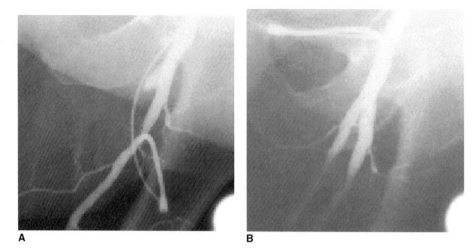

A   B

Figure 2 Antegrade sheath placement. (**A**) Angiogram demonstrating improper low insertion into the profunda femoral artery. (**B**) Repeat angiography after removal of improperly placed sheath with a suture-based closure device followed by proper placement of the sheath into the common femoral artery.

Traditionally, antegrade vascular access has often been felt to be the optimum access for tibial procedures. However, this access is associated with increased complications including retroperitoneal bleeding and errant positioning of the access sheath. Proper evaluation of the anticipated arterial puncture site with fluoroscopy may decrease inadvertently low or high punctures (Fig. 2). The use of the small diameter access needles with 0.018 wires to introduce sheaths may decrease the risk of local hematomas during antegrade vascular access. Recent experience appears to support the use of closure devices after antegrade access even after anticoagulation (17,18).

Improved technology such as non-kinking sheaths, guiding catheters, guidewires, and low profile balloons has allowed the majority of these procedures to now be performed from the lower risk contralateral femoral site. More recent downsizing of angioplasty devices now allows many of these procedures to be completed utilizing long 5-French sheaths acting as a guiding catheter.

LOCAL COMPLICATIONS

Dissection

The availability of stents has diminished the clinical impact of even large arterial dissections. Since these stents can effectively treat these dissections, most limb-threatening dissections occur either during guidewire placement or from unrecognized and untreated dissections after wire removal. Unlike the more proximal vascular beds, crossing clinically significant dissections from the opposite end of the dissection is rarely possible (Fig. 3). Coronary stents are commonly utilized for tibial artery dissections due to the lack of stents approved for tibial usage. The choice of appropriate stent can be debated. Certainly, self-expanding stents appear to be the most desirable since they cannot be crushed from outside forces. However, to date no

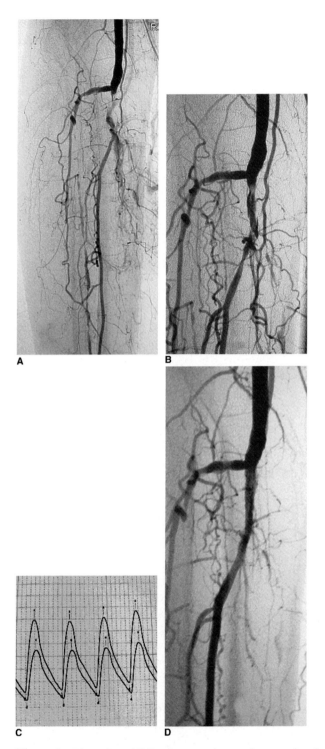

Figure 3   Dissection. (**A**) Pre-intervention angiogram showing total occlusion of the tibiope-roneal trunk. (**B**) Post-angioplasty: angiogram shows severe dissection. (**C**) Pressure gradient across dissection measured with 0.014 pressure wire. (**D**) Final result after placement of a coronary balloon expandable stent.

documented case of a tibial balloon expandable stent being crushed has been described and the technological advancements in these stents have far exceeded that of self-expanding stent technology. It has not been investigated whether there is a role for chemically covered stents such as heparin, polymer, and even drug eluting stents. Prevention of wire-induced dissection is possible by closely monitoring that the distal guidewire tip moves freely, and is always in true lumen. Sizing the balloon to native artery in appropriate fashion often allows for prevention of balloon-induced dissection.

Abrupt Thrombosis

Arterial thrombosis during angioplasty or stenting is usually due to inadequate anticoagulation or antiplatelet therapy, inadequate balloon angioplasty result, dissection, or unrecognized hypercoagulable condition. Thrombosis may also occur due to low flow state if the endovascular device, such as the guiding catheter, obstructs the arterial lumen. The patient will often present with acute deterioration in clinical status. Treatment is determined by the etiology. Dissection and inadequate luminal opening can be easily diagnosed with intravascular ultrasound and treated as described above with the placement of a stent. Inadequate heparin anticoagulation can be determined by evaluating the activated clotting at least every 60 minutes during long cases.

The prevention of subacute thrombosis has been thoroughly studied in the coronary intervention literature. Due to similar arterial diameters between coronary and tibial arteries this literature appears to be particularly relevant. Prevention of subacute thrombosis appears to be particularly low in patients treated with aspirin-plus-ticlopidine (19). It appears appropriate to recommend aspirin ticlopidine or clopidogrel for patients undergoing tibial artery intervention. The role for intravenous antiplatelet therapy such as the IIb/IIIa inhibitors awaits definition. However, there is emerging literature that supports its use especially for the treatment of visible thrombus (20).

Diagnosing an underlying hypercoagulable state first requires considering the diagnosis and then preceding to the appropriate diagnostic work-up.

Arterial Spasm

Arterial spasm rarely leads to serious complication during tibial angioplasty. However, when spasm occurs it may simulate dissection, making procedural evaluation difficult. Spasm should be prevented by routinely administering a vasodilator agent (nitroglycerine, papaverine, verapamil) intra-arterially prior to vessel intervention. Since tibial arteries are relatively straight, guidewire-induced spasm is rare.

Perforation/Rupture

Arterial perforation of the tibial arterial wall can occur from the guidewire or at the site of angioplasty/atherectomy. Overall perforation has been reported in 0–2.3% of patients undergoing endovascular procedures (9,21). Wire perforation out the side of the vessel is extremely rare unless the vessel is occluded and the wire is looped upon itself and being utilized to subintimally dissect through the total occlusion (Fig. 4). This type of perforation rarely leads to the need for surgical intervention and should be self-limited. If the wire cannot be quickly advanced into the true lumen, the next

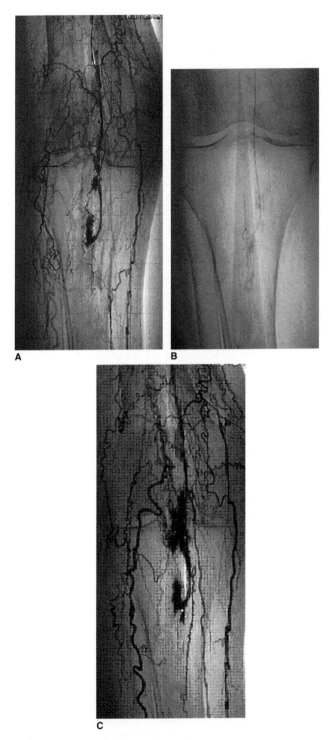

Figure 4   Perforation (**A**) Pre-intervention angiogram showing total occlusion of the distal popliteal artery. (**B**) Hydrophilic wire (0.018) looped and passing through occlusion. (**C**) Perforation of vessel with limited extravasation of contrast.

treatment response for this type of wire perforation is anticoagulation reversal followed by abandoning the procedure. However, if one is able to have the wire traverse the lesion, prolonged balloon inflation or implantation of a bare metal or polytetrafluoroethylene (PTFE)-covered stent can be utilized to seal the perforation. The other and most frequent etiology leading to guidewire perforation is the inadvertent traversal of the wire through a fragile collateral vessel. Here the clinical risk is frequently self-limited.

Balloon- or atherectomy-induced perforation with frank arterial wall rupture is of more concern since the vessel disruption is usually more significant. The etiology of balloon-induced perforation is frequently due to inappropriate over-sizing of the balloon, vessel calcification or ablative techniques that do not stay intraluminal such as laser or atherectomy. The treatment of vessel disruption ranges from prolonged balloon inflation with reversal of anticoagulation for small perforations to the placement of a PTFE covered coronary-sized stent for larger vessel rupture.

Sizing of the angioplasty balloon to a 1:1 ratio with the native vessel and predilation with an under-sized balloon in heavily calcified arteries may decrease the incidence of vessel perforation. Gentle advancement of ablative techniques decreases the likelihood of extravascular device placement.

Distal Embolization

Distal embolization to the distal tibial or pedal arteries may lead to significant symptoms, tissue loss or amputation. The etiology of embolization includes inadequate anticoagulation leading to thrombotic debris in the sheath or guiding catheter, as well as thrombus or atheromatous debris originating from the intervention site itself. Predisposing factors include inadequate anticoagulation, fresh thrombus at the arterial stenosis, and arterial ulceration. A recent increase in patient's symptoms is often a good clinical clue that a stenosis may contain significant thrombus. Athetherectomy devices may also increase the risk of distal embolization.

Cholesterol embolization is currently managed conservatively. However, the management of thrombotic distal embolization includes the use of catheter thrombectomy, mechanical thrombectomy, thrombolysis, and as last resort surgical thrombectomy. In the face of resistant debris, stenting of the debris against the arterial wall and re-establishing flow may be a useful maneuver.

The prevention of embolization includes adequate periprocedural anticoagulation and pre-angioplasty thrombolysis of acute lesions. The use of IIb/IIIa agents during rotational atherectomy has shown to significantly decrease the incidence of slow flow during coronary artery procedures, and appears justified during the use of this device in the tibial vessels as well (22).

Restenosis

Restenosis of tibial endovascular procedures appears to be high. Certainly, the length of lesion, presence of diabetes, and arterial vessel diameter are predictors of restenosis. However, when the procedural end point is limb salvage, restenosis does not appear to be a major limiting factor as long as the management includes scheduled non-invasive surveillance of the distal limb. Reintervention is usually effective in treating restenosis and maintaining clinical benefit. Whether restenosis of tibial vessels would benefit from radiation therapy as seen in the coronary vasculature is open to speculation (23).

CONCLUSION

Historically the use of endovascular procedures for the treatment of tibial arterial occlusive disease has been limited for fear of a complication leading to limb loss. This fear appears to be outdated. Adequate education leading to awareness of the complications inherent in this particular vascular bed, as well as the ability and training to recognize and treat complications should they occur, will allow for tibial intervention to be offered to patients at low risk with good clinical outcome.

REFERENCES

1. Veith FJ, Gupta SK, Wengerter KR, Goldsmith J, Rivers SP, Bakal CW, Dietzek AM, Cynamon J, Sprayregen S, Gliedman ML. Changing arteiosclerotic disease patterns and management strategies in lower-limb-threatening ischemia. Ann Surg 1990; 212(4): 402–414.
2. Schwarten DE, Cutliff WB. Arterial occlusive disease below the knee: treatment with percutaneous transluminal angioplasty performed with low-profile catheters and steerable guide wires. Radiology 1988; 169:71–74.
3. Bull PG, Mendel H, Hold M, Schlegl A, Denck H. Distal popliteal and tibioperoneal transluminal angioplasty: long-term follow-up. J Vasc Interv Radiol 1992; 3:45–53.
4. Wagner HJ, Klose KJ. Infrapopliteal angioplasty for limb-salvage: a 4-year experience. J Vasc Interv Radiol 1997; 8(suppl):247.
5. Criado FJ, Twena M, Abdul-Khoudoud O, Al-Soufi B. Below-knee angioplasty: misguided aggressiveness or reasonable opportunity? J Invasive Cardiol 1998; 10:415–424.
6. Bakal CW, Cynamon J, Sprayregen S. Infrapopliteal percutaneous transluminal angioplasty: what we know. Radiology 1996; 200:3–43.
7. Varty K, Bolia A, Naylor AR, Bell PR, London NJ. Infrapopliteal percutaneous transluminal angioplasty: a safe and successful procedure. Eur J Vasc Endovasc Surg 1995; 9:341–345.
8. Wagner HH, Rager G. Infrapopliteal angioplasty: a forgotten region? Rofo Fortschr Geb Rontgenstr Neuen Bildgeb Verfahr 1998; 168(5):415–420.
9. Matsi PJ, Manninen HI. Complications of lower-limb percutaneous transluminal angioplasty: a prospective analysis of 410 procedures on 295 consecutive patients. Cardiovasc Interv Radiol 1998; 21:361–366.
10. Burns BJ, Phillips AJ, Fox A, Boardman P, Phillips-Hughes J. The timing and frequency of complications after peripheral percutaneous transluminal angioplasty and iliac stenting: is a change from inpatient to outpatient therapy feasible? Cardiovasc Interv Radiol 2000; 23:452–456.
11. Axisa B, Fishwick G, Bolia A. Complications following peripheral angioplasty. Ann R Coll Surg Engl 2002; 84:39–42.
12. Strodon P, Matson M, Ham R. Contrast nephropathy in lower limb angiography. Ann R Coll Surg Engl 2003; 85:187–191.
13. Mintz EP, Gruberg L. Radiocontrast-induced nephropathy and percutaneous coronary intervention: a review of preventive measures. Expert Opin Pharmacother 2003; 4:639–652.
14. Baker CS, Wragg A, Kumar S, DePalma R, Baker LR, Knight CJ. A rapid protocol for the prevention of contrast-induced renal dysfunction: the RAPID study. J Am Coll Cardiol 2003; 41:2114–2118.
15. Sam AD 2nd, Morasch MD, Collins J, Song G, Chen R, Pereles FS. Safety of gadolinium contrast angiography in patients with chronic renal insufficiency. J Vasc Surg 2003; 38:313–318.
16. Sarkis A, Badaoui G, Jebara VA. Indications for gadolinium for coronary angiography. J Thorac Cardiovasc Surg 2003; 125(5):1170.

17. Duda SH, Wiskirchen J, Erb M, Schott U, Khaligi K, Pereira PL, Albes Claussen CD. Suture-mediated percutaneous closure of antegrade femoral arterial access sites in patients who have received full anticoagulation therapy. Radiology 1999; 210:47–52.
18. Khosla S, Kunjummen B, Guerrero M, Manda R, Razminia M, Ahmed A. Suture-mediated closure of antegrade femoral arteriotomy following infrainguinal intervention. Catheteriz Cardiovasc Interv 2002; 57:504–507.
19. Zidar JP. Rationale for low-molecular weight heparin in coronary stenting. Am Heart J 1997; 134(suppl):S81–S87.
20. Tong FC, Cloft HJ, Joseph GJ, Samuels OB, Dion JE. Abciximab rescue in acute carotid stent thrombosis. Am J Neuroradiol 2000; 21:1750–1752.
21. Morris CS, Bonnevie GJ, Najarian KE. Nonsurgical treatment of acute iatrogenic renal artery injuries occurring after renal artery angioplasty and stenting. Am J Roentgenol 2001; 177:1353–1357.
22. Kini A, Reich D, Marmur JD, Mitre CA, Sharma SK. Reduction in periprocedural enzyme elevation by abciximab after rotational atherectomy of type B2 lesions: results of the Rota ReoPro randomized trial. Am Heart J 2001; 142:965–969.
23. Stankovic G, Orlic D, Di Mario C, Corvaja N, Airoldi F, Chieffo A, Amato A, Orecchia R, Colombo A. Beta-radiation therapy for long lesions in native coronary vessels. A matched comparison between de novo and in-stent restenotic lesions. Cardiovasc Radiat Med 2003; 4(1):18–24.

18
Complications in Endovascular Therapy: Atherosclerotic Thoracic Aneurysm Repair

Sean P. Lyden
Department of Vascular Surgery, The Cleveland Clinic Foundation, Cleveland, Ohio, U.S.A.

Complications from endovascular repair of thoracic aneurysms can result from patient-related anatomy or device design issues. Complications can arise at the time of device delivery and placement, or during follow-up. Currently, no endoluminal graft (ELG) has been approved by the United States Food and Drug Administration to treat thoracic aortic disease. However, several devices exist in different stages of development. The AneuRx® (Medtronic AVE, Santa Rosa, California), Vanguard® (Boston Scientific, Natick, Massachusetts), and Corvita®(Boston Scientific, Natick, Massachusetts) thoracic ELGs have been in trials but development of these devices has stopped (1,2). Three devices currently under investigation in the United States and commercially available in Europe include the Thoracic Excluder® (W.L. Gore, Flagstaff, Arizona), Talent Thoracic® (Medtronic AVE, Santa Rosa, California), and Cook Thoracic endograft® (Cook, Bloomington, Indiana). Prior to initiation of trials with the aforementioned devices, many thoracic aneurysms were repaired with homemade devices, similar to that originally described by Dake (3–5). In the absence of published results from multicenter trials, defining and understanding complications from endovascular treatment of thoracic aortic aneurysm repair is relegated to review of individual reported series.

Thoracic ELGs have been used to treat both elective and ruptured thoracic aneurysms, traumatic aortic rupture, penetrating thoracic ulcers and complications of aortic dissection. Most single center case series do not discriminate results among treatment indications and combine all of these disease processes. Due to markedly differing pathophysiology, potential complications may not be similar across the various disease processes. In addition, many series do not distinguish the device associated with a complication when multiple devices were used.

Current delivery systems for thoracic ELG designs are between 20 French (F) and 27F diameters. These large devices can make passage of the ELG into the thoracic aorta a difficult problem and create complications. Vessel size and morphology can make transfemoral or even transiliac introduction of these devices impossible. Attempts to deliver an ELG through a vessel too small to accommodate the delivery system can induce dissection or rupture. Extensive medial calcification, such as that seen in patients with end stage renal disease or diabetes, increases the difficulty in obtaining access to the aorta. Since women tend to have smaller diameter vessels than men, this has led to a decreased ability to treat women and a higher prevalence of access vessel complications (6). Several case series have documented iliofemoral access-related complications in up to 28% of patients (1,2,5). Prompt recognition of access vessel injury during placement of thoracic ELG may allow endovascular salvage of the vessel using stents or stent grafts (7,8). Open repairs of damaged vessels are also frequently required. Preoperative identification of potential access difficulties is possible with scrutiny of contrast enhanced and non-contrast computerized tomography scans, in addition to liberal use of calibrated angiography and intravascular ultrasonography. Once potential access issues are identified, such as small, stenotic, or circumferentially calcified iliac arteries, consideration should be given to delivering the device through an iliac conduit. Use of iliac conduits does not increase mortality in treating abdominal aortic aneurysms with ELGs (9), and has been described in conjunction with thoracic ELGs (10,11). Once access to the aorta is achieved, complications in access can still occur due to difficulty in delivering the device across the arch. Increase in aortic length during aneurysm formation occasionally creates sharp angles at the junction of the arch and descending thoracic aorta as well as at the junction of the thoracic and abdominal aorta. Brachial-femoral through and through access is sometimes required to overcome these issues and to push a device across the arch of the aorta (12). Deployment of the sheathed devices becomes increasingly more difficult with each bend of the arterial tree crossed in reaching the intended site of implantation. Of the three commercial devices currently in use, there is marked variation in the delivery systems. The Gore Thoracic Excluder device is not manufactured within a sheath and is a very flexible design. In comparison, the Talent thoracic device is a very stiff design (7). The inflexible delivery systems may hinder access into the arch.

Distal migration during deployment can occur due to a 'windsock' phenomenon. This phenomenon is created by arterial flow pushing on only a partially opened stent graft. This problem is most pronounced when using homemade ELGs. Lowering the mean arterial pressure during deployment or inducing asystole with adenosine has been used to minimize the risk of windsock-induced migration (13–20). Design modifications to commercial devices have attempted to eliminate or minimize this problem. For example, the Gore Excluder starts to deploy from the midpoint of the device and progresses simultaneously both proximally and distally. This design lessens but does not eliminate problems from windsock. Fixation of the device to the delivery system can avoid distal migration and has been incorporated into the Cook thoracic design (4).

Atheroembolization to the cerebral, mesenteric, renal, spinal, and distal circulation may also occur with device introduction, deployment, and balloon dilatation (1,2). Avoiding balloon dilatation in the thoracic aorta may decrease the risk of atheroembolization (4). Shaggy, mobile, or circumferential thrombus increases the risk of atheroembolization, and avoiding use of thoracic ELGs in this setting may be the only means to eliminate this complication. Future prevention of embolization risk will require significant design modifications to existing devices in order to lower the delivery profile and to improve trackability.

Spinal cord ischemia has been an Achilles heel after open repair of thoracic aneurysms (21–23). Some had hoped thoracic endografts could avoid spinal cord complications by eliminating the hemodynamic alterations induced by an aortic cross-clamp (24). Yet, paraplegia does occur after ELG repair (25). A recent review cited a 1.6% incidence of paralysis in approximately 3000 worldwide cases (26). Several risk factors for the development of spinal cord ischemia have been identified. These risk factors include coverage of a long segment of the thoracic aorta with resultant loss of intercostal collaterals to the anterior spinal artery, coverage of the artery of Adamkiewicz, and prior infrarenal aortic repair (4,27,28). Drainage of cerebrospinal fluid (CSF) has been shown to reduce the risk of paraplegia in open thoracic aneurysm repair (21,22,29). Successful treatment of paralysis after thoracic ELG with CSF drainage has been reported (30–33). CSF is only used in approximately half of the reported series, and is not universally accepted as a necessary surgical adjunct to ELG repair (5–7,25,28,34). Use of somatosensory evoked potentials to predict spinal cord ischemia has also been suggested but is seldom practiced in endovascular repair (35).

Defining the risk of perioperative death for thoracic ELGs is confounded by the inclusion of ruptured aneurysms in most case series. Mortality reported for endovascular thoracic aneurysm repair has ranged from 0% to 20% (2,4,27). Emergently treated patients consistently fair worse in all series which separate out results of elective and emergent repair. It is generally believed that mortality is less with ELG than open thoracic aneurysm repair. The long-term risk of aneurysm-related death in this population remains unknown.

Success after thoracic ELG placement requires fixation to the aorta and exclusion of flow and pressure into the aneurysm sac. The inability to exclude the aneurismal segment of the aorta is a known complication of all endograft techniques. Although endoleaks were originally used to describe patterns of flow into abdominal aortic aneurysms, this classification has been applied to the thoracic aorta (36,37). Type I endoleaks are due to lack of seal at the proximal or distal fixation sites (Fig. 1). Type II endoleaks are due to branch vessel flow. Possible sources of Type II endoleaks are the subclavian artery, intercostal arteries, or the visceral vessels. Type III endoleaks are due to modular disconnections, flow between fabric pieces or fabric disruption. Type IV endoleaks are from fabric porosity within the first 30 days of implantation.

There are many possible etiologies of Type I endoleaks in thoracic ELGs. The degree of oversizing, relative to the native arterial circulation is critical. Oversizing between 10% and 20% is believed to create sufficient radial force in which to seal and avoid fabric infolding from excessive oversizing. The outward radial force generated by self-expanding stents is determined by stent diameter, height, strut thickness, and the amount of oversizing relative to the aorta. As a result of the large stent diameters used in thoracic ELGs, a larger percentage of Type I endoleaks as compared to that found with abdominal endografts might be anticipated. One series documented a Type I endoleak in 17.8% of patients (2). Yet, this high rate of Type I endoleaks has not been seen in most series. Angulation at the proximal or distal fixation site is another potential etiology of a Type I endoleak (30). The curvature of the arch of the aorta may not allow for any parallel segment in the aorta for good stent apposition to achieving a seal. Techniques to prevent Type I endoleaks include using extension cuffs to increase aortic coverage, increase radial force or increase oversizing. Another option is to deploy balloon expandable stents to increase the radial force and straighten the aorta.

Type II endoleaks have been found infrequently in thoracic endovascular aneurysm repair. Treatment of a thoracic Type II endoleak has not been reported. Intercostal endoleaks may not be treatable with microcatheter techniques due to the lack of adequate collateral pathways to access the space. Transthoracic puncture of the aneurysm sac, similar to the translumbar approach described for abdominal

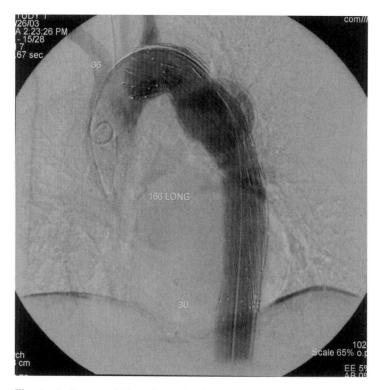

Figure 1 Image of Type I proximal endoleak after Cook thoracic endograft. This angio demonstrates flow into the aneurysm sac from the proximal attachment site and around the left subclavian orifice. The endoleak excluded by ligation of the proximal subclavian artery and carotid to subclavian artery bypass.

aneurysm endoleak management (38), may be a potential route to treat intercostal artery endoleaks.

The forces applied on a thoracic ELG due to aortic pressure are much greater than what occurs on abdominal aortic ELGs. The downward force creates a risk of migration at fixation sites or between components (25) (Fig. 2). Surveillance of the proximal and distal attachment site is needed to identify failure of the fixation mechanism. One study by Ellozy et al. found either a proximal or distal attachment site failure in 14% of patients (39). In order to avert this complication, a minimum of 20 mm of normal aorta at the proximal and distal seal zones is recommended. A minimum of 5 cm of overlap between components is also advocated to avoid modular disconnections and Type III endoleaks between components. Homemade devices have been associated with the highest degree of migration (4).

Device integrity is a common concern to all devices in the long term. This is the reason life-long surveillance is necessary. Prompt recognition allows the potential to salvage thoracic ELG prior to development of complications. Fabric and metal fractures have been identified in abdominal aneurysms and should be expected to eventually occur in thoracic ELGs as well (40,41). Fracture of the longitudinal nitinol wire, both the Gore thoracic Excluder device and Talent thoracic device, have been seen in up to 30% of implants (6). Modifications to the design of the Gore thoracic device to eliminate the longitudinal nitinol wire were implemented after

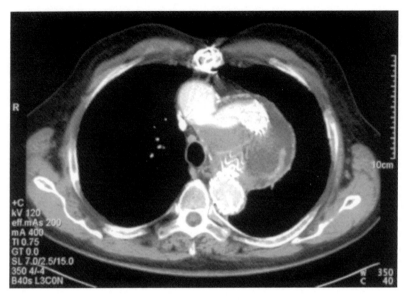

Figure 2 Image of proximal Type I endoleak. This endoleak is due to migration of a Gore thoracic endograft into the aneurysm sac.

identification of this complication. Stent strut fractures have also been identified with the Talent thoracic device. As the aortic forces exerted on thoracic ELGs are studied and better understood, design changes may eliminate material fatigue.

Prevention of aneurysm rupture is the goal in treatment of thoracic ELGs. As with abdominal ELGs, the risk of late aneurysm rupture is not eliminated by thoracic ELGs (4,39). Due to the rarity of aneurysm rupture, sac diameter stability or shrinkage has been used as a surrogate endpoint to define successful outcome. Whereas most believe that continued growth of the aneurysm sac in the absence of endoleak represents a complication and failure of the treatment, the etiology of the aneurysm growth and the associated risk of rupture in these circumstances are unknown. Changes in aneurysm diameter and the resultant complications that arise due to either shrinkage (such as device migration or kinking) or expansion will likely be device-specific as found with abdominal ELGs (42). Late erosion into adjacent structures such as the esophagus or bronchus has also been reported (27,43).

Complications of thoracic aneurysm repair may occur at the time of device placement or later. Some complications are the result of patient-specific anatomic challenges and can be minimized by good preoperative planning. Late complications are rare due to short follow-up in most series. As future generations of thoracic stent grafts are developed and enter clinical practice, new unrecognized complications will undoubtedly develop even as current complications are eliminated.

REFERENCES

1. White RA, Donayre CE, Walot I, Lippmann M, Woody J, Lee J, Kim N, Kopchok GE, Fogarty TJ. Endovascular exclusion of descending thoracic aortic aneurysms and chronic dissections: initial clinical results with the AneuRx device. J Vasc Surg 2001; 33(5): 927–934.

2. Scharrer-Pamler R, Kotsis T, Kapfer X, Gorich J, Orend KH, Sunder-Plassmann L. Complications after endovascular treatment of thoracic aortic aneurysms. J Endovasc Ther 2003; 10(4):711–718.

3. Dake MD, Miller DC, Semba CP, Mitchell RS, Walker PJ, Liddell RP. Transluminal placement of endovascular stent-grafts for the treatment of descending thoracic aortic aneurysms. N Engl J Med 1994; 331(26):1729–1734.

4. Greenberg R, Resch T, Nyman U, Lindh M, Brunkwall J, Brunkwall P, Malina M, Koul B, Lindblad B, Ivancev K. Endovascular repair of descending thoracic aortic aneurysms: an early experience with intermediate-term follow-up. J Vasc Surg 2000; 31(1 Pt 1):147–156.

5. Cambria RP, Brewster DC, Lauterbach SR, Kaufman JL, Geller S, Fan CM, Greenfield A, Hillgenberg A, Clouse WD, Evolving experience with thoracic aortic stent graft repair. J Vasc Surg 2002; 35(6):1129–1136.

6. Najibi S, Terramani TT, Weiss VJ, Mac Donald MJ, Lin PH, Redd DC, Martin LG, Chaikof EL, Lumsden AB. Endoluminal versus open treatment of descending thoracic aortic aneurysms. J Vasc Surg 2002; 36(4):732–737.

7. Criado FJ, Clark NS, Barnatan MF. Stent graft repair in the aortic arch and descending thoracic aorta: a 4-year experience. J Vasc Surg 2002; 36(6):1121–1128.

8. Alric P, Berthet JP, Branchereau P, Veerapen R, Marty-Ane CH. Endovascular repair for acute rupture of the descending thoracic aorta. J Endovasc Ther 2002; 9(suppl 2): II51–II59.

9. Abu-Ghaida AM, Clair DG, Greenberg RK, Srivastava S, O'Hara PJ, Ouriel K. Broadening the applicability of endovascular aneurysm repair: the use of iliac conduits. J Vasc Surg 2002; 36(1):111–117.

10. Yano OJ, Faries PL, Morrissey N, Teodorescu V, Hollier LH, Marin ML. Ancillary techniques to facilitate endovascular repair of aortic aneurysms. J Vasc Surg 2001; 34(1): 69–75.

11. Macdonald S, Byrne D, Rogers P, Moss JG, Edwards RD. Common iliac artery access during endovascular thoracic aortic repair facilitated by a transabdominal wall tunnel. J Endovasc Ther 2001; 8(2):135–138.

12. Al Shammari M, Taylor P, Reidy JF. Use of through-and-through guidewire for delivering large stent-grafts into the distal aortic arch. Cardiovasc Interv Radiol 2000; 23(3): 237–238.

13. Baker AB, Bookallil MJ, Lloyd G. Intentional asystole during endoluminal thoracic aortic surgery without cardiopulmonary bypass. Br J Anaesth 1997; 78(4):444–448.

14. Bernard EO, Schmid ER, Lachat ML, Germann RC. Nitroglycerin to control blood pressure during endovascular stent-grafting of descending thoracic aortic aneurysms. J Vasc Surg 2000; 31(4):790–793.

15. Diethrich EB. A safe, simple alternative for pressure reduction during aortic endograft deployment. J Endovasc Surg 1996; 3(3):275.

16. Dorros G, Cohn JM. Adenosine-induced transient cardiac asystole enhances precise deployment of stent-grafts in the thoracic or abdominal aorta. J Endovasc Surg 1996; 3(3):270–272.

17. Tanito Y, Endou M, Koide Y, Okumura F. ATP-induced ventricular asystole and hypotension during endovascular stenting surgery. Can J Anaesth 1998; 45(5 Pt 1):491–494.

18. Weigand MA, Motsch J, Bardenheuer HJ. Adenosine-induced transient cardiac arrest for placement of endovascular stent-grafts in the thoracic aorta. Anesthesiology 1998; 89(4):1037–1038.

19. Weigand MA, Schumacher H, Allenberg JR, Bardenheuer HJ. [Adenosine-induced heart arrest for endovascular reconstruction of thoracic aneurysms of the aorta]. Anasthesiol Intensivmed Notfallmed Schmerzther 1999; 34(6):372–375.

20. White GH. Transient asystole for aortic endograft deployment: a technique justified only in highly selected cases. J Endovasc Surg 1996; 3(3):273–274.

21. Coselli JS, Lemaire SA, Koksoy C, Schmittling ZC, Curling PE. Cerebrospinal fluid drainage reduces paraplegia after thoracoabdominal aortic aneurysm repair: results of a randomized clinical trial. J Vasc Surg 2002; 35(4):631–639.

22. Svensson LG, Khitin L, Nadolny EM, Kimmel WA. Systemic temperature and paralysis after thoracoabdominal and descending aortic operations. Arch Surg 2003; 138(2):175–179.

23. Coselli JS, LeMaire SA, Schmittling ZC, Koksoy C. Cerebrospinal fluid drainage in thoracoabdominal aortic surgery. Semin Vasc Surg 2000; 13(4):308–314.

24. Orend KH, Scharrer-Pamler R, Kapfer X, Kotsis T, Gorich J, Sunder-Plassmann L. Endovascular treatment in diseases of the descending thoracic aorta: 6-year results of a single center. J Vasc Surg 2003; 37(1):91–99.

25. Bell RE, Taylor PR, Aukett M, Sabharwal T, Reidy JF. Mid-term results for second-generation thoracic stent grafts. Br J Surg 2003; 90(7):811–817.

26. Dake MD. Endovascular stent-graft management of thoracic aortic diseases. Eur J Radiol 2001; 39(1):42–49.

27. Dake MD, Miller DC, Mitchell RS, Semba CP, Moore KA, Sakai T. The "first generation" of endovascular stent-grafts for patients with aneurysms of the descending thoracic aorta. J Thorac Cardiovasc Surg 1998; 116(5):689–703; discussion 703–704.

28. Gravereaux EC, Faries PL, Burks JA, Latessa V, Spielvogel D, Hollier LH, Marin ML. Risk of spinal cord ischemia after endograft repair of thoracic aortic aneurysms. J Vasc Surg 2001; 34(6):997–1003.

29. Crawford ES, Svensson LG, Hess KR, Shenaq SS, Coselli JS, Safi HJ, Mohindra PK, Rivera V. A prospective randomized study of cerebrospinal fluid drainage to prevent paraplegia after high-risk surgery on the thoracoabdominal aorta. J Vasc Surg 1991; 13(1):36–45; discussion 45–46.

30. Ortiz-Gomez JR, Gonzalez-Solis FJ, Fernandez-Alonso L, Bilbao JI. Reversal of acute paraplegia with cerebrospinal fluid drainage after endovascular thoracic aortic aneurysm repair. Anesthesiology 2001; 95(5):1288–1289.

31. Tiesenhausen K, Amann W, Koch G, Hausegger KA, Oberwalder P, Rigler B. Cerebrospinal fluid drainage to reverse paraplegia after endovascular thoracic aortic aneurysm repair. J Endovasc Ther 2000; 7(2):132–135.

32. Fleck T, Hutschala D, Weissl M, Wolner E, Grabenwoger M. Cerebrospinal fluid drainage as a useful treatment option to relieve paraplegia after stent-graft implantation for acute aortic dissection type B. J Thorac Cardiovasc Surg 2002; 123(5):1003–1005.

33. Fuchs RJ, Lee WA, Seubert CN, Gelman S. Transient paraplegia after stent grafting of a descending thoracic aortic aneurysm treated with cerebrospinal fluid drainage. J Clin Anesth 2003; 15(1):59–63.

34. Thompson CS, Gaxotte VD, Rodriguez JA, Ramaiah VG, Vranic M, Ravi R, Di Mugno L, Shafique S, Olsen D, Diethrich EB. Endoluminal stent grafting of the thoracic aorta: initial experience with the Gore Excluder. J Vasc Surg 2002; 35(6):1163–1170.

35. Bafort C, Astarci P, Goffette P, El Khoury G, Guerit JM, de Tourtchaninoff M, Verhelst R. Predicting spinal cord ischemia before endovascular thoracoabdominal aneurysm repair: monitoring somatosensory evoked potentials. J Endovasc Ther 2002; 9(3):289–294.

36. White GH, May J, Waugh RC, Chaufour X, Yu W. Type III and Type IV endoleak: toward a complete definition of blood flow in the sac after endoluminal AAA repair. J Endovasc Surg 1998; 5(4):305–309.

37. Chaikof EL, Blankensteijn JD, Harris PL, White GH, Zarins CK, Bernhard VM, Matsumura JS, May J, Veith FJ, Fillinger MF, Rutherford RB, Kent KC. Reporting standards for endovascular aortic aneurysm repair. J Vasc Surg 2002; 35(5):1048–1060.

38. Baum RA, Cope C, Fairman RM, Carpenter JP. Translumbar embolization of type 2 endoleaks after endovascular repair of abdominal aortic aneurysms. J Vasc Interv Radiol 2001; 12(1):111–116.

39. Ellozy SH, Carroccio A, Minor M, Jacobs T, Chae K, Cha A, Agarwal G, Goldstein B, Morrissey N, Spielvogel D, Lookstein RA, Teodorescu V, Hollier LH, Marin ML.

Challenges of endovascular tube graft repair of thoracic aortic aneurysm: midterm follow-up and lessons learned. J Vasc Surg 2003; 38(4):676–683.

40. Heintz C, Riepe G, Birken L, Kaiser E, Chakfe N, Morlock M, Delling G, Imig H. Corroded nitinol wires in explanted aortic endografts: an important mechanism of failure? J Endovasc Ther 2001; 8(3):248–253.

41. Riepe G, Heintz C, Kaiser E, Chakfe N, Morlock M, Delling M, Imig H. What can we learn from explanted endovascular devices? Eur J Vasc Endovasc Surg 2002; 24(2): 117–122.

42. Ouriel K, Clair DG, Greenberg RK, Lyden SP, O'Hara PJ, Sarac TP, Srivastava SD, Butler B, Sampram ES. Endovascular repair of abdominal aortic aneurysms: device-specific outcome. J Vasc Surg 2003; 37(5):991–998.

43. Ouriel K, Clair DG, Greenberg RK, Lyden SP, O'Hara PJ, Sarac TP, Srivastava SD, Butler B, Sampram ES. Endovascular repair of abdominal aortic aneurysms: device-specific outcome. J Vasc Surg 2003; 37(5):991–998.

44. Hance KA, Hsu J, Eskew T, Hermreck AS. Secondary aortoesophageal fistula after endoluminal exclusion because of thoracic aortic transection. J Vasc Surg 2003; 37(4): 886–888.

19

Complications Following Endovascular Management of Acute Distal Aortic Dissections

Roy Greenberg
Department of Vascular Surgery, The Cleveland Clinic Foundation, Cleveland, Ohio, U.S.A.

Distal aortic dissections (in relation to the origin of the left subclavian artery) are complex manifestations of a disease afflicting the aortic wall. Although chest pain and hypertension are nearly ubiquitous at the time of patient presentation, they are frequently managed without intervention solely relying on aggressive beta-blockade and other pharmacologic agents. However, patient presentation may be complicated by aortic rupture, or ischemia of the mesenteric, renal, or lower extremity circulation in 10–15% of patients with dissections. These patients require urgent therapy. Traditional treatments for acute problems with distal dissection are associated with mortality rates in excess of 50% largely due to the extent of ischemia, the quality of aortic tissue shortly after such an injury, and the magnitude of the required procedure (1–3). Endovascular treatment paradigms have replaced a significant percentage of open procedures, particularly in the setting of critically ill patients (4–7). However, despite the less invasive approach, a multitude of complications may arise as a result of the initial pathophysiologic insult or technical misadventures.

PREOPERATIVE IMAGE INTERPRETATION

Patient assessment with a high resolution cross-sectional imaging technique (CT or MRI) is mandatory prior to the determination of a therapeutic plan (8). Failure to do so may relegate the interventionalist to "guessing" what the ischemic etiology may be: branch vessel dissection versus true lumen compression, the exact location of a rupture, the luminal relationships, derivation of end-organ blood flow, and comorbid conditions that frequent the vasculature of dissection patients (concomitant occlusive or aneurysmal disease). Although contrast toxicity may be a concern in the setting of renal insufficiency, MRI studies using gadolinium, when properly performed, can supplant the need for iodinated contrast (9,10). Efforts should be directed at evaluating the aortic diameters in the arch, descending thoracic, and abdominal aorta, in addition to localizing fenestration sites (Fig. 1).

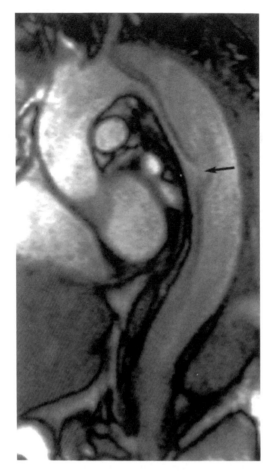

Figure 1 The dissection flap and fenestration (*arrow*) can be well visualized using MRI techniques. Careful attention to the acquisition of images, timing of contrast, and reconstruction techniques is required. *Abbreviation*: MRI, magnetic resonance imaging.

ACCESS

The choice of access sites is not straightforward in many circumstances, and must relate to a preconceived plan to enter either the true or false lumen. In contrast to most procedures, where the most easily palpable pulse becomes the puncture site of choice, in the setting of a dissection, access to the true lumen is usually established through the less pulsatile femoral artery. Frequently this requires the use of ultrasound to guide the puncture, or in the setting of a required cut-down, can be done after vessel exposure. In some dissections, it is possible to readily pass from one lumen to another from a single access site. This should be avoided when intending to place stents or stentgrafts.

ISCHEMIC COMPLICATIONS

Although this is the most frequent indication in our institution, for urgent treatment in this patient population, great variability exists with respect to the severity and location

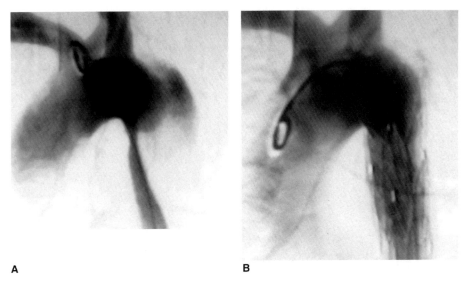

A   B

Figure 2   (**A**) A severely compressed true lumen is noted immediately distal to the left subclavian artery in a patient that presented with profound distal ischemia. (**B**) Following the placement of a homemade stent graft, complete true lumen expansion is evident. However, it is clear that the stent design is not optimal, as the proximal aspect does not conform to the arch anatomy.

of the ischemic bed, as well as the etiology of the ischemic mechanism, all of which will help to determine the type and magnitude of intervention required (11,12). Most patients presenting with ischemia following an aortic dissection suffer from proximal true lumen compression (Fig. 2A). In this circumstance, the mean pressure in the false lumen is greater than the mean true lumen pressure. Thus, the balance of space within the confinement of the aortic adventitia is given to the false lumen. A large proximal tear in the region of the left subclavian artery is usually associated with such a situation. The cause of the ischemia is hemodynamic in nature, and consequently, the treatment must address the flow of blood by limiting the false lumen inflow or increasing the potential for outflow from the false lumen. Attempts to treat true lumen compression as one may address an atherosclerotic stenosis (using stents with a high amount of radial force) are destined to fail. This relegates the interventionalist to two treatment modalities—endovascular grafting of the proximal fenestration site, or aortic fenestration above and/or below the ischemic bed with the intent of depressurizing the false lumen (stent grafting) or equalizing luminal flow (fenestration).

Endovascular Grafting

The location of the proximal tear will dictate the technology required for successful treatment. Details of techniques have been previously described (4,6,7). Dissections most frequently originate immediately distal to the left subclavian artery, a region of the aorta with dramatic tortuosity. Chosen devices must be flexible, to the point of being able to handle a right angle curve, and have a diameter matching, or slightly in excess of, the native aorta proximal to the true lumen. To accomplish the intended purpose, one must achieve a seal proximal to the fenestration, and extend the endograft into the true lumen beyond the fenestration (Fig. 2B). This will redirect flow away from the false lumen, allowing passive expansion of the true lumen. A number of mistakes can be made at this stage including:

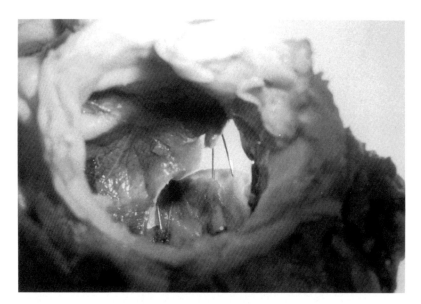

Figure 3 This homemade stentgraft was placed with an uncovered proximal Z-stent. Over time, the stent eroded through the proximal aspect of the descending thoracic aorta or distal aortic arch resulting in a fatal rupture.

1. Utilizing a device that will not conform to the shape of the arch. This will potentially result in the equivalent of a proximal endoleak, allowing continued pressurization of the false lumen. Furthermore, the desire for stiff devices (that are not precisely pre-shaped to the curve of the aortic arch) to stand up in the aorta, placing undue stress upon the superior aspect of the arch and result in late rupture (Fig. 3).
2. Undersizing the device. It is difficult to assess the desired size of an aortic prosthesis to be used in a dissection primarily because one cannot reliably predict the ultimate true lumen diameter. However, the goal is to obtain a seal proximal to the dissection, thus the device must be sized according to aortic diameter measurement immediately proximal to the primary fenestration. It may not be necessary to oversize self-expanding devices to the same extent one may do in the setting of aneurysmal disease, but undersizing a device will preclude a proximal seal and may force one to cover more of the proximal arch to obtain a seal.
3. Treating incomplete expansion with radial force. If the stentgraft appears compressed in segments, it is likely because of continued false lumen perfusion. Rather than attempting to utilize balloon expandable stents (that frequently cannot approach thoracic aortic diameters, nor can they successfully combat the compressive force generated by a patent false lumen) to augment the radial force of the repair in a given region, one should search for additional fenestrations. The treatment of additional fenestrations will allow for passive true lumen expansion. The exception to this rule is when one is confronted with a thrombosed false lumen (Fig. 4). In this circumstance, the lesion can be treated in a manner similar to an occlusive stenosis using uncovered stents to expand the true lumen.

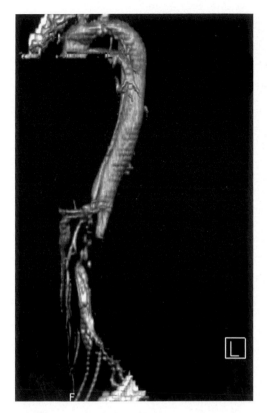

Figure 4 A CT reconstruction of a distal dissection with a prominent false lumen to the level of the visceral vessels. Distal to the visceral vessels, only the true lumen is seen. The false lumen occludes in the visceral segment, resulting in true lumen compression in a manner similar to an occlusive lesion. Stenting over the visceral segment with an uncovered stent was performed and achieved adequate mesenteric and distal blood flow.

4. Questionable lumen–wire relationship. It is absolutely critical that stentgrafts be placed into the true lumen and not the false. Should the wire inadvertently traverse a membrane, flow may be preferentially directed into the false lumen, with disastrous consequences. The use of intravascular ultrasound is extremely helpful in these circumstances and can help one definitively determine within which lumen the wire resides.
5. Discontinuous placement of stentgrafts. Although it may be necessary to treat the aorta in a segmental fashion (selectively covering fenestration sites with stentgrafts), there is considerable risk for late intrastent aortic degeneration (Fig. 5). These patients must be closely followed and treated when aortic expansion poses a significant rupture risk.

Branch Vessel Stenting

In the setting of adequate true lumen perfusion to the distal aorta when a patient clearly is suffering from ischemia, one should consider focal branch vessel flow impingement (Fig. 6). The mechanism of the branch compromise may be complex in nature. Variations have been previously described and can be grossly categorized into lesions

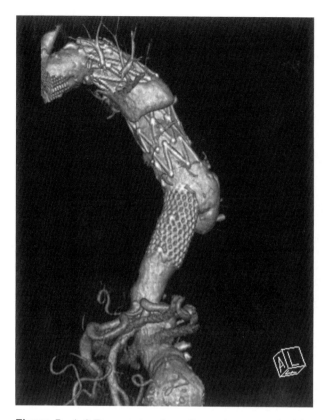

Figure 5 A 3-D reconstruction of a patient treated with segmental stentgraft for ischemia three years earlier now demonstrated marked dilation of the intra-stent aortic segments that exceeded 6 cm on cross-sectional measurements. The patient required treatment with a long segment thoracic graft to exclude the focal aneurysmal segments.

mimicking a true stenosis (a thrombosed segment of false lumen protruding into the branch) or dynamic flow limiting causes (the dissected membrane intermittently obstructing the branch orifice during systole, similar to a ball-valve effect) (11). The two etiologies are treated differently. The former can be addressed in a manner identical to fixing true atherosclerotic lesions with one caveat. Always use the true lumen as the preferred inflow site. Dynamic stenoses are more difficult to treat, and may require false lumen decompression with either stentgrafting or aortic fenestration. Again, these methods of therapy can be associated with complications including:

1. Improper identification of the etiology of ischemia. Clearly, reperfusion will not be adequate if the mechanism of ischemia is not well understood. A careful assessment of the pulsatile nature of flow into the end organ in question, coupled with intravascular ultrasound will help to delineate between the two mechanisms.
2. Derivation of inflow from the false lumen. The false lumen should not be considered an adequate source of inflow, unless a large fenestration has been created proximal to the branch. Furthermore, the false lumen never supplies tissues with blood; it must always re-enter and allow true lumen flow to supply the capillary beds. For these reasons, it is important, when

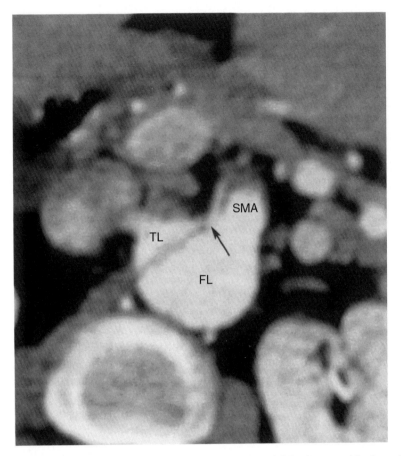

Figure 6 This CT scan demonstrates the true and false lumen with the origin of the right renal arising from the true lumen, while the SMA is split between the two lumens. This patient had focal intestinal ischemia that resulted from branch vessel dissection, rather than true lumen compression, and was successfully treated with a self-expanding stent placed into the origin of the SMA. *Abbreviations*: CT, computerized tomography; SMA; superior mesenteric artery.

stenting branch vessels, to ensure that the branch is stented into the true lumen.

3. Dissection into the distal end-organ supply. When gaining access to the distal end-organ circulation, carefully evaluate that your catheter, wire, and ultimately stent extend beyond the dissection within the branch. Thus, one always stents true lumen to true lumen.

Aortic Fenestration

Fenestrating the membrane of an acute dissection can be a challenging procedure that requires a thorough understanding of a variety of endovascular tools. The technique has been described by multiple authors, but has been supplanted, in the majority of cases, with the use of stentgrafts, yet it remains useful in some circumstances (large aortic diameters, residual ischemia following open repair of proximal dissections, or in patients with severe iliac occlusive disease) (13,14). In summary, when fenestrating a dissected membrane, one is attempting to puncture through the membrane to create a hole allowing for pressure equalization. During the course of such an endeavor, a number of issues may arise:

1. Inability to puncture through the membrane. The use of stiffer interventional systems (such as a small wire, within a microcatheter, within a standard catheter, within a guiding catheter, within a sheath) that are angled, usually allow a position to be maintained while a puncture is performed. However, undue force, improper orientation within the aorta, or poor technique can result in aortic perforation. Changing the location of the intended fenestration site, altering the angle of the system utilized, or using different puncturing equipment. Alternatively, shaped needles such as those used for TIPS or transjugular hepatic biopsy, can be employed.

2. The fenestration site closes after it is opened. The keys to successful fenestrations are the location of the hole and the size of the membranous injury created. It may not be necessary to stent across the fenestration to maintain patency, but if the membrane defect cannot be made large enough it is helpful.

3. Overaggressive or extensive fenestrations. It is possible to direct wire access from one lumen into the other and establish through and through access. At this point applying a retractive force on the wire can tear the dissected membrane. This will injure the membrane in the manner of a cheese cutter, and is very effective at rapidly establishing flow to the ischemic bed. However, the dissection flap may retract in the form of an endarterectomized segment and cause an obstructive problem distal to the fenestration. In these circumstances, one must preserve distal flow with the use of additional stents to bridge the accumulated aortic tissue.

TREATMENT OF RUPTURE

Aortic rupture following dissection is very difficult to successfully manage with endovascular techniques. Ideally, exclusion of the ruptured segment would be established by obtaining a graft to aortic wall seal above and below the rupture site. The challenge lies in the fact that most dissections traverse the visceral segment, which cannot be bridged with today's endograft technology. Continued perfusion of the false lumen following endovascular treatment of a dissection with a stentgraft can result in persistent hemorrhage or aortic growth. Thus, it would make sense to only treat focal dissections with rupture with endovascular grafting, relegating the majority of patients to open surgical repair. In these situations a few problem-solving techniques may be of assistance:

1. Inability to obtain a distal seal. If the ruptured segment is significantly proximal to the visceral vessels, combining an endovascular graft with an aortic fenestration technique may be helpful. A fenestration must be created at the intended distal landing site and extend for a length greater than the distal sealing stent. When the stentgraft is deployed, the distal stent is placed at the level of the fenestration. Following balloon expansion of such a stent, circumferential apposition of graft material can be obtained to provide a seal distal to the region of rupture.

2. Inability to locate an acceptable sealing zone. In an extensive dissection, there may not be an adequate region for establishing a seal. If the patient is incapable of tolerating a thoracotomy, aortic cross-clamping, or a period of circulatory arrest, then two choices exist:

   i. Deploy a stentgraft into the thoracic aorta across the region of suspected rupture. It is possible that the false lumen will thrombose, while the true lumen is protected from extravasation by the stent graft.

   ii. Alternatively, a mesenteric and renal bypass can be performed through a retroperitoneal incision. This is not a good technique for an unstable patient, but can be used in select circumstances to allow the distal landing site to be extended into the iliac vasculature.

PREVENTION OF LONG-TERM AORTIC DEGENERATION

The use of stentgrafts and fenestration techniques to treat acute dissection may expand the armamentarium of cardiovascular interventionalists, but also creates new problems. Aortic dilation has been noted in up to 40% of patients following dissections. However, we are unable to predict which patients will dilate and which will remain stable. Consequently, careful follow-up (including imaging studies) is mandatory for all patients with dissections. Higher rates of paraplegia have been associated with longer stentgrafts (15), but there is not enough data pertaining specifically to aortic dissections. Focal areas of dilation (Fig. 5) between devices can darken the success of the procedure. Ultimately, it is up to the interventionalist to strike a balance as to the extent of thoracic aorta to be covered with the risk of paraplegia, realizing that one may end up treating the problem in stages.

MEDICAL MANAGEMENT

The medical management of the dissection patient prior to and during an intervention is critical to optimizing results. Failure to recognize the magnitude of the ischemic injury and the potential for a significant reperfusion injury has serious consequences. The extent and duration of ischemia are critical to helping with this determination. The following suggestions can help to ameliorate medical complications:

1. Maintain adequate management of blood pressure with beta-blockade in the interventional site and post-procedure.
2. Plan for significant reperfusion injury in the setting on any ischemia. This may be associated with hyperkalemia, acidosis, and myoglobinuria, and the appropriate precautions should be taken.
3. Aggressively assess the ischemic end organ. Exploratory laparoscopy may be helpful in the setting of bowel ischemia, while fasciotomies may be of assistance following lower extremity ischemia resolution.
4. Carefully monitor the patient at all times. These interventions are best done in cooperation with a trained cardiovascular anesthesia team in an area of the hospital that lends itself to resuscitative maneuvers.

Overall, distal aortic dissections represent a complex disease process in an unforgiving patient population. Complications can relate to judgment or medical management issues, or be technical in nature. Careful attention to the pre-procedure anatomy and physiology, and familiarity with the diverse techniques available will help to limit the occurrence of poor outcomes.

REFERENCES

1. Fann JI, Sarris GE, Mitchell RS, Shumway NE, Stinson EB, Oyer PE, et al. Treatment of patients with aortic dissection presenting with peripheral vascular complications. Ann Surg 1990; 212(6):705–713.
2. Fann JI, Miller DC. Aortic dissection. Ann Vasc Surg 1995; 9(3):311–323.
3. Cambria RP, Brewster DC, Gertler J, Moncure AC, Gusberg R, Tilson MD, et al. Vascular complications associated with spontaneous aortic dissection. J Vasc Surg 1988; 7(2):199–209.
4. Greenberg RK, Haulon S, Khwaja J, Fulton G, Ouriel K. Contemporary management of acute aortic dissection. J Endovasc Ther 2003; 10(3):476–485.
5. Greenberg R, Khwaja J, Haulon S, Fulton G. Aortic dissections: new perspectives and treatment paradigms. Eur J Vasc Endovasc Surg 2003; 26(6):579–586.
6. Dake MD, Kato N, Mitchell RS, Semba CP, Razavi MK, Shimono T, et al. Endovascular stent-graft placement for the treatment of acute aortic dissection. N Engl J Med 1999; 340(20):1546–1552.
7. Nienaber CA, Fattori R, Lund G, Dieckmann C, Wolf W, von Kodolitsch Y, et al. Nonsurgical reconstruction of thoracic aortic dissection by stent-graft placement. N Engl J Med 1999; 340(20):1539–1545.
8. Hartnell GG. Imaging of aortic aneurysms and dissection: CT and MRI. J Thorac Imag 2001; 16(1):35–46.
9. Krinsky GA, Rofsky NM, DeCorato DR, Weinreb JC, Earls JP, Flyer MA, et al. Thoracic aorta: comparison of gadolinium-enhanced three-dimensional MR angiography with conventional MR imaging. Radiology 1997; 202(1):183–193.
10. Prince MR, Narasimham DL, Jacoby WT, Williams DM, Cho KJ, Marx MV, et al. Three-dimensional gadolinium-enhanced MR angiography of the thoracic aorta. Am J Roentgenol 1996; 166(6):1387–1397.
11. Williams DM, Lee DY, Hamilton BH, Marx MV, Narasimham DL, Kazanjian SN, et al. The dissected aorta: part III. Anatomy and radiologic diagnosis of branch-vessel compromise. Radiology 1997; 203(1):37–44.
12. Lee DY, Williams DM, Abrams GD. The dissected aorta: part II. Differentiation of the true from the false lumen with intravascular US. Radiology 1997; 203(1):32–36.
13. Williams DM, Brothers TE, Messina LM. Relief of mesenteric ischemia in type III aortic dissection with percutaneous fenestration of the aortic septum. Radiology 1990; 174(2): 450–452.
14. Slonim SM, Nyman U, Semba CP, Miller DC, Mitchell RS, Dake MD. Aortic dissection: percutaneous management of ischemic complications with endovascular stents and balloon fenestration. J Vasc Surg 1996; 23(2):241–251.
15. Greenberg R, Resch T, Nyman U, Lindh M, Brunkwall J, Brunkwall P, et al. Endovascular repair of descending thoracic aortic aneurysms: an early experience with intermediate-term follow-up. J Vasc Surg 2000; 31(1):147–156.

20
Complications in Peripheral Thrombolysis

Kenneth Ouriel
*Department of Vascular Surgery, The Cleveland Clinic Foundation,
Cleveland, Ohio, U.S.A.*

The principal goal of thrombolytic therapy is to dissolve intravascular thrombus. Thrombolytic agents are remarkably effective in accomplishing this goal, and they can do so in a minimally invasive fashion. Through percutaneous means alone, recanalization of an occluded bypass graft or artery can be achieved within a few hours and the thrombus can be completely dissolved over the course of 12 to 48 hours (1). Culprit stenotic lesions become readily apparent after successful thrombolytic therapy, lesions that must be addressed to diminish the risk of reocclusion (2). The unmasked lesions can frequently be repaired percutaneously. Even when open surgical revascularization is necessary, it can oftentimes be performed on an elective basis after ample time for patient preparation. Thrombolytic therapy can be employed to clear thrombus from small vessels that are inaccessible to standard balloon catheter thrombectomy, sometimes identifying target vessels for an operative bypass procedure (Fig. 1) (3). Clinical trials have proven thrombolytic therapy to be effective for the treatment of acute arterial occlusion, resulting in a reduction in mortality, limb loss, length of hospital stay, and the need for open surgical intervention (4–7).

But successful thrombolytic therapy cannot be separated from its major complication, the inextricable risk of life-threatening hemorrhage. In fact, other complications pale in comparison to bleeding, and the association between thrombolytic therapy and hemorrhage is the sole factor that has precluded the use of thrombolysis in an even broader number of patients (8). To understand the association between thrombolytic therapy and hemorrhage, it is beneficial to first consider the biochemistry underlying the mechanism of action of thrombolytic agents. The fundamental physiology of dissolving (1) pathologic intravascular thrombi, and (2) desirable plugs sealing remote sites where vascular integrity has been lost, is virtually identical. Herein lies the failure of thrombolytic therapy: how does one effect dissolution of "bad" thrombus without causing distant hemorrhage due to the dissolution of "good" thrombus sealing small vascular defects in the gastrointestinal tract, at the catheter insertion site, or, most importantly, within the calvarium.

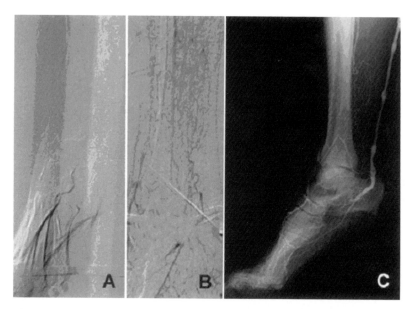

Figure 1 Thrombolytic therapy can clear thrombus from small vessels, inaccessible to balloon catheter thrombectomy. (**A**) This patient had no identifiable vessels below the popliteal, even on delayed views. (**B**) Following thrombolysis, a lateral plantar artery was identified in this patient. (**C**) A saphenous vein popliteal-plantar artery bypass was now possible.

BIOCHEMISTRY OF THROMBOLYTIC AGENTS

The sum and substance of intravascular thrombus is fibrin, a polymerized meshwork of cross-linked proteins interspersed with abundant platelets and occasional red and white blood cells. The pharmacologic goal of thrombolytic therapy is to digest this meshwork, breaking the bonds upon which the integrity of the thrombus is based. In this manner, the thrombolytic agents convert the highly insoluble fibrin-platelet mass into microscopic fragments of degenerated thrombus and, preferably, soluble breakdown products that wash into the circulation and are cleared by the kidney and liver.

It is important to emphasize that all clinically available thrombolytic agents do not degrade thrombus directly. Rather, each is a "plasminogen activator." As such, they do not directly degrade fibrinogen and without plasminogen they are inert. The thrombolytic agents comprise trypsin-like serine proteases that have highly specific activity directed at the cleavage of a single peptide bond in the plasminogen zymogen, converting it to plasmin (9). Importantly, plasmin is the active molecule that cleaves fibrin polymer to cause the dissolution of thrombus. Milstone first recognized the importance of plasminogen in 1941, when it was noted that clots formed with highly purified fibrinogen and thrombin were not lysed by streptococcal fibrinolysin unless a small amount of human serum (plasminogen) was added (10). Recognizing this direct role of plasminogen, early investigators attempted to dissolve occluding thrombi with the administration of exogenous plasmin (11). Free plasmin, when administered intravenously, is ineffective as a thrombolytic agent, accounting for the failure of these attempts. Effective thrombolysis was achieved only when *fibrin-bound* plasminogen was converted to active plasmin at the site of the thrombus (9).

The dependence of fibrinolysis on adequate circulating levels of plasminogen is best illustrated by studies of the fibrinolytic potential of blood drawn from patients receiving intravenous administration of thrombolytic agents for acute myocardial infarction (12). Blood obtained soon after the start of thrombolytic administration displayed a great degree of in vitro fibrinolytic potential. Aliquots of plasma drawn from the patients and then added to radiolabeled clots in test tubes produced rapid dissolution of the clots. By contrast, similar aliquots drawn from patients after 20 minutes of thrombolytic administration had considerably less thrombolytic potential. The explanation for this observation relates to the amount of plasminogen present in the blood. Prolonged thrombolytic administration consumed all of the endogenous plasminogen and, despite continued administration of thrombolytic agent, no further clot lysis was possible.

SAFETY OF THROMBOLYTIC AGENTS IN CLINICAL TRIALS

There exist but few well-designed clinical comparisons of different thrombolytic agents for the treatment of peripheral arterial occlusion. By contrast, the literature is replete with a broad spectrum of in vitro studies and retrospective clinical trials, most pointing to improved efficacy and safety of urokinase and alteplase over streptokinase (13–16). In an analysis of data collected in a prospective, single institution registry at The Cleveland Clinic Foundation, urokinase demonstrated a diminished rate of bleeding complications when compared with alteplase (Table 1) (17).

There have been two prospective, randomized comparisons of urokinase and alteplase. Neither was blinded. Meyerovitz and associates from the Brigham and Women's Hospital randomized 32 patients with peripheral arterial or bypass graft occlusions of less than 90 days duration to alteplase (10 mg bolus, 5 mg/hr to a maximum of 24 hours) or urokinase (60,000 IU bolus, 4000 IU/min for two hours, 2000 IU/min for two hours, then 1000 IU/min to a maximum of 24 hours total administration) (Fig. 2) (18). There was significantly greater systemic fibrinogen degradation in the alteplase group ($p = 0.01$), indicating that the fibrin-specificity of alteplase was lost at this dosing regimen. Alteplase patients achieved more rapid initial thrombolysis, but efficacy was identical in the two groups within 24 hours. The trade-off to more rapid thrombolysis was a trend toward a higher rate of bleeding complications in the alteplase-treated patients.

The second randomized comparison of urokinase and alteplase was the surgery or thrombolysis for the ischemic lower extremity (STILE) trial, a three-armed multicenter comparison of urokinase (250,000 IU bolus, 4000 IU/min for four hours, then

Table 1 Relative Rate of Complications in 627 Patients Treated with Urokinase or Alteplase between 1990 and 1998 at The Cleveland Clinic Foundation

Event	Urokinase $N = 483$ (%)	Alteplase $N = 144$ (%)	p-value
Bleeding requiring transfusion	12	23	0.004
Hematoma at catheter insertion site	22	44	<0.001
False aneurysm	1.7	2.8	Not significant
Intracranial bleeding	0.6	2.8	0.03
Death	2.7	4.2	Not significant

Source: From Ref. 17.

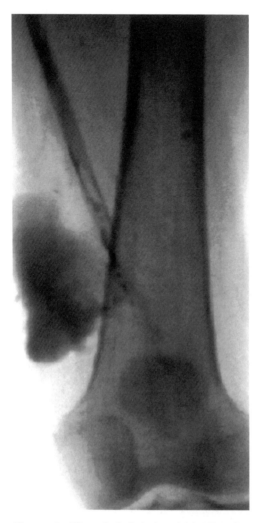

Figure 2 Thrombolytic-induced bleeding from the suture holes in a recently constructed polytetrafluoroethylene femoro-popliteal bypass graft.

2000 IU/min for up to 36 hours), alteplase (0.05–0.1 mg/kg/hr for up to 12 hours) and primary operation (Fig. 3) (19). There was one intracranial hemorrhage in the urokinase group (0.9%) and two in the alteplase group (1.5%, no significant difference). Although actual rates of overall bleeding complications and efficacy were not reported for the two thrombolytic groups, the authors remarked that there were no significant differences detected in any of the outcome variables. In a subsequent "re-analysis" of the data, reported in 1999, the frequency of complete clot lysis was similar with urokinase and alteplase at the time of the early arteriographic study (20). This recent data suggests that the rate of thrombolysis may be quite similar, in direct contradistinction to the popularly held view that alteplase is a much more rapidly acting agent.

A multicenter, blinded trial compared the results of thrombolysis with urokinase versus recombinant urokinase in 300 patients with peripheral arterial occlusion (21). These data were never published. There were no significant differences noted between the two agents. A North American multicenter trial compared three different

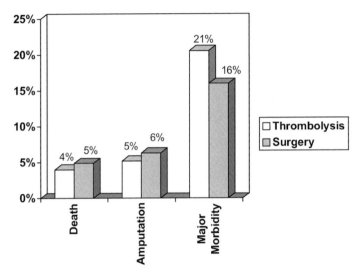

Figure 3 Complications in the STILE trial (19). Major morbidity was diminished in the surgery group, a finding that was related to a greater frequency of "on-going ischemia" in the thrombolytic group. This did not translate into differences in the more important endpoints of death and major amputation. *Abbreviation*: STILE, surgery or thrombolysis for the ischemic lower extremity

doses of prourokinase to urokinase in 241 patients with lower extremity arterial occlusions of less than 14 days duration (22). While the higher prourokinase dose was associated with slightly greater percentage of patients with complete (>95%) clot lysis at eight hours, there was a mild increase in the rate of bleeding complications compared with either the urokinase or the lower dose prourokinase groups (Table 2). The fibrinogen levels fell in the higher prourokinase group, suggesting that fibrin specificity was lost at the higher dose regimens for this compound.

PREVENTING HEMORRHAGE DURING THROMBOLYSIS: POTENTIAL FOR THE FUTURE

There are several methods to consider in the quest to diminish the rate of distant hemorrhagic complications with thrombolytic therapy. First, one might strive to

Table 2 Complications Associated with Three Escalating Doses of Prourokinase (Initiated at 2, 4, or 8 mg/hr) vs. Urokinase (Initiated at 240,000 IU/hr) in the PURPOSE Trial

Site	2.0 mg (%)	4.0 mg (%)	8.0 mg (%)	Urokinase (%)
Epistaxis	0.0	0.0	3.8	0.0
Gastrointestinal	0.0	0.0	1.9	0.0
Gums	0.0	0.0	9.6	0.0
Intracranial	0.0	0.0	0.0	0.0
Hematuria	6.6	7.3	9.6	8.3
Retroperitoneum	1.6	0.0	3.8	1.7

Abbreviation: PURPOSE, pro-urokinase vs. urokinase for recanalization of peripheral occlusions safety and efficacy.
Source: From Ref. 22.

limit the "leak" of active thrombolytic agent into the systemic circulation. In fact this was the primary reason for considering the local, catheter-directed route for low-dose thrombolysis in the 1970s and 1980s (23,24). Clearly, the intra-thrombus administration of thrombolytic agents is associated with improved efficacy (25). Whether increased safety has been achieved with this now ubiquitous method remains to be established.

The use of "fibrin-specific" agents was investigated to decrease the risk of distant bleeding (26). Fibrin-specificity is quantified by the ratio of fibrin breakdown to fibrinogen breakdown. A fibrin-specific agent degrades fibrin but not fibrinogen. This property is accomplished through a variety of mechanisms. Alteplase was the first "designer" thrombolytic agent with fibrin-specific properties (27). Alteplase binds to fibrin but not to fibrinogen and attains plasminogenolytic activity only after binding. Tenectaplase, a modified form of alteplase, has even greater fibrin specificity, with very little reduction in fibrinogen concentration during therapy (28). Nevertheless, fibrin-specificity has not resulted in a reduction in the risk of bleeding. The agents, in fact, may be associated with a greater risk of distant hemorrhage, possibly related to the production of an intermediary fibrin breakdown product, Fragment X (29). Fragment X is readily incorporated into existing distant thrombi, rendering the thrombi fragile and more susceptible to subsequent thrombolytic dissolution and hemorrhage. Interestingly, urokinase and streptokinase do not appear to generate significant quantities of Fragment X during thrombolysis, due to rapid conversion to smaller breakdown products. This mechanism might explain the putative lower incidence of distant bleeding with streptokinase and urokinase versus alteplase (30).

Limiting the use of concomitant systemic heparinization has been considered to reduce the rate of bleeding complications during thrombolytic therapy (31). The thrombolysis or peripheral arterial surgery (TOPAS) trial was initially begun using full-dose systemic heparinization (7). The rate of intracranial bleeding decreased substantially when therapeutic heparinization was deleted from the protocol. Similar results were observed when heparin was decreased in the prourokinase trials for stroke (32). Recently, a trend has emerged during peripheral arterial thrombolysis, restricting heparin administration to an infusion rate of several hundred units per hour or less (33). Further, experience from the cardiology literature suggests that bleeding complications bear a greater relationship to heparin anticoagulation than to pharmacologic thrombolysis (30).

The use of mechanical thrombectomy devices as adjuvants to pharmacologic thrombolysis holds the potential to lower the rate of bleeding complications (34–36). Recognizing the link between duration of administration and hemorrhage, bleeding complications might be lower if mechanical adjuvants diminish thrombolytic exposure (37). As well, a new mechanical thrombectomy device utilizes proximal and distal balloon occlusion to limit the distribution of thrombolytic agent to the thrombosed vascular segment. Whether these mechanical adjuvants will result in a significant reduction in the risk of bleeding remains unproved; a critical analysis is not possible without a prospective trial.

Novel agents may diminish the risk of distant bleeding. For example, the agent alfimeprase, an analogue of fibrolase, is a direct fibrinolytic with activity that is independent of plasminogen (38). Circulating alpha-2 macroglobulin inactivates alfimeprase. Systemic fibrinolysis will not occur as long as the dose of alfimeprase is kept below a threshold determined by available alpha-2 macroglobulin. Similar to alfimeprase, plasmin analogues hold promise as alternative thrombolytic agents with a decreased risk of systemic bleeding. Plasmin, while ineffective when administered systemically, retains its activity when administered directly into the thrombus (39). As well, plasmin analogues may diminish the rate of distant bleeding as a result of systemic inactivation by circulating alpha-2 antiplasmin.

NON-HEMORRHAGIC COMPLICATIONS OF THROMBOLYTIC AGENTS

There exist a wide variety of non-hemorrhagic complications associated with thrombolysis (40). Streptokinase is associated with allergic reactions in a significant percentage of patients, especially in those who have recently experienced a streptococcal infection and in those who undergo re-treatment with the agent. Urokinase may be accompanied with rigors, especially in patients for whom the agent is administered in a large bolus dose. The target vessel or bypass graft may rethrombose during thrombolytic infusion, a complication that occurs in approximately 8% of patients and seems to be reduced with heparin anticoagulation (22,31). The patient may sustain distal embolization of partially dissolved thrombus, a problem that is noted in 10–20% of patients and one that appears to be diminished in frequency when a glycoprotein IIb/IIIa inhibitor is added to the thrombolytic regimen (22,41). Of importance, amputation rate is higher when either rethrombosis or distal embolization develops during thrombolytic infusion (42). Lastly, technical complications may occur during percutaneous thrombolytic therapy, including catheter or wire perforation of the arterial wall (1%), arterial dissection (2%), pericatheter thrombosis (3%), and false aneurysm formation (1–3%) (17,22).

SUMMARY AND CONCLUSIONS

Thrombolytic therapy is associated with significant benefits to the patient, including (a) the ability to achieve restoration of blood flow in a minimally invasive fashion, (b) the identification of the culprit lesion responsible for the occlusive event, and (c) clearance of thrombus from small vessels inaccessible to balloon catheters. These benefits have culminated in a reduction in the rate of amputation and death for patients with acute limb ischemia (1,19). Complications, however, continue to occur at a relatively high frequency. Hemorrhage is the most frequent and clinically significant complication of thrombolytic therapy. The rate of hemorrhage can be diminished by avoiding therapeutic heparinization, decreasing the dose of thrombolytic agent, limiting the period of exposure, and through prudent patient selection. Even with attention to these and other measures, the rate of bleeding, distal embolization, and rethrombosis will continue to occur with some frequency. These issues should be considered when presenting the therapeutic options to a patient, carefully weighing the risks versus the potential benefits prior to embarking on a particular treatment regimen.

REFERENCES

1. Ouriel K, Shortell CK, DeWeese JA, Green RM, Francis CW, Azodo MV, Gutierrez OH, Manzione JV, Cos C, Marder VJ. A comparison of thrombolytic therapy with

operative revascularization in the initial treatment of acute peripheral arterial ischemia. J Vasc Surg 1994; 19(6):1021–1030.

2. Sullivan KL, Gardiner GAJ, Kandarpa K, Bonn J, Shapiro MJ, Carabasi RA, Smullens S, Levin DC. Efficacy of thrombolysis in infrainguinal bypass grafts. Circulation 1991; 83(suppl 2):99–105.

3. Garcia R, Saroyan RM, Senkowsky J, Smith F, Kerstein M. Intraoperative intra-arterial urokinase infusion as an adjunct to Fogarty catheter embolectomy in acute arterial occlusion. Surg Gynecol Obstet 1990; 171(3):201–205.

4. Ouriel K, Shortell CK, Azodo MV, Guiterrez OH, Marder VJ. Acute peripheral arterial occlusion: predictors of success in catheter-directed thrombolytic therapy. Radiology 1994; 193(2):561–566.

5. Comerota AJ, Weaver FA, Hosking JD, Froehlich J, Folander H, Sussman B, Rosenfield K. Results of a prospective, randomized trial of surgery versus thrombolysis for occluded lower extremity bypass grafts. Am J Surg 1996; 172(2):105–112.

6. Weaver FA, Comerota AJ, Youngblood M, Froehlich J, Hosking JD, Papanicolaou G. Surgical revascularization versus thrombolysis for non-embolic lower extremity native artery occlusions: results of a prospective randomized trial. The STILE Investigators. Surgery versus thrombolysis for ischemia of the lower extremity. J Vasc Surg 1996; 24(4):513–521.

7. Ouriel K, Veith FJ, Sasahara AA. A comparison of recombinant urokinase with vascular surgery as initial treatment for acute arterial occlusion of the legs. N Engl J Med 1998; 338:1105–1111.

8. Ricotta JJ, Green RM, DeWeese JA. Use and limitations of thrombolytic therapy in the treatment of peripheral arterial ischemia: results of a multi-institutional questionnaire. J Vasc Surg 1987; 6(1):45–50.

9. Alkjaersig N, Fletcher AP, Sherry S. The mechanism of clot dissolution by plasmin. J Clin Invest 1959; 38:1086.

10. Milstone H. A factor in normal human blood which participates in streptococcal fibrinolysis. J Immunol 1941; 42:116.

11. Cliffton EE. The use of plasmin in humans. Ann NY Acad Sci 1957; 68:209–229.

12. Onundarson PT, Haraldsson HM, Bergmann L, Francis CW, Marder VJ. Plasminogen depletion during streptokinase treatment or two-chain urokinase incubation correlates with decreased clot lysability ex vivo and in vitro. Thromb Haemost 1993; 70(6):998–1004.

13. van Breda A, Robison JC, Feldman L, Waltman AC, Brewster DC, Abbott WM, Athanasoulis CA. Local thrombolysis in the treatment of arterial graft occlusions. J Vasc Surg 1984; 1(1):103–112.

14. Ouriel K, Welch EL, Shortell CK, Geary K, Fiore WM, Cimino C. Comparison of streptokinase, urokinase, and recombinant tissue plasminogen activator in an in vitro model of venous thrombolysis. J Vasc Surg 1995; 22(5):593–597.

15. Fox D, Ouriel K, Green RM, Stoughton J, Riggs P, Cimino C. Thrombolysis with prourokinase versus urokinase: an in vitro comparison. J Vasc Surg 1996; 23(4):657–666.

16. McNamara TO, Fischer JR. Thrombolysis of peripheral arterial and graft occlusions: improved results using high-dose urokinase. AJR Am J Roentgenol 1985; 144:769–775.

17. Ouriel K, Gray BH, Clair DG, Olin JW. Complications associated with the use of urokinase and recombinant tissue plasminogen activator for catheter-directed peripheral arterial and venous thrombolysis. J Vasc Interv Radiol 2000; 11:295–298.

18. Meyerovitz MF, Goldhaber SZ, Reagan K, Polak JF, Kandarpa K, Grassi CJ, Donovan BC, Bettmann MA, Harrington DP. Recombinant tissue-type plasminogen activator versus urokinase in peripheral arterial and graft occlusions: a randomized trial. Radiology 1990; 175:75–78.

19. Anonymous. Results of a prospective randomized trial evaluating surgery versus thrombolysis for ischemia of the lower extremity. The STILE trial. Ann Surg 1994; 220(3): 251–266.

20. Comerota AJ. A re-analysis of the STILE data. Personal communication, 11-17-1990.

21. Abbott Laboratories Venture Group. A comparison of urokinase and recombinant urokinase in the treatment of peripheral arterial occlusion. Data on file, Abbott Laboratories, 1994.

22. Ouriel K, Kandarpa K, Schuerr DM, Hultquist M, Hodkinson G, Wallin B. Prourokinase versus urokinase for recanalization of peripheral occlusions, safety and efficacy: the PURPOSE trial. J Vasc Interv Radiol 1999; 10(8):1083–1091.

23. Dotter CT, Rösch J, Seaman AJ. Selective clot lysis with low-dose streptokinase. Radiology 1974; 111:31–37.

24. Katzen BT, Edwards KC, Albert AS, van Breda A. Low-dose direct fibrinolysis in peripheral vascular disease. J Vasc Surg 1984; 1(5):718–722.

25. Graor RA, Risius B, Denny KM, Young JR, Beven EG, Hertzer NR, Ruschhaupt WF, O'Hara PJ, Geisinger MA, Zelch MA. Local thrombolysis in the treatment of thrombosed arteries, bypass grafts, and arteriovenous fistulas. J Vasc Surg 1985; 2(3):406–414.

26. Hoylaerts M, Rijken DC, Lijnen HR, Collen D. Kinetics of the activation of plasminogen by human tissue plasminogen activator: role of fibrin. J Biol Chem 1982; 257:2912.

27. Lijnen HR, Van Hoef B, De Cock F, Collen D. Effect of fibrin-like stimulators on the activation of plasminogen by tissue-type plasminogen activator (t-PA): studies with active site mutagenized plasminogen and plasmin resistant t-PA. Thromb Haemost 1990; 64:61.

28. Cannon CP, Gibson CM, McCabe CH, Adgey AA, Schweiger MJ, Sequeira RF, Grollier G, Giuglianno RP, Frey M, Mueller HS, Steingart RM, Weaver WD, Van de Werf F, Braunwald. TNK-tissue plasminogen activator compared with front-loaded alteplase in acute myocardial infarction: results of the TIMI 10B trial. Circulation 1998; 98(25):2805–2814.

29. Owen J, Friedman KD, Grossman BA, Wilkins C, Berke AD, Powers ER. Quantitation of fragment X formation during thrombolytic therapy with streptokinase and tissue plasminogen activator. J Clin Invest 1987; 79(6):1642–1647.

30. The GUSTO Investigators. An international randomized trial comparing four thrombolytic therapies for acute myocardial infarction. N Engl J Med 1993; 329:673–682.

31. Ouriel K, Katzen B, Mewissen MW, Flick P, Clair DG, Benenati J, McNamara TO, Gibbens D. Initial experience with reteplase in the treatment of peripheral arterial and venous occlusion. J Vasc Interv Radiol 2000; 11:849–854.

32. del Zoppo GJ, Higashida RT, Furlan AJ, Pessin MS, Rowley HA, Gent M. PROACT: a phase II randomized trial of recombinant pro-urokinase by direct arterial delivery in acute middle cerebral artery stroke. Stroke 1999; 29:4–11.

33. McNamara TO, Dong P, Chen J, Quinn B, Gomes A, Goodwin SC, Aban K. Bleeding complications associated with the use of rt-PA versus r-PA for peripheral arterial and venous thromboembolic occlusions. Tech Vasc Interv Radiol 2001; 4(2):92–98.

34. Kasirajan K, Haskal ZJ, Ouriel K. The use of mechanical thrombectomy devices in the management of acute peripheral arterial occlusive disease. J Vasc Interv Radiol 2001; 12(4):405–411.

35. Greenberg R, Ouriel K, Srivastava S, Shortell C, Ivancev K, Waldman D, Illig KA, Green RM. Mechanical versus chemical thrombolysis: an in vitro differentiation of thrombolytic mechanisms. J Vasc Interv Radiol 2000; 11:199–205.

36. Silva JA, Ramee SR, Collins TJ, Jenkins JS, Lansky AJ, Ansel GM, Dolmatch BL, Glickman MH, Stainken B, Ramee E, White CJ. Rheolytic thrombectomy in the treatment of acute limb-threatening ischemia: immediate results and six-month follow-up of the multicenter AngioJet registry. Possis Peripheral AngioJet Investigators. Catheteriz Cardiovasc Diagn 1998; 45(4):386–393.

37. Ansel GM, George BS, Botti CF, McNamara TO, Jenkins JS, Ramee SR, Rosenfield K, Noetthen AA, Mehta T. Rheolytic thrombectomy in the management of limb ischemia: 30-day results from a multicenter registry. J Endovasc Ther 2002; 9(4):395–402.

38. Ahmed NK, Tennant KD, Markland FS, Lacz JP. Biochemical characteristics of fibrolase, a fibrinolytic protease from snake venom. Haemostasis 1990; 20(3):147–154.

39. Marder VJ, Stewart D. Towards safer thrombolytic therapy. Semin Hematol 2002; 39(3):206–216.
40. Sharma GVRK, Cella G, Parisi AF, Sasahara AA. Thrombolytic therapy. N Engl J Med 1982; 306:1268–1272.
41. Ouriel K. The RELAX Trial. Presented at the TCT Conference, Washington, D.C., September 2002.
42. Galland RB, Earnshaw JJ, Baird RN, Lonsdale RJ, Hopkinson BR, Giddings AEB, Dawson KJ, Hamilton G. Acute limb deterioration during intra-arterial thrombolysis. Br J Surg 1993; 80(9):1118–1120.

21

Endovascular Therapy for Deep Venous Occlusion

Pamela A. Flick
Department of Radiology, Concentrated Care Center, Georgetown University Hospital, Washington, D.C., U.S.A.

INTRODUCTION

The number of patients annually hospitalized in the United States with the diagnosis of deep vein thrombosis (DVT) approximates 250,000 (1). The incidence of recurrent disease and the medical cost associated with post-thrombotic complications is of the same magnitude. The cost of DVT treatment is estimated at US $1.2–2.4 billion annually (2).

Traditional therapy has included anticoagulation alone, however, as we know, this prevents only propagation of thrombus and does not restore venous patency. Extensive DVT can often result in severe debilitating symptoms, including life-threatening pulmonary embolism (PE), and later disabling post-thrombotic syndrome (PTS), making early detection of thrombus and early treatment initiation invaluable. Early detection and aggressive therapy is also advantageous in promoting the efficacy of therapy and preventing long-term impairment from thrombus propagation. Treatment strategies have the goal of alleviating patient symptoms and restoring venous patency, while maintaining vessel structural integrity (2). Strategy options are broad and include observation only with or without inferior vena cava (IVC) filter placement, systemic anticoagulation, catheter-directed thrombolysis, mechanical thrombolysis, and/or surgical thrombectomy. The limitations of anticoagulation alone and surgical thrombectomy have resulted in the introduction of mechanical and/or pharmacologic therapies with the end-result being restoration of venous patency and the elimination of thrombus. These therapies not only have the potential to restore venous valvular function and eliminate the risk of PTS, but also can effectively treat the acute event of pulmonary embolus.

Post-thrombotic sequelae are disabling, not only limiting patients' ability to work, but also significantly affecting their quality of living. A multicenter trial in the United States reported that when the disease process was followed from the time of clinical presentation, the one-year mortality was 25% of which only 2.5% died as a result of a PE (3,4). Therefore, when treating the patient with a DVT, we must learn not only to treat the acute event, but also to offer effective therapy to treat the potential long-term outcome of DVT.

PREDISPOSING FACTORS

Risk factors for venous thrombosis include conditions or events that can be categorized under Virchows' triad: hypercoagulability, injury to the vessel, and decreased blood velocity. Predisposing conditions include immobility (bed rest), pregnancy, trauma, recent surgery, neoplasm, obesity, tobacco, oral contraceptives, dehydration, and advanced age. Numerous hypercoagulable conditions which increase the risk must be considered in patients without a predisposing condition who present with new onset DVT or with recurrent rethrombosis; such conditions include protein C and S deficiencies, antithrombin III deficiency, and Factor V Leiden abnormalities (4).

SEQUELAE

The serious effects of *acute* DVT include venous ischemia, life-threatening PE, and phlegmasia cerulea dolens. Phlegmasia cerulea dolens or extensive iliofemoral thrombosis is a relatively rare condition that occurs with massive thrombus formation that has high morbidity and mortality rates, and runs the risk of limb loss (5). The most common complaint or clinical presentation for an isolated or segmental lower extremity DVT is significant pain and swelling of the affected limb. Generally, thrombus that presents distally in the infrapopliteal segment or deep calf veins tends to be less symptomatic. Of concern is the isolated calf vein thrombosis; in these patients propagation or thrombus extension has been seen to occur in 10–29% of cases (6–7). Of note, approximately 95% of patients who present with infrapopliteal DVT will lyse their clot by endogenous fibrinolysis while anticoagulated; of concern are those patients who, as stated above, continue to propagate thrombus proximally extending into the femoral and iliac veins.

PTS is a *chronic* condition that results from residual venous obstruction and valvular incompetence resulting in ambulatory venous hypertension. It is a complication that is associated with significant morbidity and socioeconomic burden (1,8–14). Those patients with both valvular incompetence and significant residual venous obstruction are those with the most severe post-thrombotic symptoms. The emergence of symptoms tends to occur within the first two years after the initial episode of acute DVT and has been approximated to occur in 20–50% of DVT patients (13). In one study, 48% of the patients treated with routine appropriate anticoagulation for their DVT developed skin changes with stasis ulceration (9a). PTS encompasses a range of symptoms that includes hyperpigmentation of the skin, leg pain or feeling of heaviness, venous claudication, edema, venous ectasia, varicosities, and skin ulceration. It is important for the clinician to distinguish between PTS and other causes of chronic insufficiency such as primary valvular insufficiency prior to selecting a treatment (1).

Although usually symptomatic, DVT can be clinically occult. Detection of an acute lower extremity DVT can be initiated by patient complaints like leg pain, edema, and skin discoloration. Strong clinical suspicion coupled with results from diagnostic radiological imaging such as ultrasound, computer topography (CT), magnetic resonance imaging, or venography will all confirm the presence of a DVT. CT findings have been shown to be better predictors of favorable outcomes of thrombolytic therapy than duration of clinical symptoms alone, though ascending venography is still considered the gold standard diagnostic method (14). Multiple segment involvement of the venous system is most commonly encountered in patients with acute DVT. The location and magnitude of the discovered clot can determine the potential for recanalization and risk for long-term debilitation or recurrence. Proximal venous thrombosis is associated with a 20–50% risk of recurrence, and iliofemoral thrombus specifically has been shown to be associated with significant post-thrombotic morbidity (8–9,15). The national multicenter Venous Registry that evaluated the impact of catheter-directed thrombolysis on DVT determined that iliofemoral DVT patients were lysed more successfully than femoro-popliteal DVT patients. The Registry analyzed the results from 312 urokinase (UK) infusions in 287 patients with symptomatic lower limb DVT. The Registry also provided additional noteworthy information such as the following: acute DVT responded better than chronic DVT, and catheter-directed therapy lysed thrombus better than systemic infusion (15–16).

MANAGEMENT

The medical community recognizes anticoagulation therapy with heparin and warfarin as the mainstay of treatment for acute DVT. In the acute episode, treating multisegment versus single segment disease remains the same in the medical community, yet the long-term outcome and complications vary greatly for these two entities. Unfractionated heparin has been shown to be effective in the prevention and treatment of DVT by reducing clot propagation and the likelihood of PE. A five- to seven-day protocol of heparin followed by at least three months on warfarin is traditionally used to maintain a therapeutic international normalized ratio of 2.0–3.0. The warfarin and heparin can be given simultaneously for approximately four days until therapeutic range is achieved. Low-molecular-weight (LMW) heparin preparations are offered as an alternative to the traditional unfractionated heparin. LMW heparin has been associated with comparable efficacy rates, less bleeding events, and lower rates of recurrence (18–21).

One of the most serious complications of DVT, pulmonary embolus, is significantly reduced in patients treated with anticoagulation therapy. PE can often be the cause for clinical presentation or can be clinically silent in DVT patients. It has been estimated that 1 in 250 patients presenting with DVT will develop a fatal PE during their three-month course of anticoagulant therapy. After anticoagulant therapy is discontinued, the risk of fatal PE is estimated at 0.3% per year (22). Despite the benefits of anticoagulation therapy, the traditional therapy has been seen as inadequate for long-segment occlusion and in addressing the long-term disability from chronic occlusion and PTS (23). Anticoagulation is dependent on the patient's own fibrinolytic system, and the extent of thrombus present can result in slow resolution of patient symptoms or propagation of the clot (2,24). Comerota and Aldridge found that of those patients evaluated with a venogram after being treated with intravenous heparin, only 4% had significant or complete lysis, 14% had partial lysis, and 82% had either no lysis or an extension of the clot (25). Also, Prandoni et al. prospectively evaluated patients being treated with anticoagulation and found that their results demonstrated a poor long-term clinical course with 30.3% of patients having recurrence (26). When the extent of the thrombus is much more involved, such as iliofemoral DVT, early recognition and local catheter-directed infusion of thrombolytics has been effective in recanalization and preservation of valvular function (15–17,24–26). Higher rates of venous recanalization and restoration of flow have been seen with systemic administration of thrombolytics when compared to standard anticoagulation. Comerota looked at 13 studies which compared standard anticoagulation therapy with systemic thrombolysis. Of the patients who had received systemic thrombolysis, 45% had complete or nearly complete resolution of thrombus, whereas 18% had partial dissolution.

As mentioned in the previous paragraph, when anticoagulation only was administered, 4% had complete lysis while 14% had partial lysis (25). There are several other studies that demonstrated the same results. More importantly, the question answered by Jeffery et al. demonstrated in a prospective randomized study that early recanalization with systemic thrombolysis of patients with an acute DVT allowed for restoration of valvular function and prevention of reflux at the popliteal valve, when reevaluated at 5 and 10 years after treatment with direct Doppler examination, foot volumetry, and photophlethymography. Therefore, thrombolysis can be utilized to reduce the formation of post-thrombotic symptoms. Meissner et al. established that early recanalization is important in preserving valvular function (17). In preventing valvular injury, the long-term disabling symptoms of PTS can be averted. Failures of recanalization when using systemic thrombolytics were secondary to the massive clot burden and the inability to get the thrombolytic agent into the thrombus. Therefore, local catheter-directed thrombolytic therapy with or without mechanical thrombectomy has become the next natural step in the treatment algorithm of DVT.

TREATMENT

Antithrombotic regimens include surgical treatment, medications that inhibit blood coagulation such as direct thrombin inhibitors, and other products like compression stockings that deal directly with venous stasis. Restoration of vein patency can now be attempted with one of the multiple agents available on today's market. Indications for *pharmaceutical thrombolysis* include the presence of thrombosis and/or symptoms for less than 14 days, symptomatic DVT, a threatened extremity (phlegmasia cerulean dolens), and no contraindications to thrombolytic therapy. Contraindications to lytic therapy include active internal bleeding, recent gastrointestinal (GI) bleed, recent stroke, major surgery/biopsy or trauma, known coagulopathy, allergy to thrombolytics, pregnancy, uncontrolled hypertension, intracerebral neoplasmor metastatic disease, and bacterial endocarditis.

Once acute iliofemoral DVT has been identified either by high clinical suspicion or through diagnostic imaging (CT, MRI, ultrasound, or diagnostic venography) a complete clinical history and physical examination should be performed, appropriate lab results gathered, and informed consent obtained. Relevant laboratory studies include blood urea nitrogen (BUN)/creatinine (Cr), coagulation studies (prothrombin time (PT)/partial thromboplastine time (PTT), fibrinogen), Hgb/Hct, and platelets. Previous imaging studies provide valuable information concerning the extent of thrombus present and indicate which route of venous access is appropriate for the case.

An additional consideration prior to lytic therapy is whether the patient requires an IVC filter placement. Filters are not routinely placed prior to thrombolysis since PE has been shown to occur infrequently with catheter-directed thrombolysis (27). However, the decision to place a filter is dependent on the extent of thrombus in the iliac veins and IVC. A large "floating" thrombus in the IVC is probable indication for an IVC filter placement (28). The filter should often be placed using the jugular approach to reduce bleeding from the insertion site while thrombolysis is in progress and also to prevent thrombus migration during placement. Temporary IVC filters may have a future role in any patient at significant risk for PE during DVT treatment.

Multiple venous access approaches have been described in the literature; these include access from the internal jugular veins, a tibial or calf vein (29), contralateral femoral vein, and ipsilateral popliteal vein. In the results of a multicenter Venous Registry, the approach most commonly used for catheter-directed thrombolysis cases was the popliteal vein approach. The retrograde passage of catheters and wires through the iliac and femoral valves can be challenging thereby making alternative access routes less desirable (16).

Ultrasound guidance (5- or 7.5-MHz linear transducer) can be used to minimize the potential complications associated with inadvertent arterial puncture or multiple attempts at accessing the vein. Additionally, a 21-gauge micropuncture needle set can be used to further reduce complications if multiple venous punctures or an inadvertent arterial stick occurs. A standard micropuncture set consists of a 21-gauge needle, a 0.018-inch diameter guidewire, and a coaxial 4- or 5-French dilator that accepts a 0.035-inch guidewire.

The extent and level of thrombus is determined by a venogram once venous access is obtained. It is recommended that an intravenous sheath be placed in the accessed vein and the occlusion crossed with a guidewire, preferably one with a hydrophilic coating, and a multiple side-holed infusion catheter. The success of catheter-directed therapy is dependent upon gaining appropriate access as well as the ability to cross the thrombosed segment of vein with both wire and catheter. The entire thrombus burden should be crossed and also lysed simultaneously, instead of repositioning the catheter with each follow-up venogram. To accomplish this, a single infusion catheter of 50 cm in length or a combination coaxial infusion system can be employed. Multiple infusion systems are on the market for both "pulse-spray" and continuous infusion catheter-directed thrombolysis. Once the infusion system is in place, the thrombolytic agent of choice can be administered. Additionally, heparin can be infused through the side-port of the introducer sheath or a bolus of heparin can be given prior to catheter placement to adequately anticoagulate the patient while the catheter is in place.

The management of patients undergoing thrombolytic therapy requires arranging for admission into an ICU or step-down unit where the patient can be monitored closely. This is dependent on the requirements for each institution while infusing thrombolytics. While on the floor, intravenous (IV), punctures and intramuscular (IM), injections should be avoided, and alternative means for blood draws should be established, i.e., peripherally inserted central catheter. Every six to eight hours laboratory values including prothrombin time, activated partial thromboplastin time, fibrinogen, hemoglobin (HGB)/hematocrit (HCT), and platelet levels are re-evaluated. Measuring fibrinogen levels can be controversial, however, some have found it to be a good parameter of active fibrinolysis. If the fibrinogen level decreases by greater than 50% of its initial value or it is less than 100 mg/dL, the thrombolytic dose is decreased by half, until the fibrinogen level returns to a value greater than 100 mg/dl. Endpoints of therapy include complete resolution (>90%) of thrombus on repeat venogram, no significant or major bleeding or no change in the thrombus burden after considerable lysis time. Repeat venograms are performed at 8 to 12 hours after initiation of lytic therapy to evaluate for restoration of patency. After completion of thrombolytics and resolution of the DVT, the vein should be evaluated for an underlying venous lesion and then treated appropriately with balloon angioplasty and/or endovascular stent placement. Immediately post-thrombosis, full-dose IV heparin is introduced and eventually the patient will receive complete anticoagulation for a three to six-month period with warfarin.

Endovascular stent placement after thrombolysis or mechanical thrombectomy has been quite successful in treating underlying venous lesions or residual occlusions after thrombolytic therapy (30,31). In lower extremity venous disease, the majority of these lesions will present on the left. Often enough they will not respond well to balloon angioplasty and reoccur immediately after treatment. The left iliac venous stenosis is commonly attributed to iliac compression syndrome, May-Thurner Syndrome, or pelvic spur syndrome (21,32–34). May-Thurner syndrome has been estimated to be present in 20% of the adult population and is thought to be the result of an intraluminal venous web or spur.

This pathology is attributed to sustained iliac artery compression of the left common iliac vein. Patel et al. evaluated the results of combined thrombolytic therapy and stent placement in May-Thurner patients and reported initial clinical success with complete resolution of symptoms (34). In patients with underlying venous disease, the location of the stent placement is a factor in establishing long-term patency. The multicenter Venous Registry reported that the stents that addressed iliac vein outflow obstruction had better patency results compared to stents placed in the femoral-popliteal veins. If the venous lesion is confined to the femoral vein, only angioplasty is recommended as femoral stents have a high propensity to rethrombosis (16). Other indications for endovenous stents, other than persistent hemodynamically significant venous stenosis or occlusion, include extrinsic compression due to tumor invasion of chronic-resistant thrombus (1). Note, currently there are no food and drug administration (FDA) approved stents for the iliofemoral venous system, however, the most effective and preferred at this time in managing balloon resistant stenoses are the self-expanding stents.

THROMBOLYTIC AGENTS

While the goals of lytic therapy are well-accepted, the available thrombolytic agents' safety and efficacy are still being compared. Available agents include Streptokinase (SK), t-PA, r-PA, and UK. SK (Streptase; AstraZeneca Laboratories, Westboro, Massachusetts) was the first thrombolytic agent to be approved for intravenous treatment of arterial and venous thrombosis and used widely in the 1970s, but now is no longer used due to its antigenicity and known risk of dangerous allergic side effects. Initial studies comparing IV SK to IV heparin in patients with acute DVT were encouraging, demonstrating significant improvement in clot lysis, and restoration of flow with thrombolytics compared to the traditional management with anticoagulation (35). Elliot et al. had 90% clot lysis in 35% of their patients, and an additional 80% clot lysis in 30% of patients treated with IV Streptokinase versus heparin (36). However, Comerota and colleagues reported a rate of only 45% partial or complete lysis with systemic infusion and had far better results with catheter-directed treatment (25,37). Due to complications associated with long infusion times and large thrombolytic doses, systemic therapy was abandoned.

UK (Abbokinase: Abbott Laboratories, Abbot Park, Illinois) was the agent of choice in the early 1990s and was used for most thrombolytic endovascular interventions. However, in 1999 UK was removed from distribution due to FDA concerns of viral contamination (38). Based on the findings of the Urokinase PE Trial and the Urokinase Streptokinase PE Trial, currently UK is the only FDA approved agent for the lysis of pulmonary emboli and is currently being reintroduced onto the market. Multiple studies have been performed illustrating the efficacy of catheter-directed thrombolysis using UK as the primary thrombolytic agent of interest. Semba and

Dake reported early awareness of the effectiveness of catheter-directed thrombolysis. They reported complete lysis in 18 of 21 (72%) patients accompanied by resolution of symptoms (24). The national multicenter Venous Registry included both acute and chronic patients treated with local catheter-directed UK. Symptoms were acute or less than 10 days in duration in 188 patients or 66%, and greater than 10 days in duration in 45 patients or 16%. They reported a technical success rate of greater than 50% lysis in 88% of patients with acute iliofemoral DVT, and in 83% of patients with femoro-popliteal thrombus. The overall patency rates at one year were 64% for patients with iliofemoral DVT and 47% for patients with femoro-popliteal disease. Predictors of success included symptoms of less than 10 days in duration, thrombus iliofemoral in location, and no prior history of DVT (16).

Alteplase (rt-PA; Activase; Genentech, Inc., San Francisco, California) is a plasminogen activator that was initially introduced as a systematic thrombolytic and became more commonly utilized after UK was taken off the market. Guidelines have been proposed for arterial use of rt-PA by an advisory panel of the Society of Cardiovascular and Interventional Radiology. These guidelines may serve as a foundation upon which to construct a protocol for catheter-directed venous thrombolysis (39). The efficacy and safety of rt-PA at different doses was further investigated after the removal of UK and similar rates were obtained. Most clinicians currently use a dose between 0.25 U/hr and 1.0 U/hr (40). Chang et al. reported 75% technical success with a pulse-spray technique administering 50 mg/day over one hour daily for a maximum of four daily doses (41).

Reteplase (r-PA; Retevase; Centacor/Johnson & Johnson, Malvern, Pennsylvania) is a recombinant derivative of rt-PA that has been approved for the treatment of acute myocardial infarction (MI) and has also emerged in the treatment algorithms for acute DVT. The results utilizing reteplase in the treatment of DVT, though anecdotal, have been promising. There have been a few studies involving reteplase therapy for DVT in the literature. Two worth mentioning were clinical studies performed by Ouriel et al. and Castaneda et al. Ouriel et al. reported that 8 of 11 patients or 72.7%, had dissolution of thrombus after receiving catheter-directed reteplase therapy, and Castaneda et al. reported a success rate of 92% using 2.5–42 U of reteplase on 25 patients with acute and chronic DVT (42,43).

When introduced, catheter-directed venous thrombolysis was well accepted due to improved clot lysis with lower complication rates and lower thrombolytic doses. The success of catheter-directed therapy is dependent upon many factors including the ability to gain appropriate access, proper patient selection, premature termination of therapy, and the ability to cross the thrombosed segment of vein (30). Although the FDA currently approves no fibrinolytic agent for catheter-directed treatment of DVT, the studies performed indicate that thrombolytics are useful in the management of DVT. Older trials comparing thrombolytic agents were based predominantly on systemic administration and often compare heparin or SK to single agents. Overall success rates of catheter-directed therapy range from 86% to 100% depending on the series. These results are based on Grossman and McPherson's review of 15 studies completed since 1991 using catheter-directed therapy for DVT. The studies reviewed were primarily UK studies and two rt-PA studies (27). Presently, there are no prospective randomized trials to compare complication rates of long-term outcomes. There was a retrospective study comparing rt-PA and UK evaluating the success and complication rates, but no significant difference was reported between the two agents. The study did associate rt-PA with lower cost and shorter infusion time (44).

COMPLICATIONS

Complications associated with thrombolysis include bleeding, PE, infection, sepsis, vessel injury, and hypersensitivity reactions to the agent. Appropriate patient selection also helps to decrease the complications. Those who would benefit the most from treatment are the younger, healthier population. Initially, in the treatment of DVT, the risk of PE was thought to be high. However, Semba and Dake monitored their patients with pre- and post-perfusion scans and found no evidence of PE (24). In the Venous Registry, 6 of 473 patients (1%) had symptomatic PE, one of which was fatal (16). IVC filter placement was evaluated in Grossman and McPherson's review of those patients who received an IVC filter prior to catheter-directed therapy; there was no single case of PE reported. In those who did not receive a filter, 0.9% or 2 of 214 patients had symptomatic PE (27).

The second major complication is bleeding. Reported rates range widely from 0% to 25% with the majority of events being minor and occurring at the puncture site (1). Major bleeds requiring blood transfusion include retroperitoneal bleeding, distant areas of hematoma formation, gastrointestinal bleeding, and intracranial hemorrhage (30). In the Venous Registry, major bleed occurred in 11% requiring blood product transfusions, and 16% minor bleeds occurred most commonly at the site of access. The risk of intracranial hemorrhage and death was 0.25% and 0.4%, respectively. Some feel that with shorter infusion times and lower thrombolytic doses decreasing the dosage of concomitant anticoagulation, complication rates will be significantly decreased (16). *Mechanical thrombectomy* devices introduced in the 1990s have been used to first debulk the thrombus prior to initiating thrombolytic agent infusion in an attempt to reduce infusion dose (45). Kasirajan et al. attempted this in a small sample group with the AngioJet thrombectomy device (Possis Medical, Inc., Mineapolis, Minnesota) and found that less of the thrombolytic agent was required (46). There are no large-scale DVT clinical trials, excluding animal model studies, with mechanical thrombectomy devices (47,48). Bleeding complications may be significantly less with combined therapy with quicker times to recanalization and decreased dose of lytic agent.

CONCLUSION

Understanding chronic venous insufficiency as well as chronic venous hypertension allows one to better understand the treatment algorithm of acute venous thrombosis. It has been established that restoring patency can alleviate patient symptoms, but achieving the goals of preserving valve function and removing venous obstruction can reduce the emergence of PTS. It has also been demonstrated that PTS can have a significant impact on patients' daily living activities and overall quality of life (1,6–8,12). Kahn and colleagues evaluated PTS patients with the Venous Insufficiency Epidemiologic and Economic Study (VEINES) quality of life and venous symptoms questionnaires. The results indicated that subjects with PTS had significantly worse disease-specific VEINES quality of life scores than those without PTS (12).

Additionally, the scores of the PTS subjects worsened significantly with the increase in the severity of the symptoms (12). It has been indicated that thrombolytic therapy is more efficacious than anticoagulation alone in preventing the formation of PTS by preserving valvular function (6). Achieving adequate thrombolysis can be facilitated by adjunctive therapy like angioplasty, stent placement, and concomitant use of mechanical thrombectomy devices. More investigation is needed to fully understand the potential of these therapies or the combination of these therapies. In the future, for those with continued valvular incompetence, percutaneous prosthetic venous valvular implants may be an alternative to chronic venous insufficiency and reflux (49). Additionally, prospective, randomized trials comparing long-term outcomes, complications, and efficacy of the various thrombolytic agents are needed to validate the role of catheter-directed thrombolysis in the treatment of acute venous thrombosis, and in the prevention of PTS.

REFERENCES

1. Sharafuddin MJ, Sun S, Hoballah JJ, Youness FM, Sharp WJ, Roh B. Endovascular management of venous thrombotic and occlusive diseases of the lower extremities. J Vasc Interv Radial 2003; 14:405–423.
2. Meissner MH, Caps MT, Bergelin RO, Manzo RA, Strandness DE Jr. Propagation, rethrombosis and new thrombus formation after acute deep venous thrombosis. J Vasc Surg 1995; 22:558--567.
3. Carson JL, Kelley MA, Duff A, Weg JG, Fulkerson WJ, Palevsky HI, Schwartz JS, Thompson BT, Popovich J Jr, Hobbins TE, et al. The clinical course of pulmonary embolism. N Engl J Med 1992 May 7; 326(19):1240–1245.
4. Kearon C. Natural history of venous thromboembolism. Circulation 2003; 107(23 suppl 1):22–30.
5. Perkins JM, Magee TR, Galland RB. Phlegmasia caerulea dolens and venous gangrene. Br J Surg 1996; 83(1):19–23.
6. Markel A, Manzo RA, Bergelin RO, Strandness DE Jr. Pattern and distribution of thrombi in acute venous thrombosis. Arch Surg 1992; 127:305–309.
7. Saarinen JP, Domonyi K, Zeitlin R, Salenius JP. Postthrombotic syndrome after isolated calf deep venous thrombosis: the role of popliteal reflux. Vasc Surg 2002; 36(5):959–964.
8. O'Donnell TF Jr, Browse NL, Burnand KG, Thomas ML. The socioeconomic effects of an iliofemoral venous thrombosis. J Surg Res 1977; 22(5):483–488.
9. Comerota AJ. Quality-of-life improvement using thrombolytic therapy for iliofemoral deep venous thrombosis. Rev Cardiovasc Med 2002; 3(suppl 2):S61– S67.
10. Johnson BF, Manzo RA, Bergelin RO, Strandness DE Jr. Relationship between changes in the deep venous system and the development of the postthrombotic syndrome after an acute episode of lower limb deep vein thrombosis: a one- to six-year follow-up. J Vasc Surg 1995; 21:307–312; discussion, 313.
11. Albrechtsson U, Anderson J, Einarsson E, Eklof B, Norgren L. Streptokinase treatment of deep venous thrombosis and the postthrombotic syndrome. Follow-up evaluation of venous function. Arch Surg 1981 Jan; 116(1):33–37.
12. Kahn SR, Hirsch A, Shrier I. Effect of postthrombotic syndrome on health-related quality of life after deep venous thrombosis. Arch Intern Med 2002; 162:1144–1148.
13. Skull KC, Nicolaides AN, Fernades JF, et al. Significance of popliteal reflux in relation to ambulatory venous pressure and ulceration. Arch Surg 1979; 114:1304.
14. Roh B, Park K, Kim E, Yoon K, Juhng S, So B, Sharafuddin MJ. Prognostic value of CT before thrombolytic therapy in iliofemoral deep venous thrombosis. J Vasc Interv Radiol 2002; 13:71–76.
15. Meissner MH. Thrombolytic therapy for acute deep vein thrombosis and the Venous Registry. Rev Cardiovasc Med 2002; 3(suppl 2):S53–S60.
16. Mewissen MW, Seabrook GR, Meissner MH, Cynamon J, Labropoulos N, Haughton SH. Catheter-directed thrombolysis for lower extremity deep venous thrombosis: report of a national multicenter registry [Published erratum appears in Radiology 1999; 213(3):930]. Radiology 1999; 211:39–49.

17. Meissner MH, Manzo RA, Bergelin RO, Markel A, Strandness DE Jr. Deep venous insufficiency: the relationship between lysis and subsequent reflux. J Vasc Surg 1993; 18:596–605; discussion, 606–608.

18. Hyers TM, Agnelli G, Hull RD, Morris TA, Samama M, Tapson V, Weg JG. Antithrombotic therapy for venous thromboembolic disease. Chest 2001; 119:176S–193S.

19. Hirsh J. Low-molecular-weight heparin: a review of the results of recent studies of the treatment of venous thromboembolism and unstable angina. Circulation 1998; 98:1575–1582.

20. Hirsh J, Warkentin TE, Shaughnessy SG, Anand SS, Halperin JL, Raschke R, Granger C, Ohman EM, Dalen JE. Heparin and low-molecular-weight heparin mechanisms of action, pharmacokinetics, dosing, monitoring, efficacy, and safety. Chest 2001; 119:64S–94S.

21. Hull RD, Raskob GE, Rosenbloom D, Lemaire J, Pineo GF, Baylis B, Ginsberg JS, Panju AA, Brill-Edwards P, Brant R. Optimal therapeutic level of heparin therapy in patients with venous thrombosis. Arch Intern Med 1992; 152:1589–1595.

22. Douketis JD, Kearon C, Bates S, Duku EK, Ginsberg JS. Risk of fatal pulmonary embolism in patients with treated venous thromboembolism. J Am Med Assoc 1998; 279: 458–462.

23. Strandness DE Jr, Langlois Y, Cramer M, Randlett A, Thiele BL. Long-term sequelae of acute venous thrombosis. J Am Med Assoc 1983; 250:1289–1292.

24. Semba CP, Dake MD. Iliofemoral deep venous thrombosis: aggressive therapy with catheter-directed thrombolysis. Radiology 1994; 191:487–494.

25. Comerota AJ, Aldridge SC. Thrombolytic therapy for acute deep vein thrombosis. Sem Vasc Surg 1992; 5:76–81.

26. Prandoni P, Lensing AW, Cogo A, Cuppini S, Villalta S, Carta M, Cattelan AM, Polistena P, Bernardi E, Prins MH. The long-term clinical course of acute deep venous thrombosis. Ann Intern Med 1996 Jul 1; 125(1):1–7.

27. Grossman C, McPherson S. Safety and efficacy of catheter-directed thrombolysis for iliofemoral venous thrombosis. Am J Roentgenol 1999; 172:667–672.

28. Norris CS, Greenfield LJ, Herrmann JB. Free-floating iliofemoral thrombus: a risk of pulmonary embolism. Arch Surg 1985; 120:806–808.

29. Cragg AH. Lower extremity deep venous thrombolysis: a new approach to obtaining access. J Vasc Interv Radiol 1996; 7:283–288.

30. Bjarnason H, Kruse JR, Asinger DA, Nazarian GK, Dietz CA Jr, Caldwell MD, Key NS, Hirsch AT, Hunter DW. Iliofemoral deep venous thrombosis: safety and efficacy outcome during 5 years of catheter-directed thrombolytic therapy. J Vasc Interv Radiol 1997 May-Jun; 8(3):405–418.

31. Nazarian GK, Bjarnason H, Dietz CA, Bernadas CA, Hunter DW. Iliofemoral venous stenoses: effectiveness of treatment with metallic endovascular stents. Radiology 1996; 2000:193–199.

32. Raju S, Owen S, Neglen P. The clinical impact of iliac venous stents in the management of chronic venous insufficiency. J Vasc Surg 2002; 35:8–15.

33. O'Sullivan GJ, Semba CP, Bittner CA, Kee ST, Razavi MK, Sze DY, Dake MD. Endovascular management of iliac vein compression (May-Thurner) syndrome. J Vasc Interv Radiol 2000 Jul-Aug; 11(7):823–836.

34. Patel NH, Stookey KR, Ketcham DB, Cragg AH. Endovascular management of acute extensive iliofemoral deep venous thrombosis caused by May-Thurner syndrome. J Vasc Interv Radiol 2000; 11:1297–1308.

35. Dotter CT, Rosch J, Seaman AJ. Selective clot lysis with low-dose streptokinase. Radiology 1974; 111:31–37.

36. Elliot EJ, Immelman PJ, Benatur MR. A comparative randomized trial of heparin versus streptokinase in the treatment of acute proximal venous thrombosis: an interim report of a prospective trial. Br J Surg 1979; 66:837–843.

37. Comerota AJ, Aldridge SC, Cohen G, Ball DS, Pliskin M, White JV. A strategy of aggressive regional therapy for acute iliofemoral venous thrombosis with contemporary venous thrombectomy or catheter-directed thrombolysis. J Vasc Surg 1994; 20(2):244–254.

38. Important drug warning: Dear Healthcare Provider (Letter). Rockville, MD: Center for Biologics Evaluation and Research, Public Health Service, Food and Drug Administration, January 25, 1999.

39. Semba CP, Murphy TP, Bakal CW, Calis KA, Matalon TA. Thrombolytic therapy with use of alteplase (rt-PA) in peripheral arterial occlusive disease: review of the clinical literature. J Vasc Interv Radiol 2000; 11:149–161.

40. Ouriel K. Safety and efficacy of the various thrombolytic agents. Rev Cardiovasc Med 2002; 3(suppl 2):S17–S24.

41. Chang R, Cannon RO III, Chen CC, Doppman JL, Shawker TH, Mayo DJ, Wood B, Horne MK III. Daily catheter-directed single dosing of t-PA in treatment of acute deep venous thrombosis of the lower extremity. J Vasc Interv Radiol 2001; 12:247–252.

42. Ouriel K, Katzen B, Mewissen M, Flick P, Clair DG, Benenati J, McNamara TO, Gibbens D. Reteplase in the treatment of peripheral arterial and venous occlusions: a pilot study. J Vasc Interv Radiol 2000; 11:849–854.

43. Castaneda F, Li R, Young K, Swischuk JL, Smouse B, Brady T. Catheter-directed thrombolysis in deep venous thrombosis with use of reteplase: immediate results and complications from a pilot study. J Vasc Interv Radiol 2002 Jun; 13(6):577–580.

44. Sugimoto K, Hofmann LV, Razavi MK, Kee ST, Sze DY, Dake MD, Semba CP. The safety, efficacy, and pharmacoeconomics of low-dose alteplase compared with urokinase for catheter-directed thrombolysis of arterial and venous occlusions. J Vasc Surg 2003; 37(3):512–517..

45. Vedantham S, Vesely TM, Parti N, Darcy M, Hovsepian DM, Picus D. Lower extremity venous thrombolysis with adjunctive mechanical thrombectomy. J Vasc Interv Radiol 2002; 13:1001–1008.

46. Kasirajan K, Gray B, Ouriel K. Percutaneous AngioJet thrombectomy in the management of extensive deep venous thrombosis. J Vasc Interv Radiol 2001; 12:179–185.

47. Trerotola SO, McLennan G, Davidson D, Lane KA, Ambrosius WT, Lazzaro C, Dreesen J. Preclinical in vivo testing of the Arrow-Trerotola percutaneous thrombolytic device for venous thrombosis. J Vasc Interv Radiol 2001; 12:95–103.

48. Sharafuddin MJ, Hicks ME, Jenson ML, Morris JE, Drasler WJ, Wilson GJ. Rheolytic thrombectomy with use of the AngioJet-F105 catheter: preclinical evaluation of safety. J Vasc Interv Radiol 1997; 8:939–945.

49. Pavenik D, Machan L, Urhida B, et al. Percutaneous prosthetic venous valves: current state and possible applications. Tech Vasc Interv Radiol 2003; 6(3):137–142.

50. Kahn SR, Hirsch A, Shrier I. Effect of postthrombotic syndrome on health-related quality of life after deep venous thrombosis. Arch Intern Med 2002; 162(10):1144–1148.

22

Thrombotic and Embolic Complications of Endovascular Therapy of Cerebrovascular Disease

Alex Abou-Chebl
Interventional Neurology, Section of Stroke and Neurological Intensive Care,
The Cleveland Clinic Foundation, Cleveland, Ohio, U.S.A.

Christopher Bajzer
Department of Cardiovascular Medicine, The Cleveland Clinic Foundation,
Cleveland, Ohio, U.S.A.

INTRODUCTION

The goal of endovascular therapy in the treatment of cerebrovascular disease is to modify the disease state in order to decrease the risk of subsequent brain injury or death. The performance of endovascular therapy for cerebrovascular disease is associated with risks for brain injury and death due to unintended complications. The formation of thrombus and/or distal embolization of thrombus or atheromatous tissue into the cerebrovascular arterial system can result in brain injury or death. The cause of unintended thrombosis in the setting of endovascular therapy for cerebrovascular disease is best understood by recalling Virchow's classic triad. Virchow initially described the classic triad of conditions predisposing to the formation of intravascular thrombosis (originally in veins): stasis of blood flow, endothelial injury, and hypercoagulable states. Obviously, if an intravascular thrombus is occlusive or near occlusive to blood flow, this will result in brain injury, and depending upon the extent and severity of the brain injury, potentially death. Embolism is the movement of material which may consist of thrombus, atheromatous debris, or other tissue from an upstream location in an artery to a downstream location where it ultimately lodges. The ultimate distal destination of the embolic material and the degree of occlusion of the blood vessel at its destination will determine the extent and severity of brain injury that results. It is easy to understand that during the manipulation of endovascular devices in the vascular space that operator-induced movement of such devices can dislodge an existing thrombus or atheromatous tissue or other tissue. It is also easy to understand how body motion including pulsatile hemodynamics of blood flow can dislodge endovascular devices or existing thrombus that formed as a result of manipulating an endovascular device. This section will review the cause and incidence of thrombotic and embolic complications of endovascular treatment of cerebrovascular disease. This section will also briefly review the prevention, detection, and treatment of thrombotic and embolic complications of endovascular treatment of cerebrovascular disease.

ETIOLOGY AND INCIDENCE

Catheters and Devices

The placement of a catheter in the endovascular space provides a non-endothelial covered surface to activate the coagulation cascade for the formation of thrombus. Studies have been performed on the thrombogenicity of diagnostic and interventional catheters in humans. The incidence of thrombus formation on the catheter surface is proportional to the length of time that the catheter is in contact with blood elements. In a recent study, catheters with the smoothest surface characteristics were the most thrombogenic. Endovascular catheters are available using different polymers for their structural composition. In this recent study, there was no correlation between the surface chemical composition and thrombogenicity. However, it was noted that catheters based primarily on polyethylene were slightly less thrombogenic compared to catheters composed mostly of a polyamide polymer.

The incidence of thrombus formation due to endovascular intervention or equipment placement in the vascular space can only be approximated. This approximation is based on clinical data on the incidence of clinical syndromes such as transient ischemic attack (TIA) and/or stroke, and has been compiled in the setting of diagnostic cerebral angiography. The incidence of TIA or stroke in the setting of diagnostic cerebral angiography has been reported to be within the range of 0–1.5% of procedures. Catheter thrombosis with subsequent embolization is not the sole reason for the incidence of these clinical events. Other causes include the embolization of air, crystallized contrast or other foreign debris introduced by poor angiographic technique, or the limitation of cerebral blood flow due to vasospasm or dissection. The actual incidence of thrombus formation associated with diagnostic catheters and other endovascular devices remains unknown. A recent study demonstrated that in the absence of a systemic anticoagulant, thrombus formation with occlusion of the lumen of the catheter was observed in 44% of 50 cm length catheters through which arterial blood from a test subject was allowed to freely flow until a threshold of 15 minutes or 30 mL of blood was reached. The occlusion time ranged between 3 minutes and 15 minutes. The average time to catheter occlusion was $8\frac{1}{2}$ minutes. The use of therapeutic anticoagulation during endovascular intervention is obligatory and mitigates this complication risk.

Using clinically detected syndromes of TIA or stroke unfortunately underestimates the true incidence of embolic events associated with diagnostic and interventional cerebral angiography. Recent studies using diffusion weighted (DWI) magnetic resonance imaging (MRI), which is exquisitely sensitive for brain infarcts, had attempted to quantify so-called "clinically silent" cerebral embolic events. In one study, DWI imaging was performed prior to and after 66 diagnostic and 34 interventional cerebrovascular procedures. No abnormalities were observed on the pre-procedural DWI MRI studies. DWI imaging lesions consistent with embolic events were observed in 17 of 66 of the diagnostic cases, and 6 of 34 of the interventional procedures. There were no new clinical neurological deficits after any of the angiographic procedures. The appearance of the DWI MRI evidence of embolic events correlated with the amount of contrast required for the procedure, as well as the total fluoroscopy time, the number of catheters utilized, and the difficulty of the placement of catheters into the cerebrovascular anatomy.

Angioplasty and Stents

The goal of both stand-alone angioplasty as well as angioplasty and adjunctive stenting is to apply an internal compressive force to a blood vessel at the location of a pathologic reduction of the cross sectional area of the blood vessel lumen. Inherent in the performance of stand-alone angioplasty or angioplasty and stenting is the resultant endothelial injury with disruption of the endothelial surface of the blood vessel. In addition, the subendothelial vascular elements are uncovered and are placed in contact with the blood stream. This disruption of the intimal surface of the blood vessel precipitates the coagulation cascade and the result is formation of thrombus. This thrombus can either be partially or totally occlusive and in certain settings the thrombus fragments result in thromboembolism. The incidence of thrombosis to any degree in the setting of angioplasty, as well as angioplasty and stenting, is likely 100%. The incidence of clinically relevant thrombosis and/or thromboembolism is substantially less frequent. Clinical endpoints of stroke or TIA can be used as a surrogate endpoint for clinically relevant thrombosis or thromboembolic events occurring in relation to balloon angioplasty and stenting. A self-reported global carotid artery angioplasty and stent registry is maintained and has been reported in the literature and updated every few years. In a recent update of the self-reported global carotid artery stent registry, the 30-day stroke rate was 3.93%, and the 30-day TIA rate was 2.45% for a combined 30-day neurological event rate of 6.38%. Similar data is available for carotid angioplasty alone and derived from a report of the CAVATAS-I study. In this study, 74% of patients undergoing endovascular treatment of carotid stenosis received stand-alone angioplasty without any mechanical emboli protection. The 30-day stroke and death rate was 5.9% and the 30-day any neurological event and death rate was 10%. Statistics for angioplasty or angioplasty and stent thrombosis or thromboembolic events are not known with precision. It is known however that long lesions measuring >15–20 mm and lesions containing an intraluminal filling defect, i.e., thrombus, are associated with an increased risk of thromboembolism during carotid artery stenting.

A systematic study of balloon angioplasty or balloon angioplasty and stenting in other locations in the cerebral vasculature such as the intracranial circulation does not exist. However, data pooled from several studies have shown an ischemic stroke rate that has ranged from 0% to 50% with an average perioperative ischemic stroke risk of 13–16% (1–8). Given the anatomic size similarity of the intracranial vessels to the coronary vessels, and the fact that the equipment initially designed for coronary use including coronary angioplasty balloons and coronary stents are utilized for angioplasty and stenting in the intracranial vessels, one could hypothesize that the risk of clinically relevant intervention site thrombosis or thromboembolic events in the cerebrovascular vessels would be similar to the incidence of the enzymatically proven myocardial infarction after intervention on comparable coronary vessels. Following this hypothesis, the estimated event rate would be in range of 3–25%. To date, no biomarkers for cerebral ischemia or anoxic injury are available for routine clinical use.

Covered Stents

The use of endovascular placed covered stents to treat cerebrovascular pathology such as vascular aneurysm is gaining in both interest and utilization. The increasing number of case reports and case series of the use of covered stents to treat spontaneous and iatrogenic dissecting aneurysms in the cerebral vasculature provide evidence. As interest and incidence of use of these devices increase, so does the understanding of complications associated with the use of these devices. It stands to reason that the placement of a large surface area of material devoid of endothelial tissue within the vascular space will promote the formation and propagation of thrombus, in spite of use of anticoagulation or antiplatelet therapy. Technical issues with device sizing and placement can result in clefts or folds in the luminal surface, which can promote blood stasis and subsequent thrombosis. Case reports of incidents of thrombosis of covered stents used to treat aneurysms have recently appeared in the literature.

Coil Embolization

Another strategy for the treatment of cerebrovascular aneurysms is the utilization of detachable coils placed in the aneurysm sac for the purpose of promoting thrombosis of the aneurysm sac. In theory, the complete thrombosis of the aneurysm sac up to and including the neck of the aneurysm as it originates from the parent vessel will then allow re-endothelialization of the parent vessel across the purposefully occluded aneurysm neck. The purpose of such therapy is to exclude the aneurysm sac from communication with parent vessel, and the blood pressure present in the parent vessel, which would cause further growth and potential rupture of the aneurysm sac itself. Coil embolization of cerebrovascular aneurysms has been demonstrated to be successful in greater than 70% to almost 100% of cases, varying in success rate due to aneurysm anatomy and technical success in completely occluding the aneurysm sac and neck with coils. A recent histopathological study of aneurysms, obtained primarily at autopsy or surgery, after being treated with Guglielmi detachable coils has been reported. Interestingly, 50% of aneurysms that had been deemed on angiography to be successfully closed showed tiny open spaces between the coils at the aneurysm neck on gross pathologic examination. In very large aneurysms, clot organization can be delayed and/or incomplete with spaces persisting between the coils, and an incomplete membranous covering in the region of the neck of the aneurysm was frequently observed. A recent case series of coil embolization of cerebral aneurysms with Guglielmi detachable coils reported 4.3% incidence of thrombus formation observed angiographically at the interface between the coiled aneurysm neck and the parent artery. The observation of this thrombus propagation prompted additional therapy with anticoagulation with either heparin or the combination of heparin and a GPIIb/IIIa antagonist and successfully prevented any clinically recognizable thromboembolic complication. A thromboembolic complication was encountered in only 2.4% of cases.

Contrast Material

The introduction of contrast material into the vascular space for the purpose of radiological imaging is also associated with the incidence of thrombus formation and thromboembolism. Isosmotic contrast material is most commonly utilized for cerebral angiography and interventions due to its decreased propensity to cause depolarization of nervous tissue, which causes patient discomfort. Among the low osmolality contrast media currently commercially available, there are choices of ionic versus nonionic contrast media. Nonionic contrast material also has a lower tendency to depolarize nervous tissues in comparison with ionic contrast material. However, nonionic contrast material is more thrombogenic than ionic contrast material. In a recent study of patients undergoing cerebral angiography, catheter clot formation was found in 4.8% of patients utilizing ionic contrast (ioxaglate) versus 22% of patients receiving nonionic contrast material (iopamidol or iohexol). It is routine in many high volume centers to add a small aliquot of heparin to the supply bottle of nonionic contrast media in order to reduce its thrombogenicity. This is often used in conjunction with procedural anticoagulation administered for diagnostic angiography and/or endovascular intervention.

Embolism

Embolization of either a formed thrombus or atheromatous or other tissue material into the cerebral vasculature is a major etiology of complications associated with endovascular treatment of cerebrovascular disease. For this reason, a great deal of effort has been expended in the detection, prevention, and treatment of embolic events during endovascular intervention in the cerebral vasculature.

Detection

Clinically detectable signs and symptoms of brain dysfunction are the most coarse detection tool for the presence of embolization complicating an endovascular procedure, but are of course the most relevant since, as will be discussed shortly, not all lesions cause clinical dysfunction. A well-trained clinician can, in the absence of any other information, generally localize the portion of the brain that is dysfunctional through a focused neurological examination. Angiography is a very useful tool in diagnosis of embolization occurring at the time of endovascular intervention. However, the search for angiographic evidence of embolization is usually clinically driven at the time the procedure is performed. Routine performance of cerebral angiography prior to and post endovascular intervention can be helpful in identifying episodes of embolization that are not immediately clinically manifest at the time of the endovascular intervention. In patients undergoing endovascular intervention, a thorough pre-operative angiogram is a must so that if any clinical deficits develop, subtle arteriographic findings suggestive of embolism such as branch occlusions, delayed transit time, arterio-venous shunting, or dye hang-up can be more easily detected by comparing with the baseline study. Additionally, intracerebral hemorrhage (ICH) may rarely occur intra-procedurally, and if significant enough, a hematoma may cause a shift of the normal arterial pattern due to its mass effect; this is more easily identified if a baseline study is available for comparison. Transcranial Doppler (TCD) interrogation of an intracranial vessel downstream of the target of endovascular intervention is a very useful tool in identifying embolization during the interventional procedure. Many case series have been reported in the literature in the setting of many different types of endovascular interventions. A common recurring theme throughout all of these literature reports is that embolization, as detected by TCD, is ubiquitous in almost all endovascular interventions. In a study of TCD monitoring during 40 carotid angioplasty and stent procedures without emboli protection, and 75 carotid endarterectomy (CEA) procedures without emboli protection, TCD was able to detect embolization in 92.5% of carotid artery angioplasty and stenting (CAS) cases with only 10% of cases having clinically evident neurological symptoms. In the same study, 61.3% of endarterectomy patients had detectable embolization by TCD with only a 1.3% rate of clinically evident neurological deficit. MRI with DWI imaging is a useful tool in the detection of subclinical embolization during cerebrovascular procedures. In a recent series of 70 carotid angioplasty and stent procedures without embolic protection, DWI MRI was performed prior to and 24 hours post-procedure. Ninety-nine percent of the patients in this study had no neurological deficits post procedure. However, 29% of the patients had new signal abnormalities on the post procedure DWI imaging study ipsilateral to the procedural carotid. In this same study, 9% of patients had new signal abnormalities on the DWI images contralateral to the procedural carotid. This again was hypothesized to be related to embolization from catheter manipulation in an area upstream of the contralateral carotid such as the aortic arch. Unfortunately, because of the absence of any clinical symptoms, the prognostic value of the discovered DWI imaging signals remains unknown.

The prevention of thrombotic and thromboembolic complications is a major goal of adjunctive drugs and devices used in endovascular interventions in the cerebral vasculature. The foundation of prevention of both thrombosis as well as thromboembolic complications is the use of antiplatelet therapy. Current standard of care for angioplasty and angioplasty and stent procedures in the cerebral vasculature is the use of a combination of antiplatelet therapies including aspirin and a dihydropyridine antagonist such as ticlopidine or more recently clopidogrel. The precise dosing regimen of antiplatelet therapy is a matter of long-standing investigation and continued debate. It appears to be a moving target as better understanding of the pharmacology and pharmacodynamics of the antiplatelet agents and their effects on platelets in individual patients is better understood. For example, by convention and using science and clinical trial data extrapolated from coronary interventional studies, carotid angioplasty and stenting is performed with the use of aspirin at 325 mg daily, and dihydropyridine antagonist such as clopidogrel at 75 mg daily. Prior treatment with both agents is preferred and has been dictated by experimental protocols so that a steady state therapeutic drug level is established prior to the endovascular procedure (9).

Other antiplatelet therapies such as the infusion of platelet glycoprotein IIb/IIIa receptor antagonists have a less clear role in the prevention of thrombosis and thromboembolic complications in endovascular intervention. Conflicting data exists on the use of the GPIIb/IIIa inhibitor abciximab as an adjunct to carotid angioplasty and stenting without mechanical emboli protection. In a study of 151 patients undergoing carotid angioplasty and stenting without mechanical emboli protection at The Cleveland Clinic Foundation, the safety of abciximab was demonstrated. All patients received pre-procedural antiplatelet therapy with aspirin and either clopidogrel or ticlopidine. Intra procedural heparin was utilized with weight-adjusted dosing. Eighty five percent of patients received traditional coronary intervention dosing of abciximab at 0.25 mg/kg bolus plus 0.125 mcg/kg/min infusion for 12 hours. The patients receiving abciximab had a lower rate of 30-day stroke and death, but a higher rate of intracranial bleeding (0.6%). However, in another study, 74 patients underwent carotid angioplasty and stenting without mechanical emboli protection, and no benefit of abciximab was demonstrated. In this study, all patients again received antiplatelet therapy with aspirin and in this case clopidogrel. Intra procedural heparin was also administered on a weight-adjusted basis. Half of the patients were randomized to receive abciximab at a 0.25 mg/kg intravenous bolus only, without an infusion. The 30-day TIA, stroke, and death rate was numerically higher in the abciximab treated group compared with control. The findings did not reach statistical significance due to small sample size.

The adjunctive use of GPIIb/IIIa antagonists has also been described to treat the complication of thrombus formation in the parent artery during Guglielmi detachable coil treatment of intracranial aneurysms. The use of GPIIb/IIIa antagonists in addition has also been demonstrated in case reports and case series to effectively treat recurrent thrombosis despite other anticoagulation in the setting of balloon angioplasty and/or stenting of the intracranial arteries. Case reports are starting to emerge on the local infusion of a combination of heparin and a thrombolytic, as well as a GPIIb/IIIa inhibitor for the treatment of ischemic stroke due to thrombosis or thromboembolism as a complication of an endovascular intervention.

Mechanical Embolic Protection in Cerebrovascular Intervention

Within the last several years, we have entered the era of mechanical emboli protection in cerebrovascular intervention. Mechanical devices have been invented and refined for use in the internal carotid artery (ICA) in order to prevent the distal embolization of any thrombotic, atheromatous, or other tissue embolic material into the end-organ vascular bed while allowing an endovascular procedure to be performed safely upstream of the device. Emboli protection devices utilize three different strategies to achieve their purpose of emboli prevention. The first strategy is interruption of blood flow with subsequent aspiration of a static column of blood to remove any embolic debris prior to reestablishing blood flow. The second strategy is the intravascular positioning of a downstream filter device which will allow blood elements to traverse the filter but not larger debris or elements which are captured and retained upstream in the filter device. The third strategy would be to reverse flow in a blood vessel so that any embolic particles liberated would be removed outside of the body by filtration prior to returning blood into the vascular circuit. For the obvious benefit that it permits uninterrupted antegrade blood flow, the utilization of the second strategy of a filter interposed in a segment of the downstream blood vessel to capture any embolic material liberated is the most common strategy clinically utilized to date. A recent report of the utilization of such a filter demonstrated that in approximately 73% of cases of carotid angioplasty and stenting, the macroscopic debris was retrieved within the filter upon removal from the blood stream. While most of this debris consists of small particulate material, a large number of patients will have very large particles trapped within the filter, some measuring 4–5 mm (Fig. 1). For reference, it is important to note that the terminal ICA measures 3–3.5 mm in diameter and the middle cerebral arteries (MCA) measure between 2 mm and 3 mm in diameter. When examined microscopically, 84% of cases have visible debris. Clinical evidence is accumulating in the support of carotid angioplasty and stenting with emboli protection as being competitive with surgical CEA and in certain instances superior to surgical treatment. The SAPPHIRE trial, which recently completed its one-year follow-up, demonstrated the superiority of carotid angioplasty and stenting with distal embolic protection over CEA in patients at high surgical risk. CEA had a 12.6% rate of death, stroke, or myocardial infarction at a 30-days compared with carotid angioplasty and stenting with emboli protection, which had a rate of 5.8%. The ACCULINK for revascularization of carotids in high risk patients (ARCHeR) registry of carotid angioplasty and stenting with embolic protection demonstrated a 30-day death, stroke, or myocardial infarction rate of

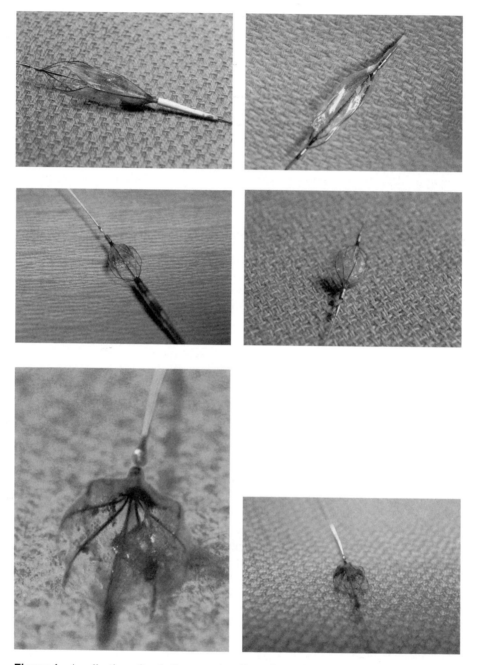

Figure 1 A collection of emboli prevention filters from different patients containing various quantities and sizes of embolic debris. As a reference, note that the diameter of the various filter devices in this series is 6 mm.

7.8%, which is equivalent to the registry arm of the SAPPHIRE study. Despite the rationale for use and the demonstrated safety and efficacy of use of emboli protection devices, debate still exists whether such devices reduce the risk of periprocedural complications. Recently, a clinical alert from the endarterectomy versus angioplasty in patients with symptomatic severe carotid stenosis (eva-3S) trial was reported. The data and safety monitoring committee halted the strategy of carotid angioplasty and stenting without emboli protection. This arm was halted on the basis of a statistically significant higher rate of procedural stroke in carotid angioplasty and stenting without cerebral protection compared with carotid angioplasty and stenting with cerebral protection. Specifically, in the 15 patients undergoing carotid angioplasty and stenting without benefit of emboli protection there were 13.3% strokes in comparison with the 5.2% procedural stroke rate seen in the cohort of 58 patients undergoing carotid angioplasty and stenting with emboli protection devices. The data and safety monitoring committee calculated that the number of patients needed to undergo unprotected carotid angioplasty and stenting to result in a solitary person harmed by stroke due to the absence of emboli protection was six.

Treatment

Treatment of unintended thrombus formation or embolization of either thrombus and/or tissue material during endovascular intervention is a study of strategies in evolution. Clearly, any strategy demonstrating the successful ability to prevent unintended thrombus formation and/or embolic events is both more desirable and more successful than the treatment of a clinical consequence of thrombus formation and/or embolic event resulting in injury to the brain. If preventative measures have failed and a patient develops a clinical deficit that is associated with an angiographic abnormality, some sort of intervention is generally warranted. The limiting factor in the treatment of all ischemic strokes, whether spontaneous or iatrogenic, is the risk of ICH. All cerebrovascular interventions carry a risk of ICH and will be discussed in the section on hemorrhage; the therapeutic options and prognosis if a hemorrhage develops are quite poor. This cannot be emphasized enough in particular since ICH can develop spontaneously after an ischemic insult, even without treatment.

The foundation of adequate treatment of a complication of thrombosis or embolization during endovascular therapy in the cerebral vasculature is to ensure adequate platelet inhibition and to prevent further clot formation and propagation. In a patient undergoing endovascular treatment who is inadequately pretreated with either aspirin or dihydropyridine platelet antagonist such as ticlopidine or clopidogrel, this may mean administering an intravenous antiplatelet agent such as glycoprotein IIb/IIIa inhibitor. Adequate anticoagulation with heparin is usually confirmed by blood testing to insure that the activated clotting time or activated partial thromboplastin time is in a therapeutic range, usually 2–2.5 times normal/baseline. With adequate antiplatelet therapy and anticoagulation, there is reasonable protection against the further development of propagation of thrombus in the setting of initial thrombus formation or an embolic event. Often, if the embolic occlusion is in a small cortical branch rather than in the main trunks of the arteries of the Circle of Willis, anticoagulation is sufficient treatment. Although heparin does not have a thrombolytic effect it can shift the coagulation/thrombolysis cascade in favor of thrombolysis, thus facilitating rapid recanalization. In such cases the prognosis for spontaneous recovery is excellent since cortical branch occlusions do not cause a severe deficit and the risk of more aggressive treatment with thrombolytics or GPIIb/IIIa antagonists is higher than the potential benefit. In cases of more significant embolization with major arterial occlusion such as occlusion of the ICA terminus, MCA trunk or its first order divisions, vertebral artery (VA) or BA, a moderate or severe deficit is often present (10). Spontaneous recanalization is unlikely in this setting and the prognosis without treatment is poor. For such patients, the administration of a thrombolytic agent has demonstrated benefit if administered within six hours of an ischemic complication. Several different thrombolytic agents have demonstrated efficacy using strategies of administering these agents intravenously or locally at the site of thrombus. Case reports have demonstrated the efficacy of such treatment of complications of endovascular intervention (Fig. 2). At the other extreme are patients who develop clinical deficits without any obvious angiographic occlusion or slow flow. For those patients the prognosis for recovery is excellent and no specific intervention is warranted except for close monitoring for deterioration. It has been our experience that even patients who develop deficits following carotid artery stenting but whose angiogram is normal will do very well clinically (unpublished data).

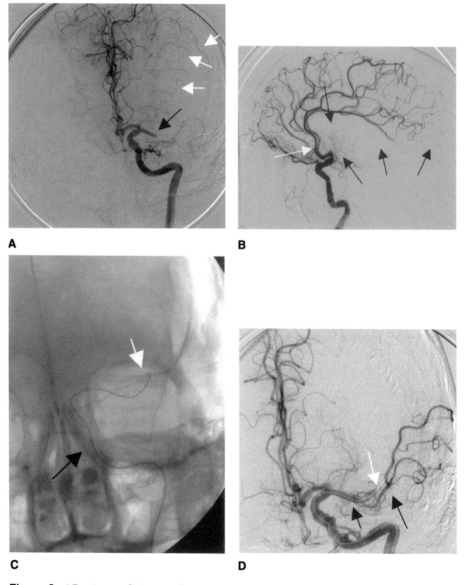

Figure 2 (*Caption on facing page*)

Although most emboli during angiography or endovascular intervention are likely to be thrombi composed of fibrin, platelets, and red blood cells it is not always the case, particularly following angioplasty and stenting. In the setting of atheromatous embolization or other tissue embolization there is the same need to prevent the formation and propagation of thrombus at the site where the embolus lodges due to the thrombogenic nature of the embolic material itself. However, the administration of a thrombolytic agent will do little or nothing in terms of resolving the ischemic consequences of the terminal lodging of an embolic particle, which is not composed of fibrin clot. In such cases, mechanical removal or fragmentation and removal will be necessary to reestablish unrestricted blood flow in the affected blood vessel. This has been demonstrated to be successful in case reports using angioplasty guidewire, snares, and small lumen diameter catheters specially designed for mechanical thrombolysis and thrombectomy. With rare exception it can be difficult if not impossible to tell by angiography alone what an embolism is composed of. Our approach, therefore, has been to use multiple treatments with emphasis on the modality that seems to be safest or most likely to work for that particular circumstance (Figs. 2 and 3). When assessing whether a patient should receive endovascular rescue and the nature of the rescue treatment, i.e., thrombolysis or GPIIb/IIIa antagonists or snaring, several factors have to be taken into consideration, including: patient factors, blood/thrombus factors, and anatomical factors. Patient factors such as increasing age (particularly age >80 years old), underlying cognitive dysfunction, hyperglycemia (particularly if profound), hypertension (particularly if extreme and long standing),

---

Figure 2A–H (*Facing Page*) Cerebral angiographic images of a 59-year-old man who developed sudden left hemiparesis and global aphasia within seconds of withdrawal of a pigtail catheter from the left ventricle after completion of a ventriculogram. A JR-4 catheter was quickly used to engage the left CCA, a DSA angiogram was performed. An AP cranial view. (**A**) shows complete occlusion of the left middle cerebral artery (MCA) from its mid portion (*black arrow*) with slow pial collateral flow from the left anterior cerebral artery (ACA)(*white arrows*). The lateral projection (**B**) shows complete loss of the cortical branches of the MCA (*black arrows*) and filling of only the ACA territory (*white arrow*). The patient received a bolus of 4000 units heparin and a #6F Envoy™ Guide catheter was advanced over an angled hydrophilic 0.035-inch wire into the distal cervical LICA. Through the guide catheter a 0.014-inch, floppy tipped, hydrophilic microwire was advanced into the distal MCA (*white arrow in* **C**) over which a #2.3F microcatheter (*black arrow*) was advanced into the mid MCA. Through the microcatheter the patient received 1 U of reteplase and 1 mg of abciximab. A repeat angiogram five minutes after the infusion showed recanalization of the MCA trunk (*short black arrow in* **D**) and a nearly complete recanalization of the superior division of the MCA (*long black arrow in* **D** *and white arrows in* **E**) (see page 348 for **E–H**). The inferior division of the MCA remained occluded (*white arrow in* **D**) and on the lateral projection there is no filling of its distal territory (*black arrows in* **E**). The microcatheter was then advanced over the 0.014-inch wire into the inferior division (*white arrow in* **D**) and an additional 1 U of reteplase followed by 5 mg of abciximab (1/4 bolus) were infused into the inferior division. Fifteen minutes later a repeat angiogram shows complete recanalization of the inferior division (*black arrow in* **F** *and black arrows in* **G**) except for a persistent filling defect in a single inferior parietal cortical branch (*white arrow in* **F**). The lateral angiogram in G shows hyperemia of the cortex of the inferior division (*small white arrows*), which is typical after a period of ischemia followed by recanalization. The procedure was terminated at that point and no further pharmacotherapy was given. The patient was observed closely in an intensive care unit where his systolic blood pressure was kept below 130 mmHg. By the next morning he had only minor difficulty finding words and by the second day his neurological exam was normal as was a CT scan of the brain (**H**).

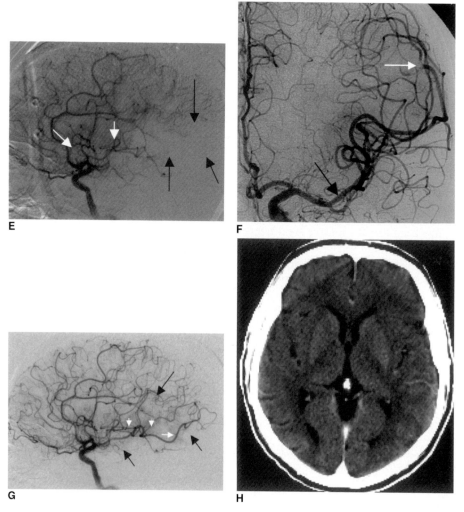

Figure 2 (*Continued*)

pre-existing ischemia (particularly if recent and the infarct is large), and increasing
duration of ischemia all increase the risk of ICH and a poor outcome even with
revascularization (11). Blood factors such as excessive anticoagulation with heparin,
adequate platelet inhibition with oral agents or GPIIb/IIIa antagonists, thrombocytopenia, or other bleeding disorders can increase the risk of ICH. Thrombus factors
such as the size of the thrombus and the size of the vessel affected, plus the possible
composition of the thrombus all affect the likelihood of success with each intervention, as well as the risk of complications. For example, small distal cortical branch
occlusions are associated with a good prognosis even without treatment, but occlusion of the anterior choroidal artery, even though it is <0.5 mm in diameter, is associated with a severe deficit and occlusion of the ICA, and is associated with a high
mortality, approaching 80%, and a low chance for recanalization even with aggressive measures. Anatomical factors such as aortic arch or great vessel tortuosity,
proximal stenoses, distal tortuosity or extensive atherosclerosis can all increase the

difficulty of an endovascular rescue and can make delivery of angioplasty balloons, stents or even microcatheters impossible, and can increase the risk of complications, particularly vessel perforation. All of these factors must be considered.

If endovascular rescue is planned, stable access to the affected artery is critical. If there is proximal tortuosity even to a moderate degree, a long sheath, typically a #7 or #8F 80 cm sheath, should be placed in the distal common carotid artery or subclavian artery proximal to the VA, whichever is appropriate. A #6F diagnostic guide is then advanced over a hydrophilic 0.035-inch curved wire into the distal cervical ICA or the distal cervical VA to just before the first turn at the second vertebral body. If a fresh stent has been placed in the artery with the occlusion, then the interventionalist must weigh the risk of crossing the stent with a large caliber guide catheter and the potential for producing more embolization without crossing the stent with the guide catheter and the potential for losing support and not being able to deliver the necessary equipment distally. Once the guide catheter is in place, a hydrophilic, soft tipped, 0.014-inch microwire is used to cross the culprit lesion, whether it is dissection, embolism or thrombotic occlusion. The microwire is placed distally enough to offer sufficient support so as to allow tracking of a microcatheter (typically #2.3F) or coronary balloon dilation catheter (typically 1.5–2 mm ×8–10 mm) into the lesion. With selective delivery of a microcatheter, thrombolytic agents can be given directly into a thrombus. If a balloon catheter is used, angioplasty can be performed to mechanically disrupt the thrombus or to dilate a stenosis or dissection. If a dissection is present, placement of a stent can tack down the intimal flap and restore flow, but if there is a perforation with subarachnoid hemorrhage (SAH), placing a stent may make matters worse since deployment of the stent will stretch the artery even more, potentially increasing the perforation. More detail can be found in a variety of references on the subject of endovascular rescue as a full discussion is beyond the scope of this work (10–16). The important lesson is that all equipment must be accurately sized for the cerebral vessel being treated, and it is often better to err on the side of undersizing balloon catheters and stents because of the fragility of the intracerebral vessels. Careful attention must also be paid to the small vessels that originate off the distal ICA and VA, but in particular the perforating vessels originating off the MCA and BA must not be cannulated with the wire.

In some instances of carotid artery stenting, ischemia develops because of slow flow through an emboli prevention filter. This occurs when embolization, usually after stent delivery, is so exuberant that the emboli prevention filter will become clogged with debris resulting in effective occlusion of the ICA with minimal or no antegrade flow. Vasospasm often occurs around the filter devices, some filter types more than others, and this may result in closure of the device (unpublished data). When either of these circumstances occurs the intervention should then be treated as a case performed with the balloon occlusion type emboli prevention device, i.e., time becomes critical because the entire ipsilateral cerebral hemisphere may be ischemic. Post-dilation should be done quickly, if at all, and most importantly, before capture of the filter, an aspiration catheter must be used to aspirate the stagnant column of blood, which presumably contains particulate debris or thrombi that could embolize if the filter is captured without aspiration—extending from the proximal end of the filter device to the common carotid bifurcation. This can be performed with a #5F multipurpose diagnostic catheter with endholes or using a specially designed aspiration catheter (Export™). Also, nitroglycerin 200–400 μg can be given directly into the carotid artery to relieve the vasospasm. Once aspiration of 50–60 cc of blood has been performed then the filter device can be captured. Although this

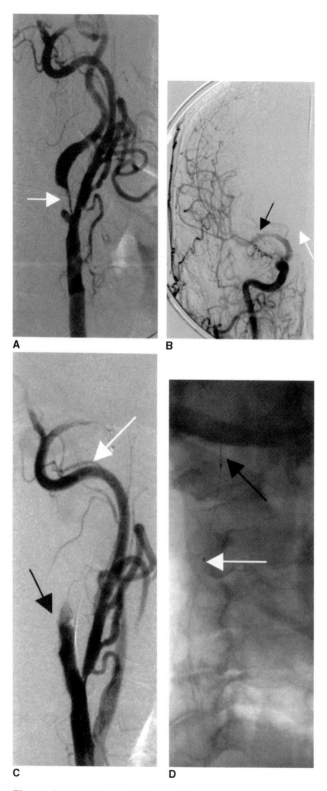

Figure 3 (*Caption on facing page*)

technique is quite effective, distal embolization to the cerebral vasculature is not uncommon in such cases and the interventionalist must be prepared for endovascular rescue (Fig. 3).

Figure 3A–K (*Facing Page*) Images from an 81-year-old man who had recurrent right hemispheric TIAs, poorly controlled hypertension and diabetes, and unstable angina that underwent RICA stenting. Image **A** shows an ipsilateral oblique subtracted angiogram of a right common carotid artery injection. There is a severe, long, tubular, ulcerated stenosis of the ICA origin (*arrow*). Intracranial views (**B**) show marked reduced filling of the right MCA (*black arrow*) and no filling of the ACA (*white arrow*). CAS was performed with an emboli prevention device. After post-dilation of the stent but before retrieval of the filter device, an oblique angiogram shows markedly reduced flow through the RICA. In **C** note the nearly complete filling of the external carotid artery (*white arrow*) and the stasis of contrast within the ICA bulb (*black arrow*). The patient became slightly confused with dysarthria and mild left sided weakness. An Export aspiration catheter (*white arrow in* **D**) was advanced over the filter wire and used to aspirate 60 cc of blood from the ICA from just below the filter (*black arrow*) to the bulb. After aspiration flow into the ICA was much improved and so the filter was retrieved. Upon examination of the filter it was filled with multiple small and several very large particles, which were yellowish and globular and had a greasy consistency (**E**). (**E–H**, see page 352; **I–K**, see page 353). A repeat angiogram showed excellent flow into the ICA (*black arrow in* **F**) with good opposition of the stent and no residual stenosis but with some irregularity of the stent margins (*white arrow in* **F**). The patient's confusion and strength improved slightly but he remained moderately aphasic. An AP intracerebral angiogram of the RICA (**G**) showed markedly improved filling of the MCA (*black arrows*) and its branches, as well as filling of the ACA (*black arrowheads*) and even flow into the contralateral ACA (*white arrow*). Careful examination however, showed an occlusion of an inferior division of the MCA (*white arrowhead in* **G**).This was best seen on the lateral angiogram in the late arterial-capillary phase (**H**). There is stasis and abrupt cutoff of the dye column (*white arrow*), an area of no flow with no cortical blush (*black arrows*), as well as retrograde pial collateral flow (*arrowheads*). Because of the irregularity of the stent margins a #6F guide catheter was not placed through the stent so as not to dislodge more emboli. Furthermore because of the fatty consistency of the debris in the filter, it was felt that thrombolytics would not be effective and with his significant hypertension, hyperglycemia, and risk for HPS thrombolytics were also considered to be relatively contraindicated. A mechanical approach with more aggressive platelet inhibition was considered a better option. The patient received a full dose bolus of intravenous abciximab and a coronary balloon dilation catheter was advanced into the MCA (*gray arrow in* **I**) over a hydrophilic soft tipped wire that was placed through the occluded segment (*white arrow in* **I**); note the stagnant dye column proximal to the embolism (*arrowhead in* **I**). After several inflations there was no change in the occlusion. The wire balloon was exchanged for a microcatheter that was passed through the occluded segment and the wire was replaced with a 2 mm gooseneck snare (*arrow in* **J**). The snare was withdrawn into the occlusion and engaged and then removed together with the microcatheter. Although there was no embolism visible on the snare, there was slight improvement in antegrade flow. One more pass with the snare and repeat angioplasty did not improve flow further, therefore the procedure was terminated. The patient was placed in an intensive care unit on a continuous infusion of nitroprusside. He made a gradual improvement over the following 24 hours and a follow-up CT scan of the brain revealed a small sized peri-insular infarct (*white arrow in* **K**) with a small amount of asymptomatic hemorrhagic conversion (*black arrow in* **K**). The patient was discharged the next day with a mild deficit with strict parameters for the monitoring and control of his blood pressure.
Abbreviations: CAS, carotid artery angioplasty and stenting; RICA, right internal carotid artery. CT, computerized tomography; MCA, middle cerebral artery; ICA, internal carotid artery; ACA, anterior cerebral artery.

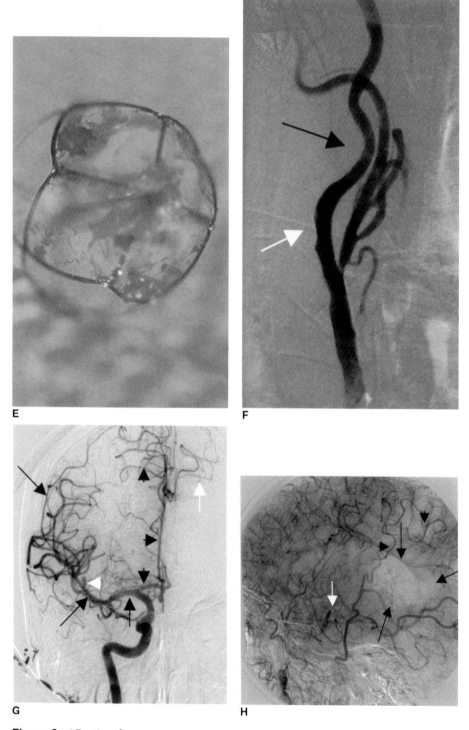

Figure 3 (*Continued*)

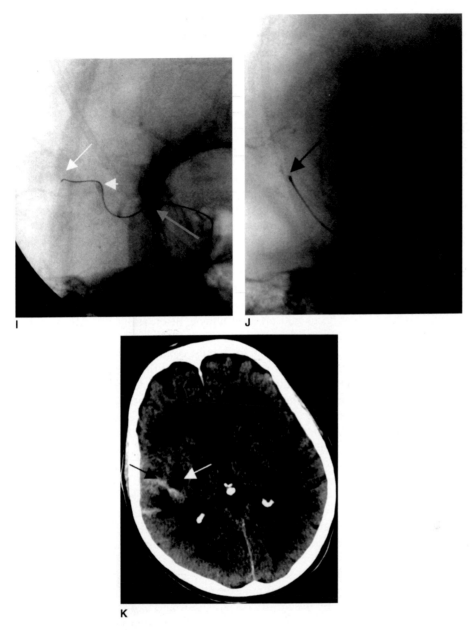

I   J

K

Figure 3   (*Continued*)

HEMORRHAGIC COMPLICATIONS

The most dreaded complication of any cerebrovascular intervention, whether surgical or endovascular is intracranial hemorrhage (ICH). The dread is justified. The prognosis of ICH is very poor and there is little that a surgeon or interventionalist can do if hemorrhage occurs. As a consequence, prevention and early detection are absolutely critical. Unfortunately, the available data on the risks of ICH following endovascular interventions are limited as compared with the available data on ischemic complications. Nonetheless, much is known about non-iatrogenic ICH mechanisms and management and this knowledge is helpful in the management of these complications following endovascular treatment.

INTRACRANIAL HEMORRHAGE (ICH)

ICH can be caused by a variety of mechanisms and each mechanism causes hemorrhage into different intracranial compartments. The clinical presentation, treatment and prognosis for ICH depends on which part of the brain is affected and therefore the compartment into which the hemorrhage occurs. ICHs can occur in the epidural space, the subdural space, the subarachnoid space, the brain parenchyma, intraventricularly, or a combination of the above. Epidural and subdural hematomas are primarily traumatic in origin but in the case of the latter may be related to anticoagulation or even spontaneous. Subdural hematomas have not been reported as complications of endovascular procedures except those procedures dealing with dural arteriovenous fistulas and the like. The remaining three types of hemorrhage have been associated with endovascular interventions. Subarachnoid hemorrage (SAH) is most commonly traumatic but is also the primary manifestation of rupture of congenital or acquired cerebral aneurysms and arteriovenous malformations (AVMs) and can complicate intracranial endovascular interventions. Intraparenchymal, or intracerebral hemorrhage (ICH) as it is also referred to, is most commonly due to hypertension but can be caused by a wide variety of mechanisms. ICH is the most common hemorrhage complicating endovascular interventions. Intraventricular hemorrhage is very rare and is most commonly attributed to hypertension or anticoagulation and has rarely been reported following extracranial endovascular interventions (17).

ICH causes brain dysfunction and injury differently than ischemia does. Brain ischemia is most often a result of occlusion of a feeding artery, i.e., the occlusion is proximal to the brain territory supplied by that artery, which leads directly to neuronal injury. In addition, recanalization can lead to reperfusion injury, which in turn can cause oxidative injury and apoptosis, potentiating the ischemic injury. In contrast, hemorrhage causes brain dysfunction by several local tissue effects and global intracranial pressure (ICP) changes. Intraparenchymal hematomas cause increasing amounts of pressure and compression on the surrounding brain tissue as they expand. A hemorrhage itself does not cause as much neuronal injury as does a similarly sized infarct; this is because the blood tends to dissect along tissue planes and displaces normal tissue. As the hematoma expands, ever increasing tissue displacement causes some damage by disruption of capillaries and axons. Eventually, local perfusion is affected and some ischemia does occur in addition to the direct injury. If a hematoma is large enough it can then cause an elevation of ICP. Since cerebral perfusion pressure is determined by the difference between mean arterial pressure (MAP) and ICP, very high ICP can greatly decrease cerebral perfusion. This can result in global ischemia and eventually brain death when ICP equals MAP. In addition, if a hematoma is strategically placed, e.g., temporal lobe, and it is large enough, it can cause massive tissue shift leading to herniation and further brain injury. All of these processes can occur rapidly following the onset of the hemorrhage and are the reason for the high acute mortality associated with hemorrhage.

The above mechanisms of injury play a role to varying degrees depending on the compartment into which the hemorrhage occurs. In intraparenchymal hemorrhage all of the above apply with tissue disruption occurring first, followed by local mass effects and only in very large hematomas or those occurring in confined cavities, e.g., cerebellar hemorrhage, do ICP and CPP become affected. The hematoma tends to expand over the course of only minutes and up to a few hours. The expansion of the hematoma is limited by the surrounding brain tissue, which offers resistance to the bleeding. Tissue perfusion and mass effect are the major issues that must be addressed in acute ICH. By contrast in cases of aneurismal hemorrhage, which occurs most commonly into the subarachnoid space, the ruptured vessels tend to be the large arteries at the base of the brain. Bleeding is rapid in this setting and ICP can rise quickly leading to rapid CPP compromise. As a consequence, 40% of patients with aneurismal SAH die immediately. ICP and blood pressure are the major parameters that must be controlled after SAH. Mass effect can occur following SAH with very localized and flocculated hematomas, particularly those in the Sylvian fissure. However, mass effect is not as important with SAH as are the delayed effects of blood within the subarachnoid space, namely vasospasm and hydrocephalus.

INTRAPARENCHYMAL HEMORRHAGE

Cervical internal carotid interventions for the prevention of ischemic stroke are the most common cerebrovascular procedures, both surgical and endovascular. Complications of CEA usually take the form of ischemic injury from embolization or hypoperfusion; however, a small percentage of patients experience neurological injury due to post-procedural hyperperfusion syndrome (HPS) and ICH. The term "hyperperfusion hemorrhage" was initially coined by Sundt and colleagues; however, reports of ICH following CEA first appeared in the 1960s (18,19). Over the past several decades, HPS has become increasingly recognized as a complication of CEA (20–30). Hyperperfusion is the primary mechanism of ICH following CEA. As with CEA, the reported nervous system complications of CAS have until recently consisted primarily of ischemic injuries. As endovascular techniques and technology have improved however, fewer ischemic complications have been reported and several case reports and small case series have reported the occurrence of ICH following CAS. Furthermore, as the use of emboli capture devices increases it is foreseeable that hemorrhagic complications, specifically those due to the cerebral HPS will become major causes of morbidity and mortality following endovascular carotid artery revascularization. Although no prospective large series have been reported, a large series of patients from The Cleveland Clinic Foundation have been studied and a more accurate picture of the incidence of hyperperfusion and ICH has emerged (31).

HPS and ICH are not unique to extracranial carotid interventions and some reports have documented the occurrence of both following intracranial and vertebrobasilar interventions (1,7,32–37). Unfortunately, intracranial angioplasty and stenting interventions are very rare and fewer than 500 cases have been reported in the medical literature. Very small sample size and widely variable patient populations and interventional techniques plague what data are available. As a result only broad generalizations can be made about HPS and ICH following these procedures. Practically speaking however, the clinical presentation and the management of patients who develop ICH following intracranial interventions are the same as for those who develop ICH following extracranial interventions, with the exception of a higher risk of SAH with intracranial interventions.

EPIDEMIOLOGY

The risk of hyperperfusion and ICH following endovascular procedures has been studied best following extracranial internal carotid interventions (17,31,38–43). Based on the largest study of this patient population, HPS occurred in 1.1% of patients and ICH developed in 0.6% (31). Smaller series have reported rates of HPS as high as 5% (38,44,45). Besides smaller numbers, these earlier series included heterogeneous patient populations including patients with intracranial interventions and even some patients who had multiple, combined interventions. Also, the patients in these series were not treated with emboli prevention devices and they received very high doses of heparin intra-procedurally, well above the most commonly used dosing regimens. Nonetheless, these numbers are in keeping with those observed following CEA, following which the incidence of HPS is between 2% and 6% and ICH between 0.3% and 1.2% (21,24–30,45). Once HPS develops, the risk of ICH has been estimated to be as high as 40% following CEA and in the series of CAS patients by Abou-Chebl et al. the risk was 60% (3/5) (31,46,47). In that series isolated headache was not consistently recorded so the overall risk of ICH if HPS develops is likely overestimated. What appears to be clear is that ICH is not more likely to occur following CAS than it is following CEA despite the use of more potent antiplatelet agents. Even in early studies of CAS that utilized platelet GPIIb/IIIa receptor antagonists, the risk of ICH was only 0.66% (41).

Hyperperfusion and ICH tend to be delayed following CAS, occurring from six hours to four days after the intervention (31,44,45). Following CEA, ICH typically occurs between the 2nd and 17th post-operative day, with a peak incidence between the 3rd and 5th postoperative days; however, cases have been observed shortly after surgery (25).

Despite the relatively low incidence, ICH remains a significant prognostic finding. In one series, two of three (66%) patients with ICH died (31). For comparison, ICH following CEA is associated with a 37–80% mortality rate. Of survivors, 20–37% have a poor recovery (24,25,27,28,30).

CLINICAL PRESENTATION

Postoperative hypertension often precedes the onset of neurological symptoms and although it appears to be a critical component in the pathophysiology of hyperperfusion, it is not essential (25,26,48). A throbbing, unilateral headache in the facial, temporal, or retro-orbital distribution ipsilateral to the side of the intervention is the most common presentation of hyperperfusion, and this may be the only manifestation of the syndrome (24,25,49). This headache is migraine-like in quality and is frequently associated with nausea and vomiting. Other symptoms commonly associated with HPS include focal deficits and seizures (focal or generalized) (25,26,48). Focal deficits and seizures may occur from an ICH but they may also occur with subcortical white matter edema or even in the absence of abnormalities on cerebral imaging studies (50). Among those patients who develop an ICH, headache (60%) and hypertension (80%) are often the first symptoms. The clinical syndrome which has been observed following CAS is similar to that described above (31,38,44,45).

ICH often causes a rapidly progressive focal deficit that is often (~70%) associated with a severe headache, nausea, and vomiting. The focal deficits are variable and depend on the location of the hemorrhage. The ICH syndrome seen in patients following CAS or interventions on the intracranial ICA or MCA is due to injury to surpratentorial structures supplied by those vessels, namely the basal ganglia and the frontal, temporal, and parietal lobes. The symptoms can include any combination of hemiparesis progressing to hemiplegia, hemisensory loss, cognitive dysfunction with aphasia (left cerebrum) or neglect (right cerebrum), or visual field deficits. The thalamus, brainstem, and cerebellum are supplied by the vertebrobasilar circulation and should not be predisposed to hyperperfusion or ICH following CAS except in very unusual circumstances or in patients who have interventions on those vessels. Hemorrhage into the regions of brain supplied by these vessels can cause a wide variety of symptoms, but altered consciousness and coma are more common and occur earlier in the course than they do in patients with anterior circulation hematomas. Ocular-motor abnormalities and bilateral sensory-motor deficits are typical of posterior circulation lesions.

What distinguishes ICH from ischemia clinically is the progression of deficits over minutes or hours. With ischemia, particularly if embolic in cause, deficits are almost instantaneous in onset and may come and go. Hemorrhage causes progressive symptoms as the hematoma expands and the symptoms rarely if ever come and go. In addition, ICH is often accompanied by progression to a state of depressed consciousness, which is often preceded by increasing headache, nausea, and vomiting. The headache is caused by the mass effect and elevation in ICP or by direct irritation of the meninges if subarachnoid or intraventricular extensions occur. The nausea and vomiting are a result of elevated ICP. In virtually every case of ICH, whether due to hyperperfusion or not, hypertension will be present to some degree, sometimes to profound levels. If the hypertension is associated with bradycardia in patients with a depressed level of consciousness, marked elevations in ICP should be suspected and a grave prognosis portended; this is the so-called "Cushing's Response" and occurs because the elevated ICP leads to brainstem ischemia. Focal or generalized seizures may occur either early or late in the course of lobar hemorrhages.

RISK FACTORS FOR HPS

The first study to systematically review HPS was conducted by Sundt and colleagues who reported on five patients with postoperative ICH (46). Their study was based on a review of 1,145 consecutive CEA procedures monitored intra-operatively with electroencephalography (EEG) and cerebral blood flow measurements. Of their 5 patients with ICH, four died. In addition, eleven patients developed postoperative seizures. The majority of these adverse events were observed in patients with a >100% increase in intra-operative cerebral blood flow (CBF). Furthermore, most of these patients were in the pre-defined "major neurological risk" group, i.e., patients with both slow flow and small-vessel occlusions by cerebral arteriography suggesting chronic or ongoing ischemia. They concluded, therefore, that these postoperative complications were due to hyperperfusion.

Subsequent research has confirmed Sundt and colleagues' premise, and risk factors for developing the HPS following CEA have been identified (20,25,26,46, 48,49,51,52). The most important risk factor appears to be the presence of a severe ICA stenosis (25,46,49). Contributing risk factors include severe contralateral ICA disease, poor collateral flow, hypertension, the use of postoperative anticoagulants, and recent cerebral ischemia. Although the technical aspects of CAS and CEA are markedly different, the resultant changes in cerebrovascular physiology are similar.

Understanding the underlying pathophysiology of HPS following CEA has given essential insight into the syndrome following CAS.

The results of the largest study of HPS following CAS indicate that the risk factors for HPS following CAS are the same as those following CEA (31). All of the patients in that study had hypertension, a severe carotid stenosis of >90% severity (mean 95.6% ±3.1%) and the presence of poor collateral blood flow because of a contralateral ICA stenosis of >80% severity or contralateral ICA occlusion. Data from other, smaller series have also shown that the treatment of a severe >90% stenosis and hypertension are important risk factors for the development of HPS and ICH (38,44,45). In some series the risk of ICH was very high compared to the risk following CEA and compared to the results of the larger series by Abou-Chebl et al. These differences can possibly be explained by the smaller numbers of patients in these other series as well as major differences in the technique of CAS. In these series, distal emboli prevention devices were not used, which could theoretically increase the risk of ICH because recent ischemia is a risk factor for the development of ICH (38,44,45). These devices reduce the risk of embolization during CAS and can reduce the risk of stroke by 50% (53–57). In addition, in one study a heparin infusion was given for 12 hours following the intervention (44). In the series by Abou-Chebl et al. heparin was used intra-procedurally only, as this is the most common practice at most large volume centers performing CAS (53–56). Some have reported an elevated risk of ICH with the concomitant use of parenteral platelet glycoprotein IIb/IIIa receptor antagonists and endovascular procedures (7,37,43). Still other series have not shown an increased risk (1,41,58,59). Again, the apparently discrepant results can be explained by differences in study size and the patient population studied. It is likely that in select patients GPIIb/IIIa receptor antagonists are unsafe, yet in others their use may be appropriate. Their use in patients who have had a recent stroke, who have hypertension, and who are undergoing endovascular intervention under full dose heparin and adequate treatment with aspirin and clopidogrel may in fact increase the risk of ICH. Patients with intracranial atherosclerosis may be another population at increased risk of ICH with the use of these drugs (7,37). At this point in time the only statement that can be made regarding GPIIb/IIIa receptor antagonists is that their use may increase the risk of ICH and they should be used judiciously, primarily in patients who have not been adequately treated with oral antiplatelet medications.

Several reports have shown that ICH is more likely in patients who undergo CEA within 6 weeks of a stroke (19,60,61). In such patients, the ICH occurs as a result of the combination of increased blood flow and the anticoagulation used during the CEA in the presence of the underlying endothelial and vascular injury induced by the infarct. This is a reperfusion injury that is related to hyperperfusion. The surgical dictum has been that patients with symptomatic stenoses should have delayed revascularization by 6 weeks following an infarct, to decrease the risk of ICH. Similarly, patients with recent stroke are often excluded from treatment trials of CAS because of the risk of ICH. While these are prudent approaches, it is important to keep in mind that data from the North American Symptomatic Carotid Endarterectomy Trial have shown that delaying surgery does not increase the risk of ICH in patients who have small and non-disabling strokes and may place the patients at an increased risk of having recurrent ischemic strokes (62). The decision to delay surgery must be weighed against the risk of recurrent stroke. In general, younger patients with small strokes and who have severe stenoses, i.e., >70%, should have early revascularization because their risk of ICH is low, particularly if they are not profoundly hypertensive. In addition, patients who have recurrent TIA or small strokes due to a severe stenosis should be considered for early revascularization because their risk of ischemic stroke is more than twice that of patients who present with a single event (63). On the other hand, patients with large strokes and severe deficits and those who are older or who have profound hypertension may be better treated in a delayed fashion. Certainly patients who have frank hemorrhagic conversion of an ischemic infarct should not have early carotid revascularization either with CEA or CAS. The significance of petechial hemorrhage as seen on CT scan is unclear and unless the patient is at very high risk for recurrent stroke, revascularization should probably be delayed. It should be noted however that when evaluated pathologically, hemorrhagic conversion is found to varying degrees in the vast majority of embolic infarcts.

PATHOPHYSIOLOGY OF HPS AND ICH

The underlying etiology of the HPS appears to be impaired autoregulation of cerebral blood flow (21,22,45,64). The chronic low-flow state induced by a severe stenosis with poor collateral blood supply results in a compensatory dilatation of cerebral vessels distal to the stenosis; this is the normal response of cerebral arteries and arterioles to low perfusion pressure and is termed *cerebral autoregulation* (Fig. 4). With chronic dilatation however, it is theorized that the cerebral vessels lose their ability to autoregulate vascular resistance in response to changing flow rates, particularly if the changes are rapid. Following a successful recanalization treatment, surgery or PTA/stenting, the perfusion pressure to the cerebral territory distal to the

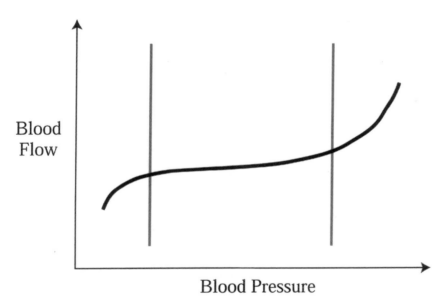

Figure 4 Cerebral autoregulation curve. At most MAP values cerebral blood flow remains constant. At the extremes of very low or very high pressures common carotid artery (CBF) can drop precipitously causing ischemia or rise dangerously increasing the risk of hemorrhage. In patients who have impaired autoregulation, the relationship between blood pressure and CBF becomes linear so that even blood pressures that are normal may be associated with very elevated CBF.

treated stenosis is greatly increased. Cerebral blood flow is greatly increased as a consequence and the chronically dilated arteries and arterioles cannot constrict. This results in loss of vessel integrity with a breakdown in gap junctions, which can lead to cerebral edema and ICH (46). This model is supported by results from animal studies as well as findings of non-invasive testing and post-mortem examinations in patients.

Using an elegant cat model with surgically created carotid-jugular fistulas to induce chronic ischemia, Sakaki and colleagues confirmed that disordered autoregulation is a critical component in the pathogenesis of the HPS (65). Some workers have postulated that neuroeffector mechanisms may be at the root of the disordered autoregulatory response (66). These are intriguing theories since they suggest that pharmacological manipulation with receptor blockers or ganglionectomy may be therapeutic options to prevent or treat HPS. Also, if this theory is correct, intracranial ICA or vertebrobasilar interventions may be less likely to cause hyperperfusion hemorrhage since they do not cause dysautonomia due to irritation/injury of the carotid sinus.

In a study of 96 patients undergoing CEA, Jørgensen and Schroeder used TCD to follow patients perioperatively (67). They observed that lowering systemic blood pressure in those patients with both clinical and TCD findings of hyperperfusion resulted in lower MCA velocities and clinical improvement (Fig. 5). Changes in MCA velocity correlate well with changes in cerebral blood flow (CBF), making it a quick and safe alternative to other tests of CBF such as acetazolamide-SPECT and Xenon-CT scanning (67–70). Although these tests of CBF are important diagnostic tools in confirming the presence of hyperperfusion, they may play a more pivotal role in screening preoperative patients to better quantify the overall risk of developing HPS and ICH.

Studies of CBF during CEA, surgery have shown that flows are dynamic and vary during the surgical procedure. Patients who are intolerant of carotid clamping, either by manifesting clinical deficits or slowing on an EEG, have poor collateral blood supply and will show decreased CBF or MCA velocities on clamping (71). Furthermore, these patients have been found to be at particular risk for developing elevated CBF and TCD velocities postoperatively (46,49). One study observed a correlation between the magnitude of decrease in MCA velocities with clamp application, and the degree of elevation in MCA velocities following clamp release (71). Following the release of the carotid clamp, elevations in MCA velocities tended to reach supra-normal levels. These elevated velocities normalized within 10 minutes and this was felt to be a transient, post-ischemic response due to poor collateral blood supply. The authors termed this phenomenon the "primary hyperemic response." The term "secondary hyperemic response" was reserved for those patients with persistently elevated MCA velocities that peaked within 6 to 12 hours. The finding of a secondary hyperemic response was confined to those patients with evidence of impaired cerebrovascular reserve prior to surgery. Although cross clamping does not occur during CAS, there are brief episodes of cessation of flow that may induce physiological changes similar to those observed with clamping during CEA, particularly if massive embolization results in clogging of the filter pores. CAS patients frequently manifest transient signs of hemispheric or even global ischemia during angioplasty, particularly during angioplasty of the carotid bulb. In a similar study employing preoperative acetazolamide-TCD in 36 CEA patients, all three patients with an abnormal preoperative response to acetazolamide developed elevated MCA velocities postoperatively (49). Furthermore, all three patients developed an ipsilateral, severe, throbbing headache; however, none progressed to ICH.

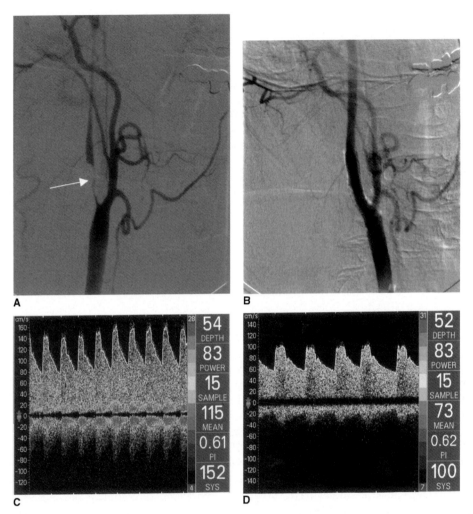

Figure 5 Right anterior oblique common carotid artery angiogram (**A**) of an 81-year-old woman with a right hemispheric stroke, shows a "string sign" severe stenosis of the right internal carotid artery (RICA) origin (*arrow*). The contralateral ICA had an 80% stenosis (*not shown*). The patient underwent successful angioplasty and stenting of the RICA (**B**). On post-operative day #1 the patient began to complain of an ipsilateral throbbing headache. Systolic arterial pressures were in the 140–150 mmHg range. Urgent TCD ultrasonography showed elevated velocities in the right middle cerebral artery (**C**) with MFV of 115 cm/s. The patient was treated with antihypertensive medications with a drop in arterial pressures into the 90–100 mmHg range and resolution of the headache. (**D**) Follow-up TCD shows a marked improvement in MFV with a mean of 73 cm/s. The patient was observed one more day and discharged with no recurrence of symptoms with frequent blood pressure monitoring.

Jansen and colleagues corroborated these findings in a TCD study of 233 consecutive CEA patients (46). In their study, five patients developed a postoperative ICH. Although the only preoperative predictor of ICH in this study was the presence of a contralateral occlusion, the investigators observed a striking relationship between postoperative elevations in MCA velocity and the development of ICH. They found that postoperative increases in MCA velocity to >175% of their preoperative values, in conjunction with >100% increases in the pulsatility index, had a 100% positive predictive value for ICH. The negative predictive value for these findings was also quite high at 99%. Although these findings were striking, they were confounded by the fact that 60% of the patients who developed ICH were receiving concomitant anticoagulation therapy compared to only 23% of those who did not develop an ICH. In aggregate, the aforementioned trials suggest that patients with evidence of impaired cerebrovascular reserve preoperatively and/or elevated MCA velocities postoperatively, are a high-risk population for developing hyperperfusion injury and ICH.

Only a few post-mortem analyses have been reported in patients who died of HPS and ICH. These have shown changes similar to those found in brain tissue surrounding arterio-venous malformations and in brains of patients with hypertensive encephalopathy, i.e., fibrinoid necrosis, thrombosis of cerebral arterioles, micro-infarcts and petechial hemorrhages (20,23,50). These findings support the model of disordered autoregulation and hypertensive injury as the causes of HPS and ICH. There are no reported postmortem studies in patients who developed ICH following CAS but the pathological changes are likely similar to those associated with ICH and HPS complicating CAS.

CLINICAL COURSE AND PROGNOSIS

As detailed earlier, the progression of HPS to ICH is associated with an extremely poor prognosis. If ICH develops, aggressive supportive measures may succeed in keeping the patient alive; however, there will almost certainly be significant residual neurological deficits. It is imperative, therefore, that patients at high risk be identified and appropriate preventative measures taken. The development of isolated HPS is in some respects a benefit since it heralds that ICH is imminent and allows for adequate preventative measures to be taken. The critical component of perioperative management is vigilant monitoring and control of systemic blood pressure (20,23,25,28, 46–48,50,67). Several studies have shown that blood pressure control prevents the onset of HPS and the progression to ICH if HPS does develop. It has been suggested that blood pressures in the "normal" range may be deleterious in patients at high risk for HPS and some patients may in fact require systolic pressures below 90 to avert ICH (25,28,67). This is analogous to the normal pressure breakthrough phenomenon, the putative cause of ICH following surgical treatment of AVMs of the brain. In general, blood pressures should be rapidly reduced until clinical symptoms resolve. Headache, rather than an arbitrary MAP value, is the best clinical guide of response to blood pressure control. Each patient is unique and the threshold for HPS and ICH is different between patients.

TCD ultrasound may assist in guiding blood pressure management. If elevated MCA mean flow velocities (MFV) are detected, then the MAP should be lowered so that MFVs normalize. Normalization of the MFV has been associated with a reduced risk of ICH (47,67). The choice of antihypertensive agents is somewhat arbitrary, but in general hydralazine should be avoided since it may paradoxically increase cerebral blood flow, which could theoretically potentiate the hyperperfusion (47). Given that neuroeffector mechanisms may play a role in the pathogenesis of HPS, beta and alpha-adrenergic blockers may have a dual effect of lowering pressures and ameliorating the dysautonomia. Careful monitoring of blood pressures should continue for at least two weeks following the procedure, even if the patient has been discharged.

This can be successfully accomplished using either home nursing visits or over-the-counter automated blood pressure monitors.

If symptoms of HPS develop suddenly or if headache is associated with nausea and vomiting, focal neurological deficits, seizures, or alteration of awareness, an urgent computed tomography (CT) scan of the brain without contrast should be obtained. Computerized tomography scanning is the most sensitive tool for the detection of ICH. In patients who develop symptoms within hours of CAS, the presence of contrast can confound the interpretation of the CT and the reading radiologist should be made aware. If there is no evidence of ICH then the patient should be transferred to an intensive monitoring unit and aggressive measures as described above should be taken to control blood pressure. Rarely, patients will have evidence of white matter edema or even focal cortical abnormalities (50). In those patients, the treatment approach is unchanged but more careful clinical observation with frequent neurological assessments should be undertaken to monitor for evidence of new or worsening focal deficits or seizures. Acute infarction from embolism may sometimes cause headaches similar to the hyperperfusion headache and when white matter or cortical edema is present it may be difficult to differentiate embolic, ischemic injury from hyperperfusion. Infarction is frequently accompanied by focal deficits whereas most patients with HPS do not have focal deficits. Furthermore, in patients with HPS who also have focal deficits but no ICH, the deficits will be more likely to fluctuate with blood pressure changes; and unlike patients who have focal deficits due to ischemia whose deficits may improve with higher blood pressures, the deficits in patients with HPS may actually improve as blood pressures are lowered. In this setting the measurement of CBF may be very helpful. Patients with ischemic injury will not typically have increased CBF and may of course have decreased CBF. Isolated cerebral white matter edema without ICH is reversible with effective treatment of hyperperfusion; corticosteroids are not indicated and will not be of benefit.

Seizures are treated symptomatically. In general a single seizure, particularly if focal and not associated with a focal neurological deficit or underlying structural abnormality on brain imaging, does not require antiepileptic drug treatment. In such patients the treatment of the hyperperfusion will decrease the risk of seizures, and persistent seizures are unlikely in the absence of focal brain lesions. On the other hand, patients who do have focal abnormalities or deficits are more likely to develop recurrent seizures and they should be treated with antiepileptics. Oral agents such as phenytoin or carbamazepine are preferred but they are associated with more side effects than newer agents such as levetiracetam. Parenteral antiepileptics such as intravenous phenytoin or phenobarbital or benzodiazepines should be reserved for patients who are in convulsive status epilepticus, i.e., patients with continuous seizure activity lasting more than 10 minutes or those who do not awaken between seizures.

The management of anticoagulation/antithrombotic therapy if symptoms of HPS develop in the postoperative period is unclear, but several authors have advocated discontinuing all such treatments following CEA unless absolutely necessary (25,47). Discontinuation of the antiplatelet treatments following CAS is potentially dangerous since acute stent thrombosis is very likely until the stent is covered with endothelium, which is not sufficiently complete until 14 days post-procedure. Furthermore, the risk of ICH due to the effects of antiplatelet agents has not been established. The high incidence of ICH in those patients who develop HPS supports the withholding of antiplatelet treatments until blood pressure control is established and symptoms resolve. In the series of patients described by Abou-Chebl et al. two patients who developed HPS were aggressively treated with antihypertensive treatments and their aspirin and clopidogrel were withheld until the symptoms resolved (31). In both patients the clinical symptoms of HPS resolved within hours to one day, and the antiplatelet treatments were resumed within 1–2 days. Since the antiplatelet effect of aspirin is permanent and the clinical effect of clopidogrel lasts five to seven days, one or two missed doses in this circumstance is unlikely to be of consequence. There are no data to support this approach and an argument can be made that withholding antiplatelets for one to two days may not have a significant effect on decreasing the risk of bleeding for the same reasons that it does not increase the risk of stent thrombosis. This issue cannot be resolved without further study and clinical judgment is the best guide. Patients who have profound hypertension or hypertension that is difficult to control may be at high risk of ICH so their antiplatelet treatments should be withheld until their symptoms resolve; on the other hand patients who respond quickly, i.e., within hours, to treatment with well controlled blood pressures may be at very low risk of ICH so they can continue to receive antiplatelets.

If ICH does develop then antithrombotics/anticoagulants should be withheld and reversed if possible. If ICH develops or is suspected while a patient is receiving heparin or anticoagulation with other anticoagulants then the agent should be stopped immediately. The agent should also be chemically reversed. In the case of unfractionated heparin, protamine sulfate can rapidly reverse the anticoagulant effect. Warfarin must be reversed with fresh-frozen plasma and/or cryoprecipitate. Other agents such as the direct thrombin inhibitors bivalirudin and argatroban do not have antidotes but have short half-lives. The anti-platelet agents are more problematic because there are no antidotes for their effects. Even platelet transfusions are ineffective with these agents which are present in plasma; unbound to platelets in sufficient concentrations they will inhibit the transfused platelets. Nonetheless, in cases of rapid deterioration, urgent platelet transfusion should be considered, particularly if neurosurgical evacuation is planned.

The presence of ICH on a CT will almost always be accompanied by focal deficits. The hemorrhages in patients with HPS can be deep, i.e., in the basal ganglia, or superficial, i.e., lobar. The prognosis and treatment of patients with ICH will depend on several factors. Hemorrhages that are deep, those that are large, particularly those >40 cc in volume, and those with intraventricular extension carry a worse prognosis (72,73). Older patients do not fare as well as younger patients. The mainstay of treatment is supportive care and anticipation of the mass effect and delayed consequences of ICH (74,75). Ideally, all patients with ICH should be observed in an intensive care unit staffed by physicians and nurses familiar with the management of patients with neurological disorders. Blood pressure control remains the mainstay of patient management. In the setting of ICH, aggressive lowering of blood pressure may actually potentiate neuronal injury, but because of the potential for spread of the ICH blood, pressures should be quickly lowered as in other patients with HPS. In patients with smaller hematomas or those without any mass effect, close observation with blood pressure control may be sufficient. Prophylactic treatment for seizures with phenytoin should be given to those patients with cortical lesions and should be continued for one to three months.

Altered awareness and a depressed level of consciousness, particularly if occurring within hours of onset herald progression due to increased mass effect and/or elevated ICP and carry a worse prognosis (76,77). These effects can be delayed by up to 72–96 hours after the ICH as edema develops in the surrounding brain tissue further exacerbating the mass effect and ICP. Such patients should have endotracheal tubes placed for airway control. ICP and mass effect control become critical in these patients. The medical treatments of mass effect and elevated ICP are temporizing measures only and are not always effective. Only surgical excision or drainage has a more durable effect. The decision to undergo surgery however cannot be made lightly in this patient population because of its unproven benefit in most cases, and the need for the maintenance of the potent and irreversible antiplatelet effects of aspirin and clopidogrel to avoid thrombosis of a newly placed stent. Surgical decompression and intraparenchymal hematoma removal require an open craniotomy with excision of injured brain. The surface of the brain is covered with arteries and veins and the risk of bleeding is high even in the absence of antiplatelet medication effects. Rebleeding into the surgical bed or the development of significant sub/epidural hematomas are real concerns and most neurosurgeons will not operate without withholding of antiplatelet agents and transfusion of platelets. Unfortunately, the effects of aspirin and clopidogrel cannot be reversed even with platelet transfusions, although transfusions may give a temporary benefit intra-operatively (see above).

Even if surgery could be performed safely it is not clear that hematoma removal is of benefit (78–80). While it is true that relief of the mass effect does have a benefit in terms of survival, neurological outcomes are not improved by surgery. The reason for this is that surgery requires the removal of brain tissue and in some circumstances access to the hematoma requires the traversal or removal of normal brain tissue. This is particularly the case in patients with deep hemorrhages that are surrounded by eloquent brain tissue and crucial arteries. In general, hematoma removal should be considered in patients with superficial, non-dominant, i.e., right, hemispheric lesions (Fig. 6). Dominant hemisphere lesions are associated with more disabling deficits because of their effects on language.

A purely medical approach is ideal even if the treatments are temporizing. Except in patients who have massive hematomas and markedly depressed consciousness at outset, patients for whom there is likely little that can be done, delayed edema and mass effect can be treated medically (75). Hyperventilation is the most rapid means of lowering ICP. Intracerebral blood volume and arterial tone are inversely related to the pH of the CSF, which in turn is inversely related to arterial partial pressure of CO_2 (pCO_2). In essence, as pCO_2 decreases, vasoconstriction of the cerebral vessels occurs and the intracranial blood volume decreases making more room in the cranium for other tissues/substances, in this case hematoma and edema. Hyperventilation to a pCO_2 of 25–30 mmHg will have an effect within 30–60 seconds. Unfortunately, the benefit is short lived and rarely lasts for more than a few hours. The hyperventilation must be maintained, otherwise rebound vasodilation may occur exacerbating the ICP and it must be reversed slowly to avoid rebound and elevation in cerebral blood volume and ICP. Hyperosmotic agents have a longer lasting benefit compared to hyperventilation but are more difficult to manage and do not have as rapid an onset. The prototypical agent is mannitol. Its exact mechanism of action is unclear but mannitol does decrease ICP with an effect that can last 24–48 hours. Mannitol must be dosed every four to six hours to achieve a serum osmolarity of 300–310. In urgent cases a large bolus of 75–100 gm can be given; imminent herniation can sometimes be delayed with such a large dose. Mannitol induces significant diuresis and if fluids are not replaced dehydration and hypoperfusion may result. In addition, mannitol can cause wasting of electrolytes, which must also be monitored closely.

There are simpler measures that can be used in almost all patients to control ICP. The first is the use of isotonic fluids for IV hydration, e.g., normal saline or lactated Ringer's. Hypotonic fluids can exacerbate cerebral edema and may precipitate herniation. In any patient who has elevated ICP or who is at risk, free water or $\frac{1}{2}$ or $\frac{1}{4}$ normal saline solutions should be avoided, particularly in the first 72–96 hours. Elevation of the head of the bed, sedation and avoidance of irritating/painful stimuli will also help control elevated ICP. Corticosteroids should not be used for preventing edema or decreasing mass effect. Their effect is delayed for at least eight hours and therefore is not helpful in patients with ICH who have rapid changes in ICP. Furthermore, corticosteroids are effective for limiting vasogenic edema from tumors but are not particularly effective for the cytotoxic edema associated with neuronal injury. The other effects of corticosteroids, i.e., hyperglycemia and increased susceptibility to infection, may actually worsen the neurological prognosis. The anti-inflammatory effect of steroids may be of theoretical benefit in decreasing oxidative injury, but this advantage is outweighed by their numerous side effects.

Besides delayed cerebral edema, obstructive hydrocephalus may be a delayed consequence of ICH if there is intraventricular or subarachnoid extension. The diagnosis and management of hydrocephalus will be discussed further in the section on SAH.

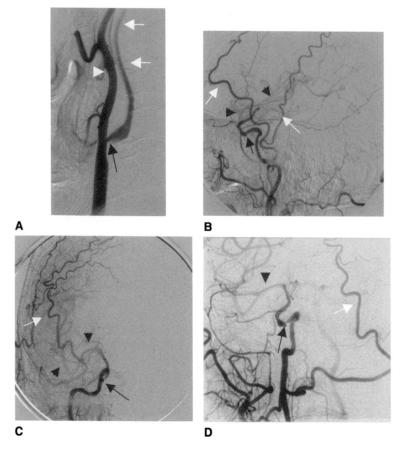

A   **B**

C   **D**

Figure 6 (*Caption on facing page*)

SUBARACHNOID HEMORRHAGE (SAH)

SAH has been reported following intracranial angioplasty and stenting and to a lesser degree following extracranial interventions (38,42–45,81). The higher incidence with intracranial interventions has to do with the fact that the intracranial vessels, amenable to endovascular intervention all lie within the subarachnoid space—with the exception of the petrous and cavernous portions of the ICA. Perforation of these vessels—and sometimes even of the petrous and cavernous ICA if mural injury is extensive—will cause SAH. The causes of injury include wire perforation, through and through dissection or vessel rupture. Wire perforation and vessel rupture occur during the intervention. The former occurs if a non-floppy wire is used, if the wire tip enters one of the small perforating branches of the MCA or BA, or if the tip lifts up a plaque and punctures through. Although dissection typically occurs during the PTA/stenting procedure, the SAH may be delayed for minutes to hours. Vessel rupture occurs if the PTA balloon or stent are oversized or if the vessel is heavily calcified and rigid. Clinical manifestations of both are immediate. If the patient is awake,

---

Figure 6A–L (*Facing Page*) A 51-year-old male who presented recurrent right hemispheric transient ischemic attacks despite medical therapy. Non-invasive studies suggested the presence of an occlusion or severe stenosis of the right ICA. In **A**, an oblique angiogram of the CCA shows a moderate stenosis of the ICA origin (*black arrow*) with markedly reduced flow into and small caliber of the cervical ICA (*white arrows*), compared with the ECA (*arrowhead*). The severity of the ICA origin stenosis was not enough to account for the slow flow so a detailed evaluation of the intracranial ICA was performed which revealed a severe, eccentric stenosis of the cavernous segment of the ICA (*black arrows in* **B, C**), which was the likely cause of the TIAs. The stenosis was seen best in a contralateral oblique view (*black arrow in* **D**). The ipsilateral MCA filled to a minimal degree from the ICA; compare the superficial temporal artery-filling pattern (*white arrows in* **B, C, D**) with the filling pattern of the MCA (*arrowheads in* **B, C, D**). Using a modification of the technique described in the text, a #6F sheath was placed in the distal CCA but a guide catheter was not placed in the ICA because of the severity of the origin stenosis. After placing a 0.014-inch microwire in a second order MCA branch (*white arrow in* **E**) (**E–H**, see page 368; **I–L**, see page 369), a 2 mm coronary balloon catheter was inflated in the stenosis (*black arrow in* **E**) with improved filling of the MCA (*white arrow in* **F**) and a fair angiographic result, but with a persistent ulceration and subtle dissection flap (*black arrow in* **F**). To insure persistent patency a 2.5 mm coronary stent was advanced into the stenosis but it could not be advanced enough to assure coverage of the entire lesion, in part because it would "catch" on the edge of the ulceration (*arrow in* **G**). On the second attempt the patient developed a retro-orbital headache. After stent delivery system removal, an oblique angiogram showed perforation of the ICA with the formation of a carotid-cavernous sinus fistula (CCF)(*arrow in* **H**). The heparin was reversed with protamine and the balloon catheter was re-introduced and inflated three times for two minutes each within the cavernous segment. After the third inflation an angiogram showed that the CCF had resolved (*arrow in* **I**). With adequate antegrade flow, the procedure was terminated and the patient was neurologically intact. Later that evening he developed alcohol withdrawal symptoms with profound agitation and hypertension that was difficult to control except with several parenteral medications and sedation. The next AM the patient developed a sudden headache and progressive left hemiparesis and was taken for an urgent CT scan, which revealed a large lobar hemorrhage (*black arrows in* **J**) with some subarachnoid extension (*white arrows in* **J**). Within 12 hours, the patient developed clinical and radiographic signs of herniation (*arrows in* **K**) due to edema. Because of the location of the hematoma (see text), surgical evacuation was performed with removal of the skull on that side (*arrows in* **L**). The patient made a rapid recovery in the first post-operative week and was discharged to rehabilitation with a moderate but improving left hemiparesis.

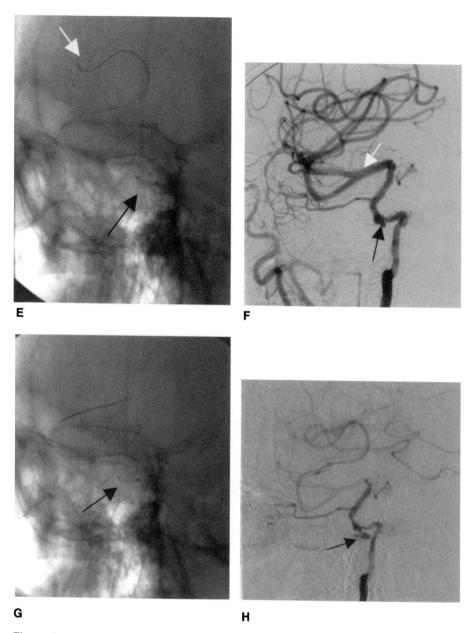

E   F

G   H

Figure 6 (*Continued*)

sudden severe headache, nausea and vomiting, and neck stiffness occur and are often associated with a sudden rise in arterial blood pressure; if the patient is sedated under general anesthesia the clinical manifestations may be limited to bradycardia or hypertension. Immediate angiography will often show extravasation of contrast into the subarachnoid space or surrounding cavernous sinus (Fig. 6).

If extravasation of contrast into the subarachnoid space is noted, the procedural anticoagulation must be stopped and reversed immediately. If unfractionated heparin is used then sufficient protamine sulfate should be used to fully reverse the

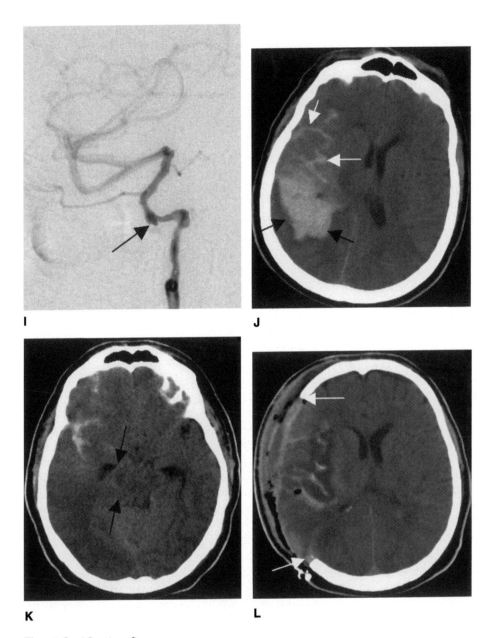

Figure 6   (*Continued*)

anticoagulation. Other agents cannot be reversed. Coincident with reversal of anti-coagulants, the patient's blood pressure must be lowered to below 140/90 and lower if the patient can tolerate it. Depending on the location of the perforation, an appropriately-sized coronary balloon catheter should be placed within the vessel at the perforation site and inflated gently to tamponade the bleeding. The balloon should stay inflated for several minutes but the inflation time should be adjusted depending on whether the patient can tolerate the cessation of flow. This technique does carry the risk of acute thrombosis of the vessel, but with adequate platelet inhi-bition the risk should be small. If bleeding is not controlled immediately, the patient's neurological status may deteriorate quickly as ICP rises. Eventually the bleeding will stop but it may be too late at that point. Airway control should be achieved quickly in these cases and immediate neurosurgical consultation obtained.

The delayed consequences of SAH include hydrocephalus and vasospasm. The latter typically occurs following aneurismal SAH and has not been studied or reported following endovascular interventions, but it may occur if sufficient quantities of blood are present in the subarachnoid space. Vasospasm causes clinical signs and symptoms by causing ischemia (82). The onset of vasospasm is often delayed until the 4th day following the hemorrhage and peaks in severity by days 10–14, decreasing rapidly thereafter. The symptoms tend to be progressive rather than abrupt in onset, but may progress quickly, and they may be focal or global. Frank infarction often occurs if vasospasm is unrecognized, but may be prevented by so-called "triple-H-therapy" where the three H's are hypertension, hypervolemia, and hemodilution. The aim of this approach is the maintenance of cerebral perfusion. TCD ultrasound and angiography are the mainstays of diagnosis. Although it has not been reported following SAH due to an endovascular procedure, it is likely appropriate to monitor MFVs by TCD in all such patients. If the vessel cannot be insonated or MFVs begin to rise with or without clinical deficits, repeat angiography may be warranted to search for vasospasm. If the ruptured vessel has been repaired and vasospasm is found, careful triple-H therapy should be considered. Angioplasty is an option but may not be appropriate if the vasospasm is in the vessel that caused the hemorrhage. A full discussion of the management of vasospasm is beyond the scope of this text, and the management of such patients is best left in the hands of a neuro-intensivist with experience managing SAH.

Hydrocephalus can occur within the first day if large enough quantities of blood find their way into the ventricular system or the basal subarachnoid spaces (75,82). Often the hydrocephalus is delayed for days or even weeks. A depressed level of consciousness or increased confusion are the usual presenting signs of hydrocephalus. Rarely, signs of downward herniation such as downward deviation of the eyes as occurs with midbrain tectum compression can herald the onset of hydrocephalus. A CT scan is the test of choice if hydrocephalus is suspected. The treatment of hydrocephalus is almost always surgical but, rarely, patients with mild and slowly developing symptoms may be treated with the carbonic anhydrase inhibitor acetazolamide. This agent decreases the production of cerebrospinal fluid and can reverse hydrocephalus. For most patients however, hydrocephalus develops over hours to a few days with marked depression in alertness. In these patients ventricular drainage via ventriculostomy can be lifesaving. Although the procedure can be done at the bedside, there is a risk of ICH and subdural hemorrhage particularly in patients being treated with anticoagulants and antiplatelet agents. The prognosis if hydrocephalus occurs is dependent on the overall status of the patient. If it develops early (<10 days) in the course and is diagnosed and treated rapidly with a ventriculostomy, most patients will have a good prognosis and can be weaned off of the ventriculostomy. Late hydrocephalus, however, will almost always require permanent ventricular drainage.

CONCLUSION

In summary, the HPS is a recognized complication of cerebrovascular revascularization. High-risk patients include those with a severe stenosis, poor intracerebral collaterals primarily due to contralateral stenosis or occlusion, hypertension, and persistently elevated MCA velocities following the procedure. Careful screening to identify high-risk patients, vigilant perioperative monitoring for signs of HPS, aggressive management of postoperative blood pressure, and the avoidance of prolonged/excessive anticoagulation therapy are all-important steps in both preventing and minimizing the impact of this potentially devastating complication. SAH on the other hand is rare following cervical interventions, and is more common with intracranial interventions. It is often a devastating complication and is best avoided by meticulous technique and a thorough understanding of the unique qualities of the intracranial vessels and circulation.

REFERENCES

1. Connors JJ III, Wojak JC. Percutaneous transluminal angioplasty for intracranial atherosclerotic lesions: evolution of technique and short-term results. J Neurosurg 1999; 91(3): 415–423.
2. Mori T, Mori K, Fukuoka M, Arisawa M, Honda S. Percutaneous transluminal cerebral angioplasty: serial angiographic follow-up after successful dilatation. Neuroradiology 1997; 39(2):111–116.
3. Mori T, Fukuoka M, Kazita K, Mori K. Follow-up study after intracranial percutaneous transluminal cerebral balloon angioplasty. AJNR Am J Neuroradiol 1998; 19(8):1525–1533.
4. Takis C, Kwan ES, Pessin MS, Jacobs DH, Caplan LR. Intracranial angioplasty: experience and complications. AJNR Am J Neuroradiol 1997; 18(9):1661–1668.
5. Mori T, Kazita K, Chokyu K, Mima T, Mori K. Short-term arteriographic and clinical outcome after cerebral angioplasty and stenting for intracranial vertebrobasilar and carotid atherosclerotic occlusive disease. AJNR Am J Neuroradiol 2000; 21(2):249–254.
6. Ramee SR, Dawson R, McKinley KL, Felberg R, Collins TJ, Jenkins JS, Awaad MI, White CJ. Provisional stenting for symptomatic intracranial stenosis using a multidisciplinary approach: acute results, unexpected benefit, and one-year outcome. Catheteriz Cardiovasc Interv 2001; 52(4):457–467.
7. Levy EI, Horowitz MB, Koebbe CJ, Jungreis CC, Pride GL, Dutton K, Purdy PD. Transluminal stent-assisted angioplasty of the intracranial vertebrobasilar system for medically refractory, posterior circulation ischemia: early results. Neurosurgery 2001; 48(6):1215–1221.
8. Gomez CR, Misra VK, Liu MW, Wadlington VR, Terry JB, Tulyapronchote R, Campbell MS. Elective stenting of symptomatic basilar artery stenosis. Stroke 2000; 31(1): 95–99.
9. Bhatt DL, Kapadia SR, Bajzer CT, Chew DP, Ziada KM, Mukherjee D, Roffi M, Topol EJ, Yadav JS. Dual antiplatelet therapy with clopidogrel and aspirin after carotid artery stenting. J Invasive Cardiol 2001; 13(12):767–771.
10. Furlan A, Higashida R, Wechsler L, Gent M, Rowley H, Kase C, Pessin M, Ahuja A, Callaham F, Clark WM, Silver F, Rivera F. Intra-arterial prourokinase for acute ischemic stroke. The PROACT II study: a randomized controlled trial. Prolyse in Acute Cerebral Thromboembolism. J Am Med Assoc 1999; 282(21):2003–2011.
11. Adams HP Jr, Brott TG, Furlan AJ, Gomez CR, Grotta J, Helgason CM, Kwiatkowski T, Lyden PD, Marler JR, Torner J, Feinberg W, Mayberg M, Thies W. Guidelines for thrombolytic therapy for acute stroke: a supplement to the guidelines for the management of patients with acute ischemic stroke. A statement for healthcare professionals from a Special Writing Group of the Stroke Council, American Heart Association. Circulation 1996; 94(5):1167–1174.

12. Ferguson RD, Ferguson JG, Lee LI. Endovascular revascularization therapy in cerebral athero-occlusive disease. Angioplasty and stents, systemic and local thrombolysis. Neurosurg Clin N Am 1994; 5(3):511–527.

13. Callahan AS III, Berger BL. Intra-arterial thrombolysis in acute ischemic stroke. Tenn Med 1997; 90(2):61–64.

14. Endo S, Kuwayama N, Hirashima Y, Akai T, Nishijima M, Takaku A. Results of urgent thrombolysis in patients with major stroke and atherothrombotic occlusion of the cervical internal carotid artery. AJNR Am J Neuroradiol 1998; 19(6):1169–1175.

15. Lanzino G, Fessler RD, Wakhloo AK, Guterman LR, Hopkins LN. Successful Intra-cranial Thrombolysis for Cerebral Thromboembolic Complications Resulting from Cardiovascular Diagnostic and Interventional Procedures. J Invasive Cardiol 1999; 11(7):439–443.

16. Lee DH, Jo KD, Kim HG, Choi SJ, Jung SM, Ryu DS, Park MS. Local intraarterial urokinase thrombolysis of acute ischemic stroke with or without intravenous abciximab: a pilot study. J Vasc Interv Radiol 2002; 13(8):769–774.

17. Mori T, Fukuoka M, Kazita K, Mima T, Mori K. Intraventricular hemorrhage after carotid stenting. J Endovasc Surg 1999; 6(4):337–341.

18. Breutman ME, Fields WS, Crawford ES, DeBakey ME. Cerebral hemorrhage in carotid artery surgery. Arch Neurol 1963; 9:458–467.

19. Wylie EJ, Hein MF, Adams JE. Intracranial hemorrhage following surgical revascular-ization for treatment of acute strokes. J Neurosurg 1964; 21:212–215.

20. Bernstein M, Fleming JF, Deck JH. Cerebral hyperperfusion after carotid endarterec-tomy: a cause of cerebral hemorrhage. Neurosurgery 1984; 15(1):50–56.

21. Schroeder T, Sillesen H, Sorensen O, Engell HC. Cerebral hyperperfusion following car-otid endarterectomy. J Neurosurg 1987; 66(6):824–829.

22. Reigel MM, Hollier LH, Sundt TM Jr, Piepgras DG, Sharbrough FW, Cherry KJ. Cer-ebral hyperperfusion syndrome: a cause of neurologic dysfunction after carotid endar-terectomy. J Vasc Surg 1987; 5(4):628–634.

23. Mansoor GA, White WB, Grunnet M, Ruby ST. Intracerebral hemorrhage after carotid endarterectomy associated with ipsilateral fibrinoid necrosis: a consequence of the hyperperfusion syndrome? J Vasc Surg 1996; 23(1):147–151.

24. Connolly ES. Hyperperfusion syndrome following carotid endarterectomy. In: Loftus CM, ed. Carotid Artery Surgery. New York: Thieme Medical Publishers, 2000:493–500.

25. Ouriel K, Shortell CK, Illig KA, Greenberg RK, Green RM. Intracerebral hemorrhage after carotid endarterectomy: incidence, contribution to neurologic morbidity, and pre-dictive factors. J Vasc Surg 1999; 29(1):82–87.

26. Solomon RA, Loftus CM, Quest DO, Correll JW. Incidence and etiology of intracereb-ral hemorrhage following carotid endarterectomy. J Neurosurg 1986; 64(1):29–34.

27. Hafner DH, Smith RB III, King OW, Perdue GD, Stewart MT, Rosenthal D, Jordan WD. Massive intracerebral hemorrhage following carotid endarterectomy. Arch Surg 1987; 122(3):305–307.

28. Piepgras DG, Morgan MK, Sundt TM Jr, Yanagihara T, Mussman LM. Intracerebral hemorrhage after carotid endarterectomy. J Neurosurg 1988; 68(4):532–536.

29. Pomposelli FB, Lamparello PJ, Riles TS, Craighead CC, Giangola G, Imparato AM. Intracranial hemorrhage after carotid endarterectomy. J Vasc Surg 1988; 7(2):248–255.

30. Reith HB, Edelmann M, Reith C. Spontaneous intracerebral hemorrhage following car-otid endarterectomy. Experience of 328 operations from 1983–1988. Int Surg 1992; 77(3):224–225.

31. Abou-Chebl A, Yadav J, Reginelli J, Bajzer C, Bhatt D, Krieger D. Intracranial Hemor-rhage and Hyperperfusion Syndrome Following Carotid Artery Stenting: Risk Factors, Prevention, and Treatment. J Am Coll Cardiol 2004; 43(9):1596–1601.

32. Bando K, Satoh K, Matsubara S, Nakatani M, Nagahiro S. Hyperperfusion pheno-menon after percutaneous transluminal angioplasty for atherosclerotic stenosis of the intracranial vertebral artery. Case report. J Neurosurg 2001; 94(5):826–830.

33. Lylyk P, Cohen JE, Ceratto R, Ferrario A, Miranda C. Angioplasty and stent placement in intracranial atherosclerotic stenoses and dissections. Ajnr: Am J Neuroradiol 2002; 23(3):430–436.

34. Marks MP, Marcellus M, Norbash AM, Steinberg GK, Tong D, Albers GW. Outcome of angioplasty for atherosclerotic intracranial stenosis. Stroke 1999; 30(5):1065–1069.

35. Miao Z, Ling F, Li S, Wang M, Hua Y, Guo D, Dong Y, Song Q. Stent-assisted angioplasty in treatment of symptomatic intracranial artery stenosis. [Chinese]. Chung-Hua i Hsueh Tsa Chih [Chinese Medical Journal] 2002; 82(10):657–660.

36. Rasmussen PA, Perl J, Barr JD, Markarian GZ, Katzan I, Sila C, Krieger D, Furlan AJ, Masaryk TJ. Stent-assisted angioplasty of intracranial vertebrobasilar atherosclerosis: an initial experience. J Neurosurg 2000; 92(5):771–778.

37. Gupta R, Schumacher HC, Mangla S, Meyers PM, Duong H, Khandji AG, Marshall RS, Mohr JP, Pile-Spellman J. Urgent endovascular revascularization for symptomatic intracranial atherosclerotic stenosis. Neurology 2003; 61(12):1729–1735.

38. Schoser BG, Heesen C, Eckert B, Thie A. Cerebral hyperperfusion injury after percutaneous transluminal angioplasty of extracranial arteries. J Neurol 1997; 244(2):101–104.

39. Morrish W, Grahovac S, Douen A, Cheung G, Hu W, Farb R, Kalapos P, Wee R, Hudon M, Agbi C, Richard M. Intracranial hemorrhage after stenting and angioplasty of extracranial carotid stenosis. [Comment]. Ajnr: Am J Neuroradiol 2000; 21(10): 1911–1916.

40. Ho DS, Wang Y, Chui M, Ho SL, Cheung RT. Epileptic seizures attributed to cerebral hyperperfusion after percutaneous transluminal angioplasty and stenting of the internal carotid artery. Cerebrovasc Dis 2000; 10(5):374–379.

41. Kapadia SR, Bajzer CT, Ziada KM, Bhatt DL, Wazni OM, Silver MJ, Beven EG, Ouriel K, Yadav JS. Initial experience of platelet glycoprotein IIb/IIIa inhibition with abciximab during carotid stenting: a safe and effective adjunctive therapy. Stroke 2001; 32(10):2328–2332.

42. Al Mubarak N, Roubin GS, Vitek JJ, Iyer SS, New G, Leon MB. Subarachnoidal hemorrhage following carotid stenting with the distal- balloon protection. Catheteriz Cardiovasc Interv 2001; 54(4):521–523.

43. Qureshi AI, Saad M, Zaidat OO, Suarez JI, Alexander MJ, Fareed M, Suri K, Ali Z, Hopkins LN. Intracerebral hemorrhages associated with neurointerventional procedures using a combination of antithrombotic agents including abciximab. Stroke 2002; 33(7):1916–1919.

44. Meyers PM, Higashida RT, Phatouros CC, Malek AM, Lempert TE, Dowd CF, Halbach VV. Cerebral hyperperfusion syndrome after percutaneous transluminal stenting of the craniocervical arteries. Neurosurgery 2000; 47(2):335–343.

45. Sundt TM Jr, Sharbrough FW, Piepgras DG, Kearns TP, Messick JM Jr, O'Fallon WM. Correlation of cerebral blood flow and electroencephalographic changes during carotid endarterectomy: with results of surgery and hemodynamics of cerebral ischemia. Mayo Clin Proc 1981; 56(9):533–543.

46. Jansen C, Sprengers AM, Moll FL, Vermeulen FE, Hamerlijnck RP, van Gijn J, Ackerstaff RG. Prediction of intracerebral haemorrhage after carotid endarterectomy by clinical criteria and intraoperative transcranial Doppler monitoring: results of 233 operations. Eur J Vasc Surg 1994; 8(2):220–225..

47. Penn AA, Schomer DF, Steinberg GK. Imaging studies of cerebral hyperperfusion after carotid endarterectomy. Case report. J Neurosurg 1995; 83(1):133–137.

48. Caplan LR, Skillman J, Ojemann R, Fields WS. Intracerebral hemorrhage following carotid endarterectomy: a hypertensive complication? Stroke 1978; 9(5):457–460.

49. Sbarigia E, Speziale F, Giannoni MF, Colonna M, Panico MA, Fiorani P. Post-carotid endarterectomy hyperperfusion syndrome: preliminary observations for identifying at risk patients by transcranial Doppler sonography and the acetazolamide test. Eur J Vasc Surg 1993; 7(3):252–256.

50. Breen JC, Caplan LR, DeWitt LD, Belkin M, Mackey WC, O'Donnell TP. Brain edema after carotid surgery. Neurology 1996; 46(1):175–181.

51. Harrison PB, Wong MJ, Belzberg A, Holden J. Hyperperfusion syndrome after carotid endarterectomy. CT changes. Neuroradiology 1991; 33(2):106–110.

52. Cikrit DF, Burt RW, Dalsing MC, Lalka SG, Sawchuk AP, Waymire B, Witt RM. Acetazolamide enhanced single photon emission computed tomography (SPECT) evaluation of cerebral perfusion before and after carotid endarterectomy. J Vasc Surg 1992; 15(5):747–753.

53. Wholey MH, Wholey M, Mathias K, Roubin GS, Diethrich EB, Henry M, Bailey S, Bergeron P, Dorros G, Eles G, et Al. Global experience in cervical carotid artery stent placement. Catheteriz Cardiovasc Interv 2000; 50(2):160–167.

54. White CJ, Gomez CR, Iyer SS, Wholey M, Yadav JS. Carotid stent placement for extracranial carotid artery disease: current state of the art. Catheter Cardiovasc Interv 2000; 51(3):339–346.

55. Roubin GS, New G, Iyer SS, Vitek JJ, Al Mubarak N, Liu MW, Yadav J, Gomez C, Kuntz RE. Immediate and late clinical outcomes of carotid artery stenting in patients with symptomatic and asymptomatic carotid artery stenosis: a 5-year prospective analysis. Circulation 2001; 103(4):532–537.

56. Veith FJ, Amor M, Ohki T, Beebe HG, Bell PR, Bolia A, Bergeron P, Connors, JJ III, Diethrich EB, Ferguson RD, et Al. Current status of carotid bifurcation angioplasty and stenting based on a consensus of opinion leaders. J Vasc Surg 2001; 33(2 suppl): S111–S116.

57. Macdonald S, McKevitt F, Venables GS, Cleveland TJ, Gaines PA. Neurological outcomes after carotid stenting protected with the NeuroShield filter compared to unprotected stenting. Journal of Endovascular Therapy. Official J Int Soc Endovasc Specialists 2002; 9(6):777–785.

58. Qureshi AI, Ali Z, Suri MF, Kim SH, Fessler RD, Ringer AJ, Guterman LR, Hopkins LN. Open-label phase I clinical study to assess the safety of intravenous eptifibatide in patients undergoing internal carotid artery angioplasty and stent placement. Neurosurgery 2001; 48(5):998–1004.

59. Qureshi AI, Suri MF, Khan J, Fessler RD, Guterman LR, Hopkins LN. Abciximab as an adjunct to high-risk carotid or vertebrobasilar angioplasty: preliminary experience. Neurosurgery 2000; 46(6):1316–1324.

60. Bruetman ME, Fields WS, Crawford ES, DeBakey ME. Cerebral hemorrhage in carotid artery surgery. Arch Neurol 1963; 147:458–467.

61. Blaisdell WF, Clauss RH, Galbraith JG, Imparato AM, Wylie EJ. Joint study of extracranial arterial occlusion. IV. A review of surgical considerations. J Am Med Assoc 1969; 209(12):1889–1895.

62. Gasecki AP, Ferguson GG, Eliasziw M, Clagett GP, Fox AJ, Hachinski V, Barnett HJ. Early endarterectomy for severe carotid artery stenosis after a nondisabling stroke: results from the North American Symptomatic Carotid Endarterectomy Trial. J Vasc Surg 1994; 20(2):288–295.

63. Paddock-Eliasziw LM, Eliasziw M, Barr HW, Barnett HJ. Long-term prognosis and the effect of carotid endarterectomy in patients with recurrent ipsilateral ischemic events. North American Symptomatic Carotid Endarterectomy Trial Group. Neurology 1996; 47(5):1158–1162.

64. Schroeder T, Jorgensen LG, Knudsen L, Perko M. [Hemodynamic assessment of cerebrovascular circulation using transcranial Doppler ultrasound in patients with carotid stenosis]. Ugeskr Laeger 1990; 152(29):2110–2113.

65. Sakaki T, Tsujimoto S, Nishitani M, Ishida Y, Morimoto T. Perfusion pressure breakthrough threshold of cerebral autoregulation in the chronically ischemic brain: an experimental study in cats. J Neurosurg 1992; 76(3):478–485.

66. Macfarlane R, Tasdemiroglu E, Moskowitz MA, Uemura Y, Wei EP, Kontos HA. Chronic trigeminal ganglionectomy or topical capsaicin application to pial vessels

attenuates postocclusive cortical hyperemia but does not influence postischemic hypoperfusion. J Cereb Blood Flow Metab 1991; 11(2):261–271.

67. Jorgensen LG, Schroeder TV. Defective cerebrovascular autoregulation after carotid endarterectomy. Eur J Vasc Surg 1993; 7(4):370–379.

68. Jorgensen LG, Schroeder TV. Transcranial Doppler for carotid endarterectomy. Eur J Vasc Endovasc Surg 1996; 12(1):1–2.

69. Jorgensen LG, Schroeder TV. Transcranial Doppler for detection of cerebral ischemia during carotid endarterectomy. Eur J Vasc Surg 1992; 6(2):142–147.

70. Magee TR, Davies AH, Horrocks M. Transcranial Doppler evaluation of cerebral hyperperfusion syndrome after carotid endarterectomy. Eur J Vasc Surg 1994; 8(1):104–106.

71. Naylor AR, Whyman M, Wildsmith JA, McClure JH, Jenkins AM, Merrick MV, Ruckley CV. Immediate effects of carotid clamp release on middle cerebral artery blood flow velocity during carotid endarterectomy. Eur J Vasc Surg 1993; 7(3):308–316.

72. Dixon AA, Holness RO, Howes WJ, Garner JB. Spontaneous intracerebral haemorrhage: an analysis of factors affecting prognosis. Can J Neurol Sci 1985; 12(3):267–271.

73. Franke CL, van Swieten JC, Algra A, van Gijn J. Prognostic factors in patients with intracerebral haematoma. J Neurol Neurosurg Psychiatry 1992; 55(8):653–657.

74. Voelker J, Kaufman H. Clinical aspects of intracerebral hemorrhage. In: Welch K, Caplan L, Reis D, Siesjo B, Weir B, eds. Primer on Cerebrovascular Diseases. San Diego: Academic Press, 1997:432–436.

75. Management of nontraumatic brain hemorrhage. In: Ropper A, Gress D, Diringer M, Green D, Mayer S, Bleck T, eds. Neurological and Neurosurgical Intensive Care. Philadelphia: Lippincot Williams & Wilkins, 2004:217–230.

76. Hier DB, Davis KR, Richardson EP Jr, Mohr JP. Hypertensive putaminal hemorrhage. Ann Neurol 1977; 1(2):152–159.

77. Paillas JE, Alliez B. Surgical treatment of spontaneous intracerebral hemorrhage. Immediate and long-term results in 250 cases. J Neurosurg 1973; 39(2):145–151.

78. Juvela S, Heiskanen O, Poranen A, Valtonen S, Kuurne T, Kaste M, Troupp H. The treatment of spontaneous intracerebral hemorrhage. A prospective randomized trial of surgical and conservative treatment. J Neurosurg 1989; 70(5):755–758.

79. Auer LM, Deinsberger W, Niederkorn K, Gell G, Kleinert R, Schneider G, Holzer P, Bone G, Mokry M, Korner E. Endoscopic surgery versus medical treatment for spontaneous intracerebral hematoma: a randomized study. J Neurosurg 1989; 70(4):530–535.

80. Batjer HH, Reisch JS, Allen BC, Plaizier LJ, Su CJ. Failure of surgery to improve outcome in hypertensive putaminal hemorrhage. A prospective randomized trial. Arch Neurol 1990; 47(10):1103–1106.

81. Castriota F, Cremonesi A, Manetti R, Liso A, Oshola K, Ricci E, Balestra G. Impact of cerebral protection devices on early outcome of carotid stenting. J Endovasc Ther Official J Int Soc of Endovasc Specialists 2002; 9(6):786–792.

82. Subarachnoid hemorrhage. In: Ropper A, Gress D, Diringer M, Green D, Mayer S, Bleck T, eds. Neurological and Neurosurgical Intensive Care. Philadelphia: Lippincot Williams & Wilkins, 2004:231–242.

83. Sabiston D.C. Essentials of Surgery W.B. Saunders Company, 1987.

84. B. Olin, et al. Vascular Medicine.

85. Bailly AL, Lautier A, Laurent A, Guiffant G, Dufaux J, Houdart E, Labarre D, Merland JJ. Thrombosis of angiographic catheters in humans: experimental study. Int J Artif Organs 1999; 22(10):690–700.

86. Johnston DC, Champman KM, Goldstein LB. Low rate of complications of cerebral angiography. Routine Clin Pract Neurol 2001; 57(11):2012–2014.

87. Bendszu M, Koltzenburg M, Burger R, Warmuth-Metz M, Hofmann E, Solymosi L. Silent embolism in diagnostic cerebral angiography and neurointerventional procedures: a perspective study. Lancet 1999; 354(9190):1594–1597.

88. CAVATAS Investigators. The Carotid and Vertebral Artery Trans Luminal Angioplasty Study (CAVATAS). Lancet 2001; 357:1729–1737.

89. Topol EJ, Leya F, Pinkerton CA, Whitlow PL, Hofling B, Simonton CA, Masden RR, Serruys PW, Leon MB, Williams DO. A comparison of directional atherectomy with coronary angioplasty in with coronary artery disease. The CAVEAT Study Group. N Engl J Med 1993; 329:221–227.

90. Kocer M, Kizilkiliz O, Albayram S, Adaletli I, Kantarci F, Islak C. Treatment of iatric genic internal carotid laceration at carotid cavernous fistula with endovascular stent-graft placement. American J Neuroradiol 2002; 23(3):442–446.

91. Link J, Feyerabend B, Graberer M, Linstepet U, Brossmann J, Thomsen H, Heller M. Dacron-covered stent-grafts for the percutaneous treatment of carotid aneurysms: effectiveness and biocompatibility-experimental study in swine. Radiology 1996; 200(2): 397–401.

92. Levy EI, Boulos AS, Bendok VR, Kim SH, Qureshi AI, Guterman LR, Hopkins LN. Brainstem infarct after delayed thrombosis of a stented vertebral artery fusi form aneurysm: case report. Neurosurgery 2002; 51(5):1280–1284.

93. Nelson PK. Neurointerventional management of intracranial aneurysms. Neurosurg Clin N Am 1998; 9(4):879–895.

94. Bavinzski G, Talazoglu V, Killer M, Richling B, Gruber A, Gross CE, Plank H Jr. Gross and microscopic histopathological findings in aneurysm of the human brain treated with guglielmi detachable coils. J Neurosurg 1999; 91(2):284–293.

95. Workman MJ, Cloft HJ, Tong FC, Dion JE, Jensen ME, Marx WF, Callmes DF. Thrombus formation at the neck of cerebral aneurysms during treatment of guglielmi detachable coils. Am J Neuroradiol 2002; 23(9):1558–1576.

96. Sato E, Saito I. Risk of clot formation with ionic and nonionic contrast media in cerebral angiography, tama contrast media study group. Acad Radiol 1996; 3(11):925–928.

97. Unpublished data. The Cleveland Clinic Foundation Cardiac Catheterization Laboratory, 2004.

98. Carpenter MB, ed. The Core Text of Neuroanatomy. 3rd ed. Baltimore, Maryland: Williams & Wilkins Publishers, 1985.

99. Orlandi G, Parenti G, Bertolucci A, Puglioli M, Coloavoli P, Murri L. Carotid plaque features on angiography and asymptomatic cerebral micro-embolism. Acta Neurol Scand 1997; 96(3):183–186.

100. Gerraty RP, Bowser DN, Infeld B, Mitchell PJ, Davis SM. Microemboli during carotid angiography. Association with stroke risk factors or subsequent magnetic resonance imaging changes? Stroke 1996; 27(9):1543–1547.

101. Jordan WD Jr, Voellinger DC, Doblar DD, Plyushcheva NP, Fisher WS, McDowell HA. Microemboli detected by transcranial Doppler monitoring in patients during carotid angioplasty versus carotid endarterectomy. Cardiovasc Surg 1999; 7(1):33–38.

102. Jaeger HJ, Mathias KD, Hauth E, Drescher R, Gissler HM, Hennings S et al. Cerebral ischemia detected with diffusion-weighted MR imaging after stent implantation in the carotid artery. Ajnr: American Journal of Neuroradiology 2002; 23(2):200–207.

103. Hoffman R, et al. Stroke 2002; 33(3):725–727.

104. Woimant F, Chapot R, Mounayer C, Soria C, Merland JJ. Thrombolysis of extracranial and intracranial arteries after IV abciximab.

105. Kawon OK, Lee KJ, Han MH, Oh CW, Han DH, Koh YC. Intra-arterially administered abciximab an adjuvant thrombolytic therapy: report of three cases. Am J Neuroradiol 2002; 23(3):447–451.

106. Whitlow PL, Lylyk P, Londero H, Mandiz OA, Mathias K, Jaeger H, Parodi J, Schonholz C, Malei J. Carotid artery stenting protected with an emboli containment system. Stroke 2002; 33(4):1308–1314.

107. Jaeger H, Mathias K, Drescher R, Hauth E, Bockisch G, Demirel E, Gissler HM. Clinical results of cerebral protection with a filter device using stent implantation at the carotid artery. Cardiovasc Interv Radiol 2001; 24(4):249–256.

108. Bates MC, Dorros G, Parodi J, Ohki T. Reversal of the direction of internal carotid artery blood flow by occlusion of the common and external carotid arteries in a swine model. Catheteriz Cardiovasc Interv 2003; 60(2):270–275.
109. Angelini A, Reimers B, Della BM, Sacca S, Pasquetto G, Cernetti C et al. Cerebral protection during carotid artery stenting: collection and histopathologic analysis of embolized debris. Stroke 2002; 33(2):456–461.
110. Unpublished Data. Transcatheter Therapeutics, 2003.
111. Unpublished Data. American Heart Association Scientific Sessions, 19th November 2002.
112. Unpublished Data. American College of Cardiology Chicago at American Society of Interventional Radiology Salt Lake City the 30th of March 2003.
113. MacDonald S, McKevitt F, Venables GS, Cleveland TJ, Gaines PA. Neurologic outcomes after carotid stenting protected with a neuroshield filter compared to unprotected stenting. J Endovasc Ther 2002; 9(6):777–785.
114. Grúbe E, Colombo A, Hauptmann E, Londero H, Reifart N, Gerckens U, Stone GW. Initial multicentric experience with a novel distal protection filter during carotid stent implantation. Catheteriz Cardiovasc Interv 2003; 58(2):139–146.
115. Wilentz JR, Chati Z, Krafft V, Amor M. Ridenol embolization during carotid angioplasty and stenting: mechanisms and role of cerebral protection systems. Catheteriz Cardiovasc Interv 2002; 56(3):320–327.
116. Mas JL, Chatellier G, Beyssen D. EVA-3S Investigators. Carotid angioplasty and stenting with and without cerebral protection: clinical work from the endarterectomy versus angioplasty in patients with symptomatic severe carotid stenosis (EVA-3S) trial. Stroke 2004; 35(1):E18–E20.
117. del Zoppo GJ, Higashida RT, Furlan AJ, Pessin MS, Rowley HA, Gent M. PROACT: phase II randomize trial of bro-urokinase by direct arterial delivery in the acute middle cerebral artery stroke. PROACT Investigators. Prolyse in acute cerebral thromboembolism. Stroke 1998; 29(1):4–11.
118. Arnold M, Nedeltchev K, Mattle HP, Lohar TJ, Stepper F, Schroth G, Brekenfeld C, Sturzenegger M, Remonda L. Intra-arterial thrombolysis in 24 consecutive patients with internal carotid artery t occlusion. J Neurol Neurosurg Psychiatry 2003; 74(6):739–742.
119. Zaidat OO, Suarez JI, Santillan C, Sunshine JL, Tarr RW, Paras VH, Selman WR, Slandis DN. Response to intra-arterial and combined intravenous and intra-arterial thrombolytic therapy in patients with distal internal carotid artery occlusion. Stroke 2002; 33(7):1821–1827.
120. Wechsler LR, Jungreis CA. Intra-arterial thrombolysis for carotid circulation ischemia. Criti Care Clin 1999; 15(4):701–718.
121. Bellon RJ, Putman CN, Budzik RF, Pergolizzi RS, Reinking GF, Norbash AN. Rheolytic thrombectomy of the occluded internal carotid artery in the setting of acute ischemic stroke. Am J Neuroradiol 2001; 22(3):526–530.
122. Wholey MH, Wholey M, Eles G, Toursakissian B, Bailey S, Jarmolowski C, Tan WA. Evaluation of glycoprotein IIb/IIIa inhibitors in carotid angioplasty and stenting. J Endovasc Ther 2003; 10(1):33–41.
123. Topol EJ, Yadav JS. Circulation 2000; 101(5):570.
124. Wholey MH, Wholey M, Bergeron P, Diethrich EB, Henry M, Laborde JC, Mathias K, Myla S, Roubin GS, Shawl F et Al. Current status in cervical carotid stent placement. J Cardiovasc Surg 2003; 44:331–339.
125. Wholey MH, Wholey M, Bergeron P, Dietrich EB, Henry M, Laborde JC, et al. Current global status of carotid artery stent placement. Catheteriz Cardiovasc Diag 1998; 44(1):1–6.
126. Ohki T, Veith FJ, Grenell S, Lipsitz EC, Gargiulo N, Nckay J, Valladares J, Suggs WD, Kazmi M. Initial experience with cerebral protection devices to prevent embolization during carotid artery stenting. J Vasc Surg 2002; 36(6):1175–1185.

127. Bhatt DL, Kapadia SR, Bajzer CT, Chew DT, Ziada KM, Mukherjee D, Roffi M, Topol EJ, Yadav JS. Dual antiplatelet therapy with clopidogrel and aspirin after carotid artery stenting. J Invasive Cardiol 2001; 13(12):767–771.
128. Tong FC, Cloft HJ, Joseph GJ, Samuels OB, Dion JE. Abciximab rescue in acute carotid stent thrombosis. Am J Neuroradiol 2000; 21(9):1750–1752.
129. Rubin GS, Yadav S, Iyer SS, Vitek J. Carotid stent-supported angioplasty: under a vascular intervention to prevent stroke. Am J Cardiol 1996; 78(38):8–12.
130. Ouriel K, Yadav JS. Stents in patient's with carotid disease. Rev Cardiovasc Med 2003; 4(2):61–67.
131. Chaturvadi S, Sohib S, Tselis A. Carotid stent thrombosis: report of two fatal cases. Stroke 2001; 32(11):2700–2702.

23

Complications Associated with the Use of Percutaneous Mechanical Thrombectomy Devices

K. Kasirajan
Department of Vascular Surgery, Emory University, Atlanta, Georgia, U.S.A.

Until recently the principle methods for removing thrombi were thrombolytic drugs and open surgery. Although thrombolytic drug therapy can effectively manage many thrombotic occlusions, it does not achieve this rapidly in urgent cases or those in which symptoms appear relatively late. Additionally, the unavoidable risk of bleeding complications limits their dose and duration and, not all patients are candidates for thrombolytic therapy. On the contrary, surgical removal of thrombus results in rapid blood flow restoration, but it is relatively invasive. Thus, timing and patient safety are two factors spurring interest in alternatives for rapid and minimally invasive removal of thrombus. Hence, mechanical thrombectomy devices are gaining popularity as a useful adjunct to pharmacological thrombolysis (1,2).

Numerous percutaneous mechanical thrombectomy (PMT) devices are currently available in the United States for dialysis graft declotting, however, only two devices are approved for infrainguinal arterial use in the United States. A list of various PMT devices is given in Table 1. Many of the devices given in Table 1 are currently in their investigational phase, with minimal pre-clinical and clinical data. The devices are classified into aspiration or micro fragmentation-only devices (3). The latter embolize the micro fragments that are created by the mechanical component of the device. Since many of these devices were designed primarily for dialysis graft declotting, embolization is not seen as a device limitation. However, when used for peripheral arterial or venous application, the risk of down-stream embolization may be significant.

A few of the PMT devices also function as "wall-contact" devices. For example, the Arrow-Trerotola (Arrow International, Inc., Reading, Pennsylvania) device is a "wall-contact" device with a potential for significant endothelial damage, and may not be applicable for peripheral vascular indications.

Complications associated with use of PMT for acute peripheral arterial and venous thrombosis may be classified as device and non-device related events and, these in turn may be subdivided into local and systemic complications (Table 2).

Table 1 Percutaneous Mechanical Thrombectomy Devices

Aspiration devices	
Angiojet[a]	Possis Medical, Minneapolis, Minnesota
Trellis[a]	Bacchus Vascular, Santa Clara, California
Fino	Bacchus Vascular, Santa Clara, California
Solera	Bacchus Vascular, Santa Clara, California
Rescue	Boston Scientific, Watertown, Massachusetts
Oasis	Boston Scientific, Watertown, Massachusetts
Hydrolyser	Cordis Endovascular, Miami, Florida
Gelbfish EndoVac	NeoVascular Technologies, Brooklyn, New York
Thrombex PMT System	Edwards Life Sciences, Irvine, California
The Cleaner	Rex Medical/Boston Scientific, Waterton, Massachusetts
Xtrak Thrombectomy Device	Xtrak Medical, Salem, New Hampshire
Rotarex	Straub Medical, Wangs, Switzerland
X-Sizer	EndiCOR Medical, San Clemente, California
Micro-fragmentation devices	
Arrow-Trerotola	Arrow International, Reading, Pennsylvania
Amplatz Clot Buster	Microvena, White Bear Lake, Minnesota
Cragg Brush	Micro Therapeutics Inc., Aliso Viego, California
Casteneda Brush	Micro Therapeutics Inc., Aliso Viego, California
Ultrasound devices	
Acolysis	Angiosonics, Morrisville, North Carolina
Resolution 360 Therapeutic wire	Omnisonics, Wilmington, Massachusetts

[a]Approved for infrainguinal vascular application in the United States. *Abbreviations*: PMT, percutaneous mechanical thrombectomy.

PRECLINICAL EVALUATION OF DEVICE SAFETY

In a preclinical study comparing the three different rheolytic catheters, the Hydrolyser had the largest overall emboli weight (66.50 ± 42 mg), followed by the Angiojet (22.90 ± 9.55 mg), and the least embolic weight was observed with the Oasis catheter (1.91 ± 1.14 mg) (4). In another study evaluating the use of the Angiojet catheter particulate embolization accounted for 12% of the initial thrombus volume with 99.83% being smaller than 100 μm and none more then 1000 μm. The effluent collected did not cause any ischemic changes when injected into a normal kidney (5). Another in vitro study comparing the Angiojet with the Hydrolyser demonstrated a lower particulate embolization for the Angiojet device ($1.8\% \pm 2.9$ vs. $4.8\% \pm 6.1$) (6).

Sharafuddin et al. evaluated the extent of endothelial damage resulting from Angiojet thrombectomy in 15 canine vascular segments compared to four vascular segments subjected to Fogarty balloon pullback thrombectomy, and 10 untreated vessels (5). Comparing endothelial denudation under the scanning electron microscope, Angiojet-treated vessels had greater mean endothelial coverage ($88\% \pm 7.9\%$) compared to Fogarty balloon thrombectomy ($58\% \pm 8.0\%$, $p < 0.0002$), and no significant difference compared to untreated vessels ($89.7\% \pm 11.6\%$, $p = 0.77$). Hemolysis equivalent to that resulting from thrombolysis of 75 mL of blood was seen after a

Table 2 Complications Resulting from Use of Percutaneous Mechanical Thrombectomy Devices

Local Complications	Systemic Complications
Device related	*Device related*
Vessel dissection	Hemoglobinuria, Hemolysis
Perforation	PE
Spasm	
Embolization	
Acute rethrombosis	
Mechanical device failure	
Non-Device related	*Non-device related*
Compartment syndrome	Myoglobinuria
Ongoing ischemia	Reperfusion injury
Acute rethrombosis	Cardiac complication (MI, arrhythmias, etc.)
Amputation	Respiratory failure
Access site complications	Renal failure
Hematoma	Stroke
Infection	Death
Traumatic arteriovenous fistula	
Pseudoaneurysm	
Access vessel thrombosis	

Abbreviations: PE, pulmonary embolism.

standard pump run; however, no elevation in blood urea nitrogen or creatinine was noted. Plasma-free hemoglobin and hematocrit returned to baseline within three days.

A total of 102 arterial segments in goats were subject to Hydrolyser thrombectomy in a report by van Ommen et al. (7). The Hydrolyser catheter produced less neo-intimal hyperplasia after three weeks compared to a Fogarty balloon catheter thrombectomy ($p < 0.001$). Inner diameter of vessels larger than 3 mm showed no difference in the endothelial response to Hydrolyser thrombectomy compared to the control procedure.

Following thrombectomy with the Cragg Brush in nine canine models with occluded synthetic femoro-popliteal arterial grafts, distal emboli were noted in 67% of cases, with embolic particles up to 3 mm in diameter. Histological studies of the proximal and distal vessels at the level of the anastomoses showed vessel wall damage to the intima or media in five of nine (56%) proximal anastomoses and at seven of nine (78%) distal anastomoses (8).

The Amplatz thrombectomy device resulted in emboli particle size ranging from 13 μm to 1000 μm. No difference was noted in the embolic particle size and distribution for 30 second and 60 second activation time (9).

The author performed tests to evaluate the extent of hemolysis produced in test samples of human blood between a new mechanical thrombectomy device (Solera, Bacchus Vascular, Santa Clara, California) in comparison to the Helix Clot Buster (Microvena, White Bear Lake, Minnesota). The bench-top model consisted of three glass tubes, filled with approximately 20 mL of heparinized human blood, and then placed into $37 \pm 2°C$ waterbath positioned vertically, for each device to be evaluated. The first tube was analyzed at time 0. The second tube remained in the water bath as a negative control. The third tube was used to run the test devices. All tests were

Table 3 In Vitro Study Comparing the Extent of Hemolysis Between the Solera and the Helix Devices

Test samples	Helix		Solera	
	Hb released (mg/mL)	Hemolytic index	Hb released (mg/mL)	Hemolytic index
1	39.4	47.40%	0.254	0.18%
2	40.8	53.50%	0.123	0.09%
3	37.4	46.30%	0.224	0.15%
4	33.3	44.40%	0.31	0.21%
Mean	37.725	47.90%	0.22775	0.16%

Abbreviations: Hb, hemoglobin; mg, milligram; mL, milliliter.

performed with two separate devices and then repeated. The average absorbance reading, amount of hemoglobin released, and the hemolytic index was calculated.

The hemolytic index was calculated by the formula = (hemoglobin released/ hemoglobin present) × 100. The Helix had a 44–54% hemolysis for the one-minute run time. The Solera had <1% hemolysis for the 5- and 15-minute run time (Table 3).

COMPLICATIONS: IDENTIFICATION AND MANAGEMENT

Perforation

Vessel perforation has been reported by various authors (Table 4). Often the perforation is caused by a technical mistake during vascular access or tracking the device, and not actually related to device activation. Most perforations are small and can be managed conservatively. The perforation may be noticed when performing a completion angiogram or occasionally suspected when hemodynamic instability is unexpectedly encountered. Perforation in the suprainguinal region may cause significant blood loss and hypotension, as the retroperitoneum is not an ideal place for spontaneous tamponade. Management depends on the presence of hemodynamic instability. If patients are stable and the perforation is located in one of the infrainguinal vessels, observation alone may suffice. Occasionally, reversal of anticoagulation, and balloon tamponade may be necessary. The author has never been required to perform an open surgical exploration for infrainguinal perforations. On the contrary, suprainguinal perforations may be accompanied by significant blood loss. Once a perforation is encountered in any of the suprainguinal vessels, immediate balloon tamponade and reversal of anticoagulation is recommended. If a persistent leak is noted after balloon occlusion, one of the available covered stents may be deployed to cover the area of vessel perforation (Fig. 1A–D). The use of covered stents is the author's preferred method of management of suprainguinal perforation, since angiograms are often misleading as to the amount of blood loss in this location. Blood product transfusion may be required and a computed tomogram should be performed when the patient is thermodynamically stable. This helps for follow-up and to document the amount of blood loss.

Embolism

Distal embolization may be the most commonly encountered problem with the use of mechanical thrombectomy devices. Symptomatic embolization was observed

Table 4 Publications on Percutaneous Mechanical
Thrombectomy Devices with Reported Complications

Author	N	Complications (%)
OASIS		
Hoepfner (10)	51	Hemorrhage 8
		Embolism 4.8
		Acute occlusion 37
		Amputation 17.7
		Mortality 8
ANGIOJET		
Müller-Hülsbeck (11)	112	Embolization 9.8
		Dissection 8
		Perforation 3.6
		Amputation 1.8
		Mortality 7
Silva (12)	22	Hemorrhage 10
		Embolism 9
		Dissection 5
		Occlusion 18
		Amputation 5
		Mortality 14
Wagner (13)	50	Hemorrhage 6
		Embolism 6
		Dissection 6
		Perforation 4
		Amputation 8
		Mortality 0
Kasirajan (1)	86	Hemorrhage 3.5
		Embolism 2.3
		Dissection 3.5
		Perforation 2.3
		Amputation 11.6
		Mortality 9.3
HYDROLYSER		
Reekers (14)	28	Embolism 18
		Hemorrhage 0
		Acute occlusion 11
		Amputation 11
		Mortality 0
Henry (15)	41	Acute occlusion 12
		Embolism 2.4
		Amputation 0
		Mortality 0
AMPLATZ		
Rilinger (16)	40	Hemorrhage 2.5
		Device failure 7.5
		Embolism 0
		Amputation 5
		Mortality 0
Tadavarthy (17)	14	Hemorrhage 14.3
		Embolism 14

(Continued)

Table 4 Publications on Percutaneous Mechanical
Thrombectomy Devices with Reported Complications
(*Continued*)

Author	N	Complications (%)
Görich (18)	18	Device failure 7 Amputation 0 Mortality 0 Hemorrhage 6 Device failure 6 Amputation 6

Abbreviations: N, number of patients.

in $6.8 \pm 3\%$ of patients following use of the Angiojet for acute limb ischemia (Table 4).
The author has found a much higher incidence of distal embolization if all asymptomatic embolic events are angiographically documented. As none of the studies were
prospective, the number quoted above may be a falsely low estimate (Table 4). The
author has also noted a higher incidence of significant distal embolization if the
Angiojet is used as a stand-alone therapy (Figs. 2A–B). I currently use an

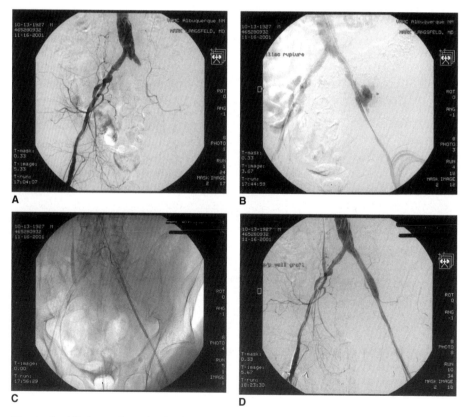

Figure 1 (**A**) Acute thrombosis of the left iliac artery at location of prior common iliac stent.
(**B**) Perforation noted after thrombus removal with a mechanical thrombectomy device.
(**C**) A covered stent (wall-graft) positioned across the site of perforation. (**D**) Completion
angiogram demonstrates good flow with no evidence of contrast extravasation.

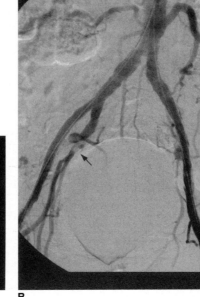

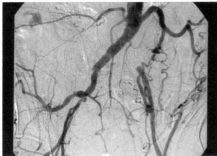

A   B

Figure 2 (A) Right external iliac and left common iliac artery occlusion. (B) Following mechanical thrombectomy and stent insertion an embolism is noted in the right internal iliac artery (*arrow*).

8–10 hour infusion of urokinase (Abbott, Abbott Park, Illinois) and subsequently use the Angiojet for removal of residual thrombus. This has helped significantly lower the incidence of down-stream embolization and also helped decrease the dose and duration of thrombolytic infusion. The reason for a lower incidence of distal embolization with preliminary thrombolytic therapy may be related to the dissolution of the soft friable thrombus that may have had a higher potential for embolization. Additionally any embolic particles may already be laced with the thrombolytic agent resulting in their spontaneous dissolution.

Clinical symptoms may depend on the size of the embolic debris and also on the status of collateral circulation. Once recognized, every effort is made to remove the embolic particle. The PMT device that was used to clear the proximal thrombus may be moved distally to reach the smaller vessels. The coronary Angiojet (XVG, Possis Medical, Minneapolis, Minnesota) can be passed as far distal as the dorsalis pedis and posterior tibial vessels into the foot for thrombus extraction. It requires the use of a coronary 0.014-inch guidewire. In patients with non-atherosclerotic native vessels, a significant amount of spasm may be noted when PMT devices are used below the level of the popliteal artery.

I routinely use intra-arterial papaverine before using PMT in the infrapopliteal location. If the PMT is unable to reach and/or remove the embolic debris and the patient has adequate distal collateral flow, a distal infusion of urokinase (Abbott, Abbott Park, Illinois) at 4000 IU/min via a catheter located in the thrombus is recommended. Occasionally, direct aspiration using 4–8 Fr catheters is helpful; smaller (4 or 5 Fr) would have to be used in the infrapopliteal location. When using salvage

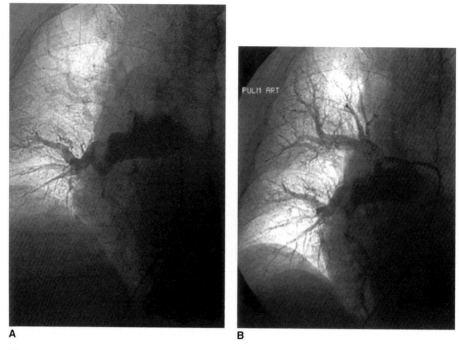

A   B

Figure 3 (**A**) Massive pulmonary artery embolism following venous thrombectomy. (**B**) Treatment of pulmonary artery embolism using the Angiojet catheter.

thrombolytic therapy, if improvement is not observed in three to four hours, or a worsening of symptoms is noted, a repeat angiogram and repositioning of the infusion catheter maybe required. If the catheter is in the correct location, aspiration thrombectomy or open surgical thrombectomy would have to be attempted for successful limb salvage.

In the venous side embolism can be of a life-threatening nature; fortunately the incidence of fatal or symptomatic pulmonary embolism (PE) is uncommon (19,20). However, I would recommend the use of temporary inferior vena cava (IVC) filters in patients with extensive caval thrombosis or free-floating thrombus in the IVC. We have encountered one PE in a patient with extensive caval thrombus. In this one patient, we used the Angiojet catheter to directly aspirate the PE, as the patient was experiencing hemodynamic instability (Fig. 3A and B). In the absence of hemodynamic compromise, use of thrombolytic agents and heparin anticoagulation is recommended. It is our practice to administer the thrombolytic agent directly into the pulmonary artery as a bolus therapy.

The use of embolic protection devices once available may help significantly reduce the incidence of embolic events. The Trellis device (Bacchus, Santa Clara, California), is currently the only PMT device with an integrated emboli protection system (the distal occlusion balloon) (21).

Spasm

PMT devices are probably most effective in synthetic graft occlusion. When used for embolic occlusions or in native vessels with minimal atherosclerotic changes, significant vessel spasm may be encountered. Although the spasm most often resolves with intra-arterial vasodilators, in the acute setting it may be difficult to distinguish a dissection from spasm. Once spasm is noted, I use catheter directed intra-arterial papaverine at the region of the spasm (Figs. 4A–F). Infusion of vasodilators proximal to the spasm may not be effective, as they have a tendency to bypass the area of spasm and pass through the collaterals. It is also important not to lose guidewire access across the region of spasm. Once spasm is encountered, I exchange for a smaller guidewire (0.014) and infuse papaverine through the catheter as it is moved from distal to proximal across the site of spasm (a proximal Y-adaptor is required for simultaneous vasodilator infusion and to maintain guideware access). If resolution of the

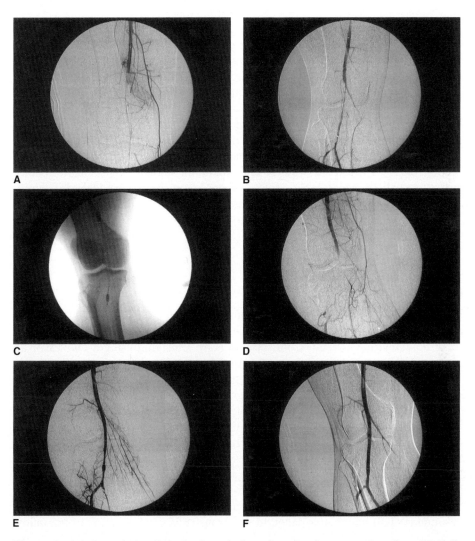

Figure 4 (**A**) Acute insitu thrombotic occlusion of popliteal artery and outflow. (**B**) Following overnight infusion of urokinase—partial resolution of thrombus in popliteal artery and significant improvement in the distal bed. (**C**) Proximal and distal occlusion balloons of the Trellis device. (**D**) Severe spasm of popliteal arterial following treatment with the Trellis-turbo. (**E**) Immediately following injection of papaverine, partial resolution of spasm. (**F**) Complete resolution of spasm after 10 minutes.

spasm is not observed at this point, gentle angioplasty with a smaller balloon may help differentiate between spasm and dissection. Papaverine and patience are often quite effective (more of the latter) for resolution of the spasm.

Dissection

Dissection results more often from catheter or device manipulation, and not directly from PMT device use. The two approved devices (Angiojet, Trellis) are relatively atraumatic to the vessel wall and dissection is not frequently encountered. If wall-contact devices such as the Arrow-Trerotola (Arrow International, Reading, Pennsylvania) are used in an "off-label" fashion there is a higher propensity for endothelial damage and vessel dissection. Dissection is visualized as an area of lower contrast density on the angiogram or occasionally an actual plane of dissection may be visible. Dissections may be classified as either flow limiting or non-flow limiting lesions. Non-flow limiting dissections (Figs. 5A–C) often do not require any invasive treatment and a short period of anticoagulation (warfarin/aspirin) for three months is often all that is required.

For larger dissections involving more than 50% of the circumference or flow limiting dissections, I attempt initial balloon dilation (leave inflated for two to three minutes). If no improvement is noted a stent may be deployed to approximate the dissection plane to the vessel wall. A self-expanding stent is often a better choice compared to balloon expandable stents, as these lesions have a tendency for significant elastic recoil. For extensive dissections, especially in the infrapopliteal region, an open surgical bypass may be required to a target vessel located distal to the site of dissection.

Acute Rethrombosis

Rethrombosis may result due to a variety of reasons (Table 5). It is recognized by the acute re-onset of symptoms or no obvious improvement immediately following a successful angiographic result. Confirmation is by reimaging using a Duplex or an angiogram. Therapy is directed at the possible etiology. The etiology for acute rethrombsis may not always be readily apparent. Following thrombus removal by the PMT, a good quality completion angiogram needs to be obtained to demonstrate the etiology for the thrombotic event. A culprit lesion is unmasked in about 70–80% of patients (Figs. 6A–B). It has been the author's experience that acute rethrombosis is not uncommon if a culprit lesion is not recognized in patients with insitu thrombotic occlusion. In the absence of an unrecognizable culprit lesion, we routinely anticoagulate these patients for life, and a hypercoagulation work-up is performed. Occasionally, a biplane angiogram may not demonstrate a culprit stenosis, and pull-back pressure measurements or the use of an intravascular ultrasound (IVUS) may better define these lesions (Fig. 7). The status of the inflow and outflow vessels are important for prolonged patency and may have to be addressed independently (Figs. 8A–B). Higher levels of heparin anticoagulation or the adjunctive use of antiplatelet agents such as GIIb-IIIa inhibitors may be warranted in some patients.

Finally, patients with extensive rethrombosis have to be investigated for the possibility of heparin-induced thrombocytopenia.

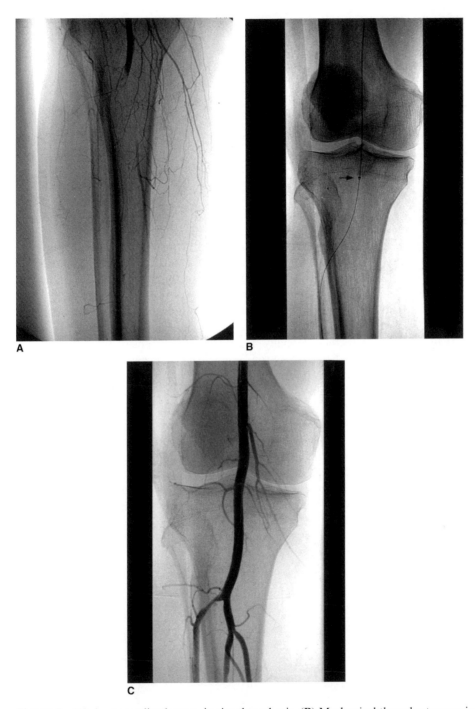

Figure 5 (**A**) Acute popliteal artery in situ thrombosis. (**B**) Mechanical thrombectomy using the e-train Angiojet catheter. (**C**) Non-flow limiting dissection seen at the origin of the anterior tibial artery.

Table 5 Possible Etiology for Acute Rethrombosis

Endothelial damage
Unrecognized culprit lesion
Hypercoagulable condition
Inadequate anticoagulation
Heparin induced thrombocytopenia
Disease- inflow or outflow vessels
Diffusely diseased native vessel or bypass conduit
Inadequate thrombus removal
Vessel dissection
Poorly expanded or malpositioned stents

Hemolysis

Due to the presence in most PMT devices of actively moving macerating components, a certain amount of hemolysis is often observed (see pre-clinical device evaluation). In the author's experience, the amount of hemolysis is directly related to the duration of device activation and the inadvertent use of the device in non-occlusive sites. Hemolysis is visible in the urine as a dark brown discoloration (hemoglobinuria). In the author's experience hemoglobinuria was not an uncommon event following use of the Angiojet catheter, especially in patients with extensive thrombus burden (Figs. 9A–B). However, hemoglobinuria as an isolated event did not result in a permanent clinical sequel. In patients with pre-existing renal failure or concomitant myoglobinuria, renal tubular necrosis may occur. Following reperfusion the sudden release of products of anaerobic metabolism results in significant fall in blood pH. Under acidic conditions myoglobin is precipitated in the renal tubules resulting in acute renal failure. Prevention is my means of adequate hydration (maintain urine output to >100 mL/hr), alkalinization of the urine, and use of mannitol. Mannitol may also have the additional beneficial effect of acting as a free radical scavenger, which is often implicated as an important intermediary in ischemia-reperfusion injury. In patients with pre-procedural elevation in creatinine, we limit the amount of contrast used,

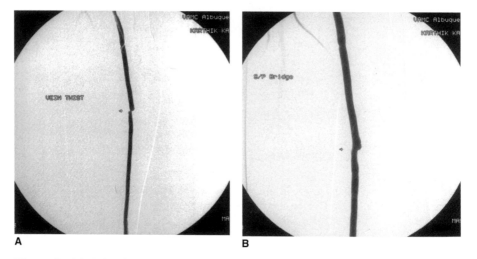

Figure 6 (**A**) Following percutaneous mechanical thrombectomy, a culprit lesion (vein graft torsion) is clearly visible. (**B**) Treatment of vein graft torsion with a self-expanding stent.

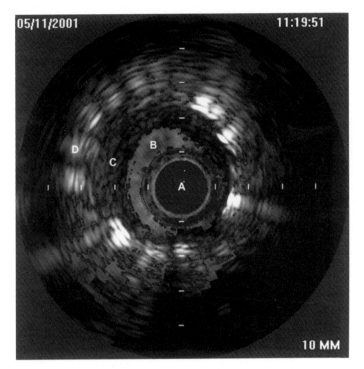

Figure 7 A culprit lesion not seen on an angiogram is visible on IVUS interrogation. (*A. IVUS catheter; B, blood flow channel; C, area of neointimal hyperplasia; D, stent struts*).

optimize the hydration status, minimize the PMT device run-time, and have recently employed routine use of fenoldepam (Abbott, Abbott Park, Illinois) at 0.1 μg/kg/min starting 20 minutes before the procedure and continuing for six hours after.

Mechanical Failure

Most PMT devices have a simple design and mechanical failure is uncommon. However, in the devices using passive aspiration, clogging of the aspiration lumen with thrombus may be encountered.

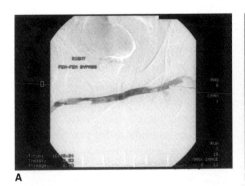
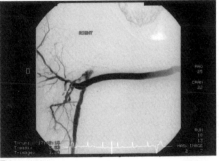

A   **B**

Figure 8 (**A**) Thrombosis of a femoral to femoral bypass graft. (**B**) Etiology for thrombosis was poor outflow due to anastomoses to deep femoral artery. This was revised by performing a jump graft to the superficial femoral artery.

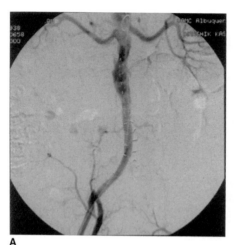
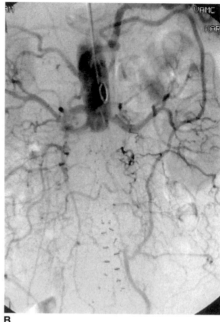

A   B

Figure 9 (**A**) Extensive thrombus burden seen with occlusion of an aortic endograft. (**B**) Massive hemoglobinuria was noted after Xpeedior (Possis Medical, Minneapolis, Minnesota) thrombectomy; this resolved with adequate hydration as no other risk factors for renal failure was present.

Devices that employ fluid jets (rheolytic catheters) for thrombus extraction are less likely to encounter this problem. Catheter clogging was occasionally encountered with the Trellis device, and seen most frequently with the Solera and the Fino devices. The inability to get adequate aspiration may be indicative of clogging of the out-flow lumen. Unfortunately, this cannot be confirmed with the device in place. If gentle flushing of the aspiration lumen does not help, the device will have to be removed for flushing out the aspiration lumen before reuse (Fig. 10). Occasionally, a new device will have to be used if the catheter cannot be adequately cleaned. Another reason for inability to aspirate may be a kink in the catheter, especially when crossing-up and over the aortic bifurcation to the contralateral limb. In this situation, use of a stiffer wire or passing the device through an up-and-over sheath is recommended.

Non-Device Related Events

Patients presenting with acute limb-threatening ischemia are often friable from a variety of systemic co-morbid conditions making them susceptible to life threatening systemic events. In the management of acute limb ischemia, attention has to be directed to life as well as limb. More than a few patients may not be ideal candidates for revascularization, as the metabolic consequence of the reperfusion may overwhelm the already compromised defense mechanisms in these patients. Patients with severe single system organ dysfunctions or two or more organ dysfunctions may be best served by primary amputation. The various systemic consequences of reperfusion will not be further discussed in this chapter as they can result from any one of the techniques that may be used for revascularization and not specific to PMT devices (22,23).

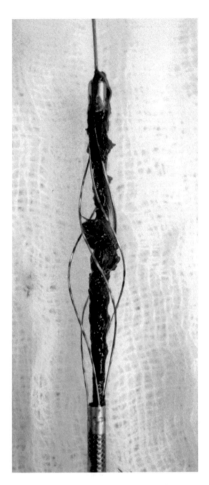

Figure 10 Clogging of the Fino (Bacchus Vascular, Santa Clara, California) catheter.

CONCLUSION

Open surgery is considered the gold standard in the management of acute vascular occlusion. All PMT devices should ideally be compared to open surgery for adequate demonstration of safety and efficacy.

Table 6 Comparison of Local Complications Between Angiojet Treatment Group and Open Surgical Treatment Group

	Angiojet	Surgery	p-value
Infection	0	11(14%)	
Dissection	2(3%)	0	
Embolism	2(3%)	1(1%)	
Hematoma	7(11%)	10(13%)	
Acute occlusion	1(2%)	8(10%)	
Perforation	2(3%)	0	
Total	11(17%)	32(41%)	0.002

Table 7 Comparison of Systemic Complications Between the Angiojet Treatment Group and the Open Surgery Group.

	Angiojet	Surgery	*p*-value
Pulmonary	1(2%)	13(16%)	
MI	2(3%)	12(15%)	
Renal	4(6%)	5(6%)	
DVT	0	2(3%)	
Myoglobinuria	4(6%)	1(1%)	
Total	8(12%)	32(41%)	< 0.001

Unfortunately, no prospective randomized trial is available or currently underway to address this issue. We performed a retrospective comparison of the use of the Angiojet catheter ± adjunctive thrombolytic therapy to open surgical revascularization (24). Overall, PMT outperformed open surgery when comparing local or systemic complication (Tables 6 and 7). Fortunately, complications with the use of PMT are uncommon, but when encountered require prompt identification and correction for optimal patient outcomes.

REFERENCES

1. Kasirajan K, Gray B, Beavers FP, Clair DG, Greenberg R, Mascha E, Ouriel K. Rheolytic thrombectomy in the management of acute and subacute limb threatening ischemia. J Vasc Interv Radiol 2001; 12:413–421.
2. Kasirajan K, Haskal Z, Ouriel K. The use of mechanical thrombectomy devices in the management of acute peripheral arterial occlusive disease. J Vasc Interv Radiol 2001; 12:405–411.
3. Kasirajan K, Marek JM, Langsfeld M. Mechanical Thrombectomy as a first-line treatment for arterial occlusion. Semin Vasc Surg 2001; 14(2):123–131.
4. Müller-Hülsbeck S, Bangard C, Schwarzenberg H, Glüer CC, Heller M. In vitro effectiveness study of the three hydrodynamic thrombectomy devices. Radiology 1999; 211:433–439.
5. Sharafuddin MJ, Hicks ME, Jennson ML, Morris JE, Drasler WJ, Wilson GJ. Rheolytic thrombectomy with the Angiojet-F105 catheter: preclinical evaluation of safety. J Vasc Interv Radiol 1997; 8:939–945.
6. Bucker A, Schmitz-Rode T, Vorwewrk D, Gunther R. Comparative in vitro study of two percutaneous hydrodynamic thrombectomy systems. J Vasc Interv Radiol 1996; 7: 445–449.
7. van Ommen VG, van der Veen FH, Geskes GG, Daemen M, Habets J, Dassen WR, Wellens HJ. Comparison of arterial wall reaction after passage of the Hydrolyser device versus a thrombectomy balloon in an animal model. J Vasc Interv Radiol 1996; 7:451–454.
8. Castañeda F, Smouse HB, Swischuk JL, Wyffels P, Patel JC, Li R. Pharmacological thrombolysis with use of the brush catheter in canine thrombosed femoropopliteal arterial PTFE bypass grafts. J Vasc Interv Radiol 2000; 11:503–508.
9. Yasui K, Qian, Nazarian GK, Hunter DW, Castañeda-Zuniga WR, Amplatz K. Recirculation-type Amplatz clot macerator: determination of particle size and distribution. J Vasc Interv Radiol 1993; 4:275–278.
10. Hoepfner W, Vicol C, Bohndorf K, Loeprecht H. Shredding embolectomy thrombectomy catheter for treatment of acute lower-limb ischemia. Ann Vasc Surg 1999; 13:426–435.

11. Müller-Hülsbeck S, Kalinowski M, Heller M, Wagner HJ. Rheolytic hydrodynamic thrombectomy for percutaneous treatment of acutely occluded infra-aortic native arteries and bypass grafts: Midterm follow-up results. Inv Rad 2000; 35:131–140.
12. Silva JA, Ramee SR, Collins TJ, Jenkins JS, Lansky AJ, Ansel GM, Dolmatch BL, Glickman MH, Stainken B, Ramee E, White CJ. Rheolytic thrombectomy in the treatment of acute limb-threatening ischemia: immediate results and six-month follow-up of the multicenter Angiojet registry. Catheteriz Cardiovasc Diagn 1998; 45:386–393.
13. Wagner H-J, Müler-Hülsbeck S, Pitton MB, Weiss W, Wess M. Rapid thrombectomy with a hydrodynamic catheter: results from a prospective, multicenter trial. Radiology 1997; 205:675–681.
14. Reekers JA, Kromhout JG, Spithoven HG, Jacobs MJ, Mali WM, Schultz-Kool LJ. Arterial thrombosis below the inguinal ligament: percutaneous treatment with a thrombosuction catheter. Radiology 1996; 198:49–53.
15. Henry M, Amor M, Henry I, Tricoche O, Allaoui M. The Hydrolyser thrombectomy catheter: a single-center experience. J Endo Surg 1998; 5(1):24–31.
16. Rilinger N, Görich J, Scharrer-Palmer R, Vogel J, Tomczak R, Krämer S, Merkle E, Brambs HJ, Sokiranski R. Short-term results with use of the Amplatz thrombectomy device in the treatment of acute lower limb occlusion. J Vasc Interv Radiol 1997; 8(3):343–348.
17. Tadavarthy SM, Murray PD, Inampudi S, Nazarian GK, Amplatz K. Mechanical thrombectomy with the Amplatz device: human experience. J Vasc Interv Radiol 1994; 5(5):715–724.
18. Görich J, Rilinger N, Sokiranski R, Kramer S, Mickley V, Schutz A, Brambs HJ, Pamler R. Mechanical thrombectomy of acute occlusions of both the superficial and the deep femoral arteries using a thrombectomy device. AJR 1998; 170:1177–1180.
19. Kasirajan K, Gray B, Ouriel K. Percutaneous Angiojet thrombectomy in the management of extensive deep venous thrombosis. J Vasc Interv Radiol 2001; 12:179–185.
20. Bo Eklof, Kasirajan K. Treating proximal deep vein thrombosis. Endovasc Today 2003; 4:17–23.
21. Kasirajan K, Ramaiah V, Diethrich EB. A novel mechanical thrombectomy device in the treatment of acute limb ischemia. JEVT. In press.
22. Kasirajan K, Ouriel K. Management of acute lower extremity ischemia: treatment strategies and outcomes. CICR 2000; 2:119–129.
23. Kasirajan K, Ouriel K. Current revascularization options for peripheral arterial disease. Prog Cardiovasc Nurs 2002; 17:26–34.
24. Kasirajan K, Ouriel K. Percutaneous mechanical thrombectomy versus open surgery in the management of acute limb-threatening ischemia. Endovasc Today. In press.

24

Percutaneous Treatment of Occluded Dialysis Fistulae

John Carlos Lantis II
Division of Vascular Surgery, College of Physicians and Surgeons, St. Luke's-Roosevelt Hospital Center, Columbia University, New York, New York, U.S.A.

Ziv J. Haskal
Division of Vascular and Interventional Radiology, College of Physicians and Surgeons, New York Presbyterian Hospital, Columbia University, New York, New York, U.S.A.

BACKGROUND

In 2001, the number of end stage renal disease (ESRD) patients in the United States was 398,553 (1). This population is expected to double by 2010 representing a growth rate of 7% per year (2,3). In the same year, 94,905 patients required renal replacement therapy for the first time (1). Most are dialyzed with hemodialysis (HD) using an arteriovenous fistula (AVF) or prosthetic arteriovenous graft (AVG). Complications of vascular access represent the single largest source of morbidity in the ESRD population, accounting for 15% of hospitalizations (4). The estimated annual cost of graft complications is $1 billion.

The native AVF is superior to AVG because of better patency and less infection. Reported primary patencies for AVF range from 85% and 54% at one and two years, compared to 40% at one year for AVG (5,6). In general, the primary patencies of AVFs exceed those of AVGs by up to 36% (7,8). Secondary patency rates range between 45% and 60% at one year, for AVF and AVG, respectively. Despite this, the United States has lagged behind Europe in the prevalence of AVF. In the United States only 24% of HD patients have AVF (0–87% by center). For new HD patients, 15% have an AVF, 24% have an AVG and 60% have a catheter placed (9).

The long term unassisted patency of AVG after angioplasty has been consistently described as 40–50% at 6 months (10–15). Success rates with percutaneous management of occluded native fistulae are less clear, though some studies report success rates of 76–100% (16). The unassisted patencies after surgical revision is even more poorly defined since in those studies it is usually cumulative patency which is reported (17–19). The Work Group that developed the Dialysis Outcomes Quality Initiative guidelines (DOQI) stated that a 50% one-year unassisted patency after surgical revision of AVG should be the goal, holding surgery to a higher standard than PTA because of the frequent use of jump grafts, thereby using up more vein (20).

PATIENT SELECTION

Prior to initiating any procedure, a complete assessment of fluid status and metabolic derangement (e.g., fluid overload preventing the patient from lying supine or hyperkalemia) should be made in each patient to insure their safe ability to undergo such procedures. The patient may require transient access at another site to facilitate pre-procedure HD. Site infections, that manifest by blanching erythema, fever, or cellulites, are a contraindication to percutaneous intervention. Technical contraindications may include: AVFs without any mature segments, large aneurysms, and known patent foramen ovale.

GENERAL CONSIDERATIONS

AVFs can be declotted for up to three weeks following thrombosis and AVGs even longer depending upon propagation of clot into the outflow vein. Treatment of the thrombosed HD access has three stages: removal or fragmentation of the clot, identification of the cause of the thrombosis, and treatment of the underlying lesion. Therefore, this chapter will be divided into sections based on these sequential phases: access, thrombus removal (mechanical and/or chemical), and treatment (PTA and/or stenting) with a comment on outcomes.

ACCESS

Complication: Inability to Access the Lesion

The standard algorithm is to puncture the AVF or AVG and place two sheaths in opposite directions (or use a single apex AVG puncture), allowing both the arterial inflow and the venous outflow to be addressed. However, some arterial anastomoses cannot be accessed by a retrograde technique.

Predisposing factors: There may be a high-grade proximal stenosis, large aneurysmal dilation of the graft, or enlarged collaterals which the wire preferentially enters.

Short and long-term consequences: Need to gain access at another site is often mandatory, and if the wire passed through the vein during manipulation there may be local hemorrhage with hematoma formation.

Management of the complication: Puncturing the brachial artery with a 3-Fr catheter can provide a roadmap or allow antegrade access to facilitate retrograde cannulation. If needed, the antegrade arterial wire can be exteriorized through the venous sheath after it is used to guide the venous catheter across the stenotic or occluded arterial anastomosis.

Prevention: Regular screening and physical examination will indicate diminished flow, thrill, and pulse, warranting surveillance venography. At intervention, detailed examination of the AVF/AVG may guide preferred access sites. This technical challenge is nevertheless rare and is almost universally surmountable.

Complication: Inability to Access the AVF

The immature fistulae can be difficult to catheterize in both patent and occluded settings.

Predisposing factors: Unused forearm fistulae are more prone to this event.

Short and long-term consequences: Failed percutaneous puncture can create a hematoma at the site, which may impair subsequent surgery. Repeated vein punctures that fail to lead to catheterization and percutaneous thrombectomy may begin bleeding once the AVF is revascularized by other means.

Management of the complication: Placing a tourniquet high on the arm will allow the basilic or cephalic vein to distend so that it can more readily be punctured in a retrograde fashion. If the arm is obese, or the fistula deep and non-palpable, sonographic puncture can be performed. In some settings, it may be impossible to catheterize the occluded immature fistula.

Prevention: Once again careful pre-procedure physical exam is paramount in assessing forearm AVFs. Identifying telltale sites of fistula puncture during routine dialysis can provide clues to access sites.

Complication: Inability to Traverse an Outflow Lesion

Rarely, an outflow vein stenosis may be difficult to traverse. Use of roadmapping and hydrophilic guidewires have made this step relatively simple. More common are difficulties recanalizing occluded outflow or central veins.

Predisposing factors: Outflow vein lesions near the graft are most typically caused by flow-induced intimal hyperplasia. In more remote veins in patients with forearm or radiocephalic fistulae, latent vein stenoses due to repeated venipuncture from blood drawing or intravenous access can create stenoses which are unmasked when exposed to the high flow of dialysis shunts. The most common cause of central vein stenoses and occlusions is prior temporary or tunneled dialysis catheter, particularly one placed in subclavian or left internal jugular veins. The incidence of venous stenoses or occlusions related to subclavian vein catheterizations is so much greater than those seen with right internal jugular veins catheters, it is arguably negligent that subclavian dialysis catheters be placed.

Short and long-term consequences: Fistula or graft revision, jump grafts, transposition, or abandonment may be necessary depending upon the response of the treated segment to angioplasty (or stent). Currently, uncovered central vein stents remain prone to intimal hyperplasia, making their use a temporizing measure, which allows the clinician to delay the need to abandon access in that extremity.

Management of the complication: Proper graft surveillance and physical examination can demonstrate signs of excessive venous hypertension within the arm, manifest by local or diffuse arm swelling, or a gradually diminishing thrill within the fistulae and graft. Early intervention can prolong access life as it is accepted that graft function is better with assisted patency than with secondary patency.

Prevention: Again, pre-procedure assessment is the key to avoiding or at least planning in advance for these hurdles.

THROMBECTOMY (MECHANICAL, THROMBOASPIRATION)

Complication: Symptomatic Pulmonary Embolism

In 1994, Trerotola et al. published an article that described intentional embolization of the AVG thrombus as a part of graft thrombectomy (21). During thrombectomy of the venous limb, an occlusion balloon was used to push the macerated thrombus prograde toward the lungs. This proved remarkably well tolerated in practice and in subsequent published series. The vast majority of patients experienced no symptoms, perhaps due to the small average AVG clot volume of 3 mL (22–24). Nevertheless, reports have described fatal pulmonary emboli, septic pulmonary embolism, or paradoxical embolis resulting in hemiplegia (23,25–28). These complications can occur immediately at the time of procedure or in the ensuing days.

Predisposing factors: Symptomatic sequelae of the passage of central venous clot occurs in patients with dilated AVFs that harbor greater than 100 mL of clot (diameter of fistula × length of fistula proximal to stenosis). Obviously, aneurysmal fistulas are more likely to exhibit this type of clot burden. Patients are much more likely to experience symptoms if they have a known patent foramen ovale or have pre-existing heart disease, lung disease or have undergone the procedure previously (27). It has been postulated that these are the underlying factors that led to death in 5% of patients undergoing the procedure in one particular study (26).

Short and long-term consequences: Although the occurrence of reported non-symptomatic pulmonary emboli when evaluated with ventilation-perfusion scintigraphy ranges from 0% to 60% (26,29), death has been reported to occur very infrequently. In one report of 43 patients who underwent pulse spray thrombolysis followed by mechanical declotting, two patients had fatal pulmonary embolisms (26). One concern is that repeated small, individually asymptomatic, pulmonary emboli can lead to eventual pulmonary hypertension or risk of sudden death after repeat thrombectomy.

Management of the complication: The management of acute clinically relevant pulmonary emboli after dialysis thrombectomy is no different than conventional management of pulmonary emboli, consisting of anticoagulation, oxygen, possible thrombolysis, and, if needed, respiratory support. One unique difference is the possibility of septic emboli from an infected graft. Antibiotic therapy is indicated in cases in which graft infection may, in retrospect, have been present. While sudden neurologic deterioration during graft thrombectomy can be due to excessive conscious sedation, the possibility of paradoxical emboli must be kept in mind. Catheter directed lysis may be used to reduce permanent neurologic injury.

Prevention: Avoiding balloon thrombectomy in patients with cardiac and pulmonary disease is prudent (26). The technique is absolutely contraindicated in patients with known anatomic right to left shunts. Patients with larger clot burdens (e.g., large clotted aneurysms, or thrombosis of the outflow venous distal to the AVG) should undergo clot aspiration, chemical thrombolysis, or mechanical thrombectomy using aspirating devices prior to undergoing venoplasty of the underlying lesion. Ultimately, the use of pure balloon thrombectomy has become a procedure of largely historic relevance, popular during the time preceding the widespread availability of mechanical thrombectomy devices and lyse-and-wait techniques (14). The routine use of Gram-positive antibiotic prophylaxis during shunt interventions is reasonable, although no studies have demonstrated reductions in the severity of very rare symptomatic septic pulmonary emboli.

Complication: Arterial Embolism

The incidence of distal artery embolization during balloon mechanical thrombectomy of AVG is 6% (30). These emboli result "asterial plug" is dislodged during artorial anastomos instrumentation, or the plug is pushed into the artery from a sudden increase in the pressure in the graft when it is flushed, or in one case report when the angioplasty balloon ruptured (31) (Figs. 1A–C). Most of these emboli are asymptomatic, however, ischemic symptoms can occur.

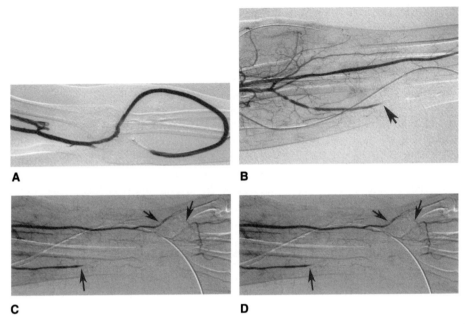

Figure 1   Distal arterial embolization. (**A**) The arterial plug is seen in place with no distal arterial flow. (**B**) Embolization into the already diseased ulnar circulation. (**C**) Further distal emboli seen within the radial artery and the palmar arch. (**D**) The hand circulation after distal lytic infusion.

Predisposing factors: Although no true factors have been identified, emboli, in general, can be presumed to occur more frequently in patients with difficult to traverse arterial anastomoses (and excessive manipulations by less experienced operators). Symptomatic emboli can be presumed to be more likely to occur in patients with underlying upper extremity peripheral vascular disease and patients with incomplete arterial palmar arches.

Short and long-term consequences: Immediate painful ischemia, manifest by pain, parathesias, pallor, poikilothermia, and paralysis, can occur acutely. In the long term, partially occlusive emboli may result in local pain, loss of motor function and muscle wasting on the hand. This iatrogenic complication may be mistaken for arterial steal as it may only occur during dialysis. Arguably, new onset of steal after thrombectomy warrants distal arteriography.

Management of the complication: Recognition of the complication is the first step in the process. Although only between 10% and 20% of recognized arterial emboli will be symptomatic, digital subtraction arteriography at the cessation of the thrombectomy through retrograde contrast injection is recommended. If distal arterial emboli are recognized, removal should be attempted even if asymptomatic in the acute setting. In the asymptomatic patient we use one of the three techniques. Passage of a 0.035-inch hydrophilic guidewire past the embolism is the first step in the treatment of this complication. Once the guidewire has passed beyond the clot, an over the wire occlusion balloon can be used to draw the embolus into the graft, releasing it into the central circulation. If this technique is not successful the "back-bleeding technique" may be employed. This involves occluding the arterial inflow above the inflow to the graft with a compliant balloon, then exercising the hand or massaging the forearm to increase retrograde pressure.

The success of this technique is based on the assumption that the collateral flow plus the exercise/massage will create enough backflow to dislodge the arterial clot into the graft (31). Accordingly, the AVF/AVG must be patent for this technique to work. Finally, local thrombolysis can be instituted using catheters introduced retrograde into the artery through the AVG. Surgical embolectomy is reserved for the symptomatic patient who has failed these percutaneous approaches.

Prevention: While chemical thrombolysis has been suggested as a safer approach than mechanical techniques, this has never been validated in a formal fashion. Further, the multiplicity of different mechanical devices makes general statements about relative risks of chemical versus mechanical approaches impossible. Ultimately, the risk of distal embolization exists with nearly all techniques because of the need to "pull" the arterial plug out of the arterial anastomosis of the AVG. In unusual, high-risk cases, embolic protection devices may have theoretic utility.

Complication: Large Residual Thrombus in Aneurysmal Dilation

The thrombi can act as a nidus for future clot formation, however, leaving them uncontained can lead to detachment, intermittent flow blockage, or complete breakage that leads to complete occlusion or pulmonary embolism.

Predisposing factors: This problem generally affects large mature AVFs that carry adherent thrombi within sections of aneurysmal dilation. Occasionally, a degenerated AVG may have a similar picture within what is really a pseudoaneurysm.

Short and long-term consequences: Not removing or trapping the clot can lead to recurrent AVF/AVG failure or pulmonary embolism.

Management of the complication: Thromboaspiration or mechanical thrombolysis in conjunction with external compression of the aneurysm can bring the clot into contact with the thrombectomy device. Methods that have been reported to deal with large amounts of residual thrombus include trapping them outside of a stent or revising the graft surgically.

Prevention: The risks of embolization are relatively small. Thus, the decision for a wait-and-see approach versus a surgical revision is an individual one.

THROMBOLYSIS

Complication: Bleeding Complications Associated with Thrombolysis

To date, no definitive studies have proven differences in bleeding risks associated with different modern thrombolytic agents used in dialysis access thrombolysis. The two most common infusion techniques are the "lyse-and-wait" and the "pulse-spray" techniques (32,33). Persistent post-procedure bleeding at the access sites are the primary complication noted in these local lytic infusion algorithms.

Predisposing factors: Local bleeding is common from old puncture sites and more likely to occur in AVGs than AVFs. Patients with numerous aneurysms have been noted to bleed more than other patients with AVFs. Higher activated clotting times related to heparin use increase bleeding risks.

Short and long-term consequences: Severe consequences are unlikely in this group unless bleeding is uncontrolled. Pressure dressings are dangerous in these settings as they may mask and contain large amounts of continued hemorrhage. Typically bleeding at the catheter removal sites is well treated with a purse string suture, topical hemostatic patches, prolonged compression, and intravenous desmopressin.

Prevention: Use of purse-string sutures may prevent this complication in most cases.

ANGIOPLASTY AND STENTING

Complication: Rupture of the Vein

Rupture of the outflow vessel can occur during PTA. In central veins, such as subclavian or superior vena cava, immediate life-threatening extravasation and hemodynamic instability can occur. In more peripheral locations, unchecked venous ruptures can lead to small or large soft tissue hematomas (Figs. 2A–C).

Predisposing factors: All outflow veins can rupture if overdilated. Immature small caliber veins or long stenotic segments may be more prone to rupture when overexpanded. Radiated veins are more prone to rupture.

Short and long-term consequences: If the subclavian or superior vena cava veins are injured, hemodynamic compromise can occur acutely. In the more peripheral setting, local hematoma formation can cause compression of the AVF and lead to an increased risk of infection and cellulitis.

Management of the complication: Central venous rupture is an emergency managed by immediate balloon tamponade. Typically, the balloon used during the initial dilation can be temporarily inflated at the rupture site. Graft-covered stents can provide definitive treatment if prolonged balloon inflation fails to resolve the complication. More peripheral extremity vein rupture during venoplasty can be treated with prolonged balloon inflation or stents. Most extravasation resolves after place-

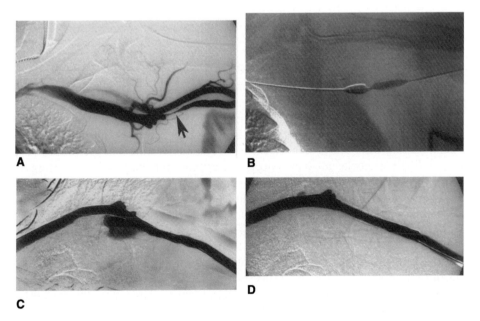

Figure 2 Axillary vein rupture. (**A**) Axillary vein stenosis. (**B**) Angioplasty of axillary vein stenosis. (**C**) Extravasation from axillary vein rupture. (**D**) Successful treatment of the rupture with an uncovered stent, no further extravasation is seen.

ment of conventional uncovered stents, perhaps due to the creation of a lower pressure flow channel through the stents, or because the injury site is "tacked down" by the stent (34) (Fig. 2D).

Prevention: A vigorous attempt not to over distend the vein is the best method to avoid this complication. Adequate assessment of the adjacent vein diameters both proximal and distal to the stenosis is necessary prior to the start of the procedure.

OUTCOMES

Complication: Failure of Treatment in Less than One Month

Several studies have compared the efficacy of various types of graft salvage procedures. Studies evaluating angioplasty versus surgical revision of grafts have shown similar one-month patencies, with no statistical difference between methods. The primary patency for a revised graft at one month is 70–85%, by either method (35,36). Surgical thrombectomy alone without surgical revision of the underlying lesion results in a 30% one-month primary patency and a 10% patency at 120 days (37). Studies evaluating the use of lytics in the declotting of thrombosed dialysis grafts exhibit similar 30-day patency rates of 70%, and a 90-day primary patency of 50% (38,39). Therefore, it would appear that a reasonable goal is a one-month patency rate of 75%, with a 50% three-month patency which exceeds the 40% benchmark set by the DOQI (40).

Predisposing factors: The group of patients most likely to experience graft failures are those with severely diseased outflow veins. These patients include: patients with forearm grafts that may have long segment disease of the veins in the upper arm and patients with a history of multiple grafts in the same site, who also show greater potential for severe venous outflow disease. In addition, patients with AVFs, on stenosis in the mid vein, particularly if accompanied by an adjacent aneurysmal dilation, are best treated by surgical revision. However, if the fistula has not been used or the procedure is being done to allow the fistula to mature, the procedure will uniformly fail.

Short and long-term consequences: Failure in the short term can lead to inadequate dialysis and recidivism. In the long term, failed dialysis access and re-intervention are very costly to the US health care system and to the patient's native venous system.

Management of the complication: Since the accepted 90-day patency after thrombectomy of an arteriovenous access is 40% (31), there is an inevitability that this complication will occur. Aggressive assessment and treatment of the venous outflow including the subclavian vein is necessary at times this may include stenting of the subclavian vein. In the patient in whom the outflow vein is tenuous, it is not unreasonable to place a tunneled dialysis catheter at the time of completion of venography, an approach championed by some authors (41).

Prevention: While prevention cannot be complete, sound clinical judgment applied to the choice of outflow vessel for the initial graft is a key component. One study has identified a better initial success rate when a more experienced operator performs thrombectomy. This increased success has been attributed to shorter procedure times that, in turn, allow for shorter periods of instrumentation within the graft (41).

More experienced operators are also more likely to recognize inadequate outflow vessels and intervene appropriately. Perfection is technically unattainable but is certainly approachable, and should be the goal of the interventionalist. The addition of oral anticoagulants in this population is associated with a very high risk of major bleeding complications in one study this therapeutic choice showed bleeding in 40% of patients over two years, resulting in 542 hospital days (42). Others have shown a similar complication rate with no improvement in graft survival (43). In the patient with recurrent thrombosis of their access, despite no radiographic abnormality, hypercoagulable work-up is warranted. A high prevalence of primary antiphospho-lipid antibody syndrome is recognized in the CRF population. Patients who have an identified hypercoagulable state should be anticoagulated appropriately; there are case reports of such therapy preventing further graft failure (44). It is interesting to note that certain drugs are associated with improved primary graft patency (calcium channel blockers), or improved secondary patency (aspirin and angiotensin-converting enzyme inhibitors). Warfarin use was associated with worse primary access patency (45).

CONCLUSION

At this time, percutaneous AVF, graft declotting, and revisions have proven a reli-able and effective method of preserving HD access function. While up to 60% of patients with arteriovenous access for dialysis will require revision yearly, it is para-mount that these procedures be performed as safely as possible. Percutaneous declot-ting, whether mechanical or chemical, is minimally invasive, spares healthy vein, is easily repeatable, and, most importantly, allows for the evaluation of the entire sys-tem from arterial inflow to the central venous system. It is our belief that applying the outlined Prevention and Management sections appropriately can further mini-mize the recognized 5% rate of morbidity associated with the above armamentarium of techniques.

REFERENCES

1. Renal Data System. USRDS 2003 Annual Data Report. Bethesda, MD: National Insti-tute of Diabetes and Digestive and Kidney Diseases.
2. Luke RG. Chronic renal failure—a vasculopathic state. N Engl J Med 1998; 339:841–843.
3. Abt Associates, Ad Hoc Committee on Nephrology Manpower Needs. Estimated work-force and training requirements for nephrologists through the year 2010. J Am Soc Nephrol 1997; 8:S1–S32.
4. Feldman HI, Held PJ, Huthcinson JT, et al. Hemodialysis vascular access morbidity in the United States. Kidney Int 1993; 43:1091–1096.
5. Hodges TC, Fillinger MF, Zwolak RM, et al. Longitudinal comparisons of dialysis access methods: risk factors for failure. J Vasc Surg 1997; 26:1009–1019.
6. Cinat ME, Hopkins J, Wilson SE. A prospective evaluation of PTFE graft patency and surveillance techniques in hemodialysis access. Ann Vasc Surg 1999; 13:191–198.
7. Ascher E, Gade P, Hingorani A, et al. Changes in the practice of angioaccess surgery: impact of dialysis outcome and quality iniative recommendations. J Vasc Surg 2000; 31:84–92.
8. Gibson KD, Gillen DL, Caps MT, et al. Vascular access survival and incidence of revi-sions: a comparison of prosthetic grafts, simple autogenous fistulas, and venous trans-position fistulas from the United States Renal Data System Dialysis Morbidity and Mortality Study. J Vasc Surg 2001; 34:694–700.
9. Pisoni RL, Young EW, Dykstra DM, et al. Vascular access use in Europe and the United States: results from the DOPPS. Kidney Int 2002; 61:305–316.

10. Glanz S, Gordon D, Butt KMH, Hong J, Adamson R, Sclafani SJA. Dialysis access fistulas: treatment of stenoses by transluminal angioplasty. Radiology 1984; 152:637–642.
11. Mori Y, Horikawa K, Sato K, Mimuro N, Toriyama T, Kawahara H. Stenotic lesions in vascular access: treatment with transluminal angioplasty using high-pressure balloons. Int Med 1994; 33:284–287.
12. Beathard GA. Percutaneous angioplasty for the treatment of venous stenosis: a nephrologists view. Semin Dial 1995; 8:166–170.
13. Gmelin E, Winterhoff R, Rinast E. Insufficient hemodialysis access fistulas: late results of treatment with percutaneous balloon angioplasty. Radiology 1989; 171:657–660.
14. Turmel-Rodrigues L, Pengloan J, Blanchier D, Abaza M, Birmele B, Haillot O, Blanchard D. Insufficient dialysis shunts: improved long-term patency rates with close hemodynamic monitoring, repeated percutaneous balloon angioplasty, and stent placement. Radiology 1993; 187:273–278.
15. Calligaro KD, Dougherty MJ. Endovascular versus surgical treatment of failed hemodialysis access. J Endovasc Ther 2003; 10:I-1–I-51.
16. Turmel-Rodrigues L, Raynaud A, Louail B, et al. Manual catheter-directed aspiration an other thrombectomy techniques for declotting native fistulas for hemodialysis. J Vasc Interv Radiol 2001; 12:1365–1371.
17. Palder SB, Kirkman RL, Whittemore AD, Hakim RM, Lazarus JM, Tilney NL. Vascular access for hemodialysis: patency rates and results of revision. Ann Surg 1985; 202: 235–239.
18. Tordoir J, Herman JMMPH, Kwan TS, Diderich PM. Long-term follow-up of the polytetrafluoroethylene (PTFE) prosthesis as an arteriovenous fistula for haemodialysis. Eur J Vasc Surg 1987; 2:3–7.
19. Etheredge EE, Haid SD, Maeser MN, Sicard GA, Anderson CB. Salvage operations for malfunctioning polytetrafluoroethylene hemodialysis access grafts. Surgery 1983; 94: 464–470.
20. http://www.kidney.org/professionals/kdoqi/guidelines_updates/doqiupva_v.html#19.
21. Trerotola S, Lund G, Scheel P, et al. Thrombosed hemodialysis access grafts: percutaneous mechanical declotting without urokinase. Radiology 1994; 191:721–726.
22. Winkler T, Trerotola S, Davidson D, et al. Study of thrombus from thrombosed hemodialysis access grafts. Radiology 1995; 197:461–465.
23. Soulen M, Zaetta J, Amygdalos M, et al. Mechanical declotting of thrombosed dialysis grafts: experience in 86 cases. J Vasc Interv Radiol 1997; 8:563–567.
24. Haage P, Vorwerk D, Wildberger J, et al. Percutaneous treatment of thrombosed primary venous arteriovenous hemodialysis access fistulae. Kidney Int 2000; 57:1169–1175.
25. Trerotola S, Vesely T, Lund G, et al. Treatment of thrombosed hemodialysis access grafts: Arrow-Trerotola percutanoeous thrombolytic device versus pulse-spray thrombolysis. Radiology 1998; 206:403–414.
26. Swan T, Smyth S, Ruffenach S, et al. Pulmonary embolism following hemodialysis access thrombolysis/thrombectomy. J Vasc Interv Radiol 1995; 6:683–686.
27. Owens C, Yaghmai B, Aletich V, et al. Fatal paradoxic embolism during percutaneous thrombolysis of a hemodialysis graft. AJR Am J Roentgenol 1998; 170:742–744.
28. Briefel G, Regan F, Petronis J, et al. Cerebral embolism after mechanical thrombolysis of a clotted hemodialysis access. Am J Kidney Dis 1999; 34:2:341–343.
29. Petronis J, Regan F, Briefel G, et al. Ventilation-perfusion scintigraphic evaluation of pulmonary clot burden after percutaneous thrombolysis of clotted hemodialysis access graft. Am J Kidney Dis 1999; 34(2):207–211.
30. Lazzaro C, Trerotola S, Shah H, et al. Modified use of the Arrow-Trerotola percutaneous thrombolytic device for the treatment of thrombosed hemodialysis access grafts. J Vasc Interv Radiol 1999; 10(8):1025–1031.
31. Trerotola S, Johnson M, Shah H, et al. Backbleeding technique for treatment of arterial emboli resulting from dialysis graft thrombolysis. J Vasc Interv Radiol 1998; 9:141–143.

32. Cynamon J, Lakritz P, Wahl S, et al. Hemodialysis graft declotting: description of the "lyse and wait" technique. J Vasc Interv Radiol 1997; 8:825–829.

33. Bookstein J, Fellmeth B, Roberts A, et al. Pulsed-spray pharmacomechanical thrombolysis: preliminary clinical results. AJR Am J Roentgenol 1989; 152:1097–1100.

34. Turmel-Rodrigues L, Pengloan J, Rodrique H, et al. Treatment of failed native arteriovenous fistulae for hemodialysis by interventional radiology. Kidney Int 2000; 57: 1124–1140.

35. Bitar G, Yang S, Badosa F. Balloon versus patch angioplasty as an adjuvant treatment to surgical thrombectomy of hemodialysis. Am J Surg 1997; 174:140–142.

36. Dapunt O, Feurstein M, Rendl KH, et al. Transluminal angioplasty versus conventional operation in the treatment of hemodialysis fistula stenosis: results from a 5-year study. Br J Surg 1987; 74:1004–1005.

37. Brotman D, Fandos L, Faust G, et al. Hemodialysis graft salvage. J Am Coll Surg 1994; 178:431–434.

38. Cohen M, Kumpe D, Durham J, et al. Improved treatment of thrombosed hemodialysis access sites with thrombolysis and angioplasty. Kidney Int 1994; 46:1375–1380.

39. Middlebrook M, Amygdalos M, Soulen M, et al. Thrombosed hemodialysis grafts: percutaneous mechanical balloon declotting versus thrombolysis. Radiology 1995; 196: 73–77.

40. Owen J, Robert J, Alexander S, et al. NKF-DOQI clinical practice guidelines for hemodialysis adequacy. Am J Kidney Dis 1997; 30(suppl):S15–S64.

41. Falk A, Mitty H, Guller J, et al. Thrombolysis of clotted hemodialysis grafts with tissue-type plasminogen activator. J Vasc Interv Radiol 2001; 12:305–311.

42. Biggers J, Remmers A, Glassford D, et al. The risk of anticoagulation in hemodialysis patients. Nephron 1977; 18:109–113.

43. Crowther M, Clase C, Margetts P, et al. Low-intensity warfarin is ineffective for the prevention of PTFE graft failure in patients on hemodialysis: a randomized controlled trial. J Am Soc Nephrol 2002; 13:2331–2337.

44. Martinez-Rubio M, Moreno-Lopez R, Lama M, et al. Primary antiphospholipid syndrome diagnosed in hemodialysis. Nefrologia 2002; 22:71–74.

45. Saran R, Dykstra D, Wolfe R, et al. Association between vascular access failure and the use of specific drugs: the Dialysis Outcomes and Practice Patterns Study (DOPPS). Am J Kidney Dis 2002; 40:1255–1263.

25

Percutaneous Treatment for Pulmonary Embolism

Matthew J. Eagleton and Lazar J. Greenfield
Section of Vascular Surgery, University of Michigan, Ann Arbor, Michigan, U.S.A.

INTRODUCTION

Pulmonary embolism (PE) secondary to deep venous thrombosis (DVT) is estimated to occur at an incidence rate of 69 cases per 100,000 and a prevalence rate of 3.5 cases per 1000 hospital admissions (1,2). The three-month mortality following PE was reported at 17.4% in the International Cooperative Pulmonary Embolism Registry, and in the Management Strategy and Prognosis of Pulmonary Embolism Registry the mortality rate rose to 31% in those patients with hemodynamic instability (3,4). The size of the embolus does not seem to affect outcome. Massive PE, as defined by angiographic pulmonary artery obstruction $\geq$50% or obstruction of two or more lobar arteries, is not associated with increased mortality unless accompanied by hemodynamic instability (5). A subset of the hemodynamically stable group with right ventricular dysfunction, however, may be at increased risk of death (6).

Anticoagulation Therapy

The mainstay of treatment for PE is initial anticoagulation with unfractionated heparin sodium. This line of therapy has been shown to prevent further thrombus formation, thrombus propagation, and recurrent venous thromboembolism while endogenous fibrinolysis attempts to decrease the clot burden (7). Early anticoagulation is a necessity as the risk of recurrent PE is highest in the preliminary hours following the initial event, and it is the most common cause of death in hemodynamically stable patients (6,8). More recent evidence suggests that treatment with low molecular weight heparins may be as efficacious as unfractionated heparin, but with a more simplified mode of administration and without the need to monitor blood levels (9).

Thrombolytic Therapy

Thrombolytic therapy offers several advantages over anticoagulation alone in the management of PE. Patients receiving thrombolytic therapy undergo faster and more complete thrombus resolution than those treated with anticoagulation alone (10,11). By perfusion scan, however, limited differences exist between the two groups after one-week time. Long term, though, more patients treated with only anticoagulation have recurrent PE and dyspnea on exertion compared with patients receiving thrombolytics (12). Those patients treated with heparin alone had elevated pulmonary artery pressures and pulmonary vascular resistance. This suggests that thrombolytic therapy may reduce the development of pulmonary hypertension. Only one study to date has shown a clear benefit in mortality in those patients treated with thrombolytics versus anticoagulation alone (13). It is suggested, however, that patients with increased mortality risk, such as those having right ventricular dysfunction, may benefit from thrombolytic therapy even if they present with hemodynamic stability (6,14). This conclusion is based on the premise that patients with right ventricular dysfunction have impending hemodynamic instability and a low tolerance for recurrent PE (15).

Patients with PE and hemodynamic instability should be treated with thrombolytic therapy barring any contraindications, although its use has not been proven to reduce mortality in hemodynamically stable patients, and its use is not without risk. Mikkola et al. in 1997 reported the complications in 312 patients who received thrombolytic therapy for PE while enrolled in five different clinical trials (16). Major bleeding complications were observed in 20% of the patients within 72 hours of thrombolytic therapy. These complications included catheter site hematoma, hematuria, and intracranial hemorrhage. Increasing age, larger body size, and the use of catheterization procedures to provide local thrombolytic therapy predisposed patients to bleeding complications.

Surgical Therapy

When medical and endovascular therapy fail, surgical pulmonary thromboembolectomy can be considered. The procedure is generally performed through a median sternotomy and the main pulmonary artery is opened to extract the clot. This procedure can be performed with or without the adjunctive use of cardiopulmonary bypass. Historically, there has been significant morbidity and mortality associated with operative pulmonary thromboembolectomy. Del Campo, in 1985, reported the results from 651 cases which demonstrated a 40% mortality rate for those procedures performed while on cardiopulmonary bypass and a 51% mortality rate in those with procedures performed without bypass (17). Gulba et al. has suggested that in some instances surgical pulmonary embolectomy is more successful than thrombolytic therapy (18). In this series, patients treated with thrombolysis had a 75% success rate and a 33% mortality rate while the surgical arm of the study had an 85% success rate and a 23% mortality rate. The groups, however, were not randomized, nor were they comparable with regard to demographics, comorbidities, and clinical scenarios. A more recent evaluation of the outcomes from acute pulmonary thromboembolectomy reports a mortality rate of only 11% (19). The success in this series is based on having an established multidisciplinary team in addition to careful patient selection. The patients in this series were not as critically ill as those reported in earlier series, as most patients underwent surgery when they demonstrated impending hemodynamic instability with moderate or severe right ventricular dysfunction (19).

ENDOVASCULAR THERAPY

Due to the high morbidity and mortality historically associated with surgical pulmonary embolectomy, alternative endovascular methods of reducing pulmonary artery thrombus burden following PE have been developed. There are three main endovascular modalities by which this is accomplished: suction thrombectomy, catheter-directed thrombus fragmentation, and mechanical thrombectomy. Suction thrombectomy involves the aspiration of thrombus into a specially designed cup, or into a guiding catheter, and then removal from the venous system. Catheter-directed thrombus fragmentation involves the simple maceration of thrombus with a pre-formed angiographic catheter or angioplasty balloon. Finally, mechanical thrombectomy devices can be broadly divided into two main categories: hydrodynamic recirculation devices and rotational recirculation devices (20). Hydrodynamic recirculation devices work on the principle of the Venturi effect. Retrograde-directed high-speed saline jets induce high shear forces that macerate the thrombus and suck it into the device. Rotational recirculation devices fragment thrombus through the use of a high-speed rotational impeller or basket that generates a hydrodynamic vortex. Many of these modalities do not totally remove the thrombus but fragment portions of it which migrate peripherally in the pulmonary circulation. The main pulmonary artery is recanalized thus improving pulmonary perfusion (21,22). The rationale for all of these devices is the rapid relief of pulmonary artery central obstruction. With an increased vascular volume in the distal pulmonary circulatory bed, redistribution of thrombus to the periphery may acutely improve cardiopulmonary hemodynamics, increase total pulmonary blood flow and decrease right heart strain (23–25).

Suction Thrombectomy

Transvenous approaches to the removal of pulmonary emboli were first described by Greenfield et al. in 1969, and the first clinical application was described in 1971 (26,27). This technique involved the use of a suction embolectomy apparatus that is inserted, under local anesthesia, through a cut-down on the femoral or internal jugular veins. If inserted via a femoral approach, Fogarty catheter thrombectomy of occluding thrombus within the ilio-femoral system may be indicated. The suction-cup tipped device is inserted through a venotomy and advanced to the pulmonary artery under fluoroscopic guidance (Fig. 1). Juxtaposition of the cup onto the thrombus is verified by the injection of a small amount of contrast. Sustained suction is then applied which holds the thrombus to the end of the cup and the catheter and thrombus are withdrawn. Multiple retrievals may be necessary (28). With the development of large sheath introducers, this procedure can be performed in a percutaneous fashion from the femoral approach. If attempted from the jugular approach in a dyspneic patient, the risk of air embolism is higher.

    Several small case series describing the results of this procedure have been reported (29,30). In 1991, Timsit et al. presented their experience with performing transvenous suction pulmonary embolectomy in 18 patients (25). In this report, 11 of 18 patients had successful removal of pulmonary emboli with a success rate of 61%. The overall mortality rate was 27%, but this decreased to 18% in those having a successful embolectomy, and rose to 43% in those in whom an embolectomy was not possible. Greenfield and colleagues, however, in 1993 presented the largest group of patients treated in this fashion (31). In this series, 46 patients underwent suction

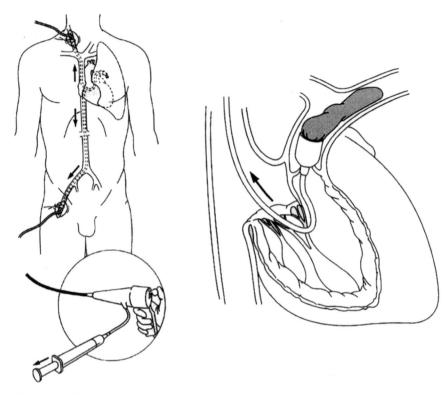

Figure 1 The embolectomy catheter introduced via a femoral approach and guided to the right side of the heart. A suction cup on the end of the catheter is used to retrieve the thrombus.

pulmonary embolectomy with a technical success rate of 76%, and a 30-day survival rate of 70%. The mean long-term survival for all patients was 46 months, and this was extended to 89 months in those having a successful procedure. Multiple complications were apparent in these studies and are depicted in Table 1. Further discussion of these complications will occur later.

Thrombus Fragmentation

The use of standard angiographic catheters to fragment and disperse pulmonary emboli has been described as a technique that is available to all angiographers in all centers as it holds the advantage of requiring no special equipment. The procedure entails gently pushing the thrombus distally by simply advancing the guidewire and catheter. This results in some initial increased pulmonary blood flow (21). The guidewire is then removed and the pre-formed angiographic catheter is allowed to reform. On withdrawal of the reformed catheter, the thrombus is fragmented further. An evolution of this concept introduced a specialized catheter that could be mechanically rotated, thus enhancing its ability to fragment the pulmonary thrombus (32). Again, the majority of the reports of clinical outcomes of this technique is comprised of case reports or series involving only a few patients (21,32,33). The only reported complication in these publications was formation of a hematoma at the venous puncture site. The largest series of patients was reported by Schmitz-Rode in 1998 (34). Ten patients underwent fragmentation of pulmonary emboli

Table 1 Complications in Larger Series Evaluating Endovascular Treatment of PE

Series	Procedure	Procedure failure	Complications					
			Deaths	Hematoma	Perforation	Recurrent DVT/PE	Pulmonary injury
Timsit et al. (1991) (n = 18)	Suction embolectomy	7/18 (39%)	5/18 (28%)	5/18 (28%)	0/18 (0%)	NR	NR
Greenfield et al. (1993) (n = 46)	Suction embolectomy	11/46 (24%)	14/46 (30%)	7/46 (15%)	2/46 (4%)	5/46 (11%)	5/46 (11%)
Schmitz-Rode et al. (1998) (n = 10)	Catheter fragmentation	3/10 (30%)	2/10 (20%)	0/10 (0%)	0/10 (0%)	NR	NR
Fava et al. (1997) (n = 16)	Fragmentation and thrombolytics	2/16 (12%)	1/16 (6%)	3/16 (19%)	0/16 (0%)	NR	NR
De Gregorio et al. (2002) (n = 9)	Fragmentation and thrombolytics	3/59 (5%)	3/59 (5%0)	8/59 (14%)	0/59 (0%)	NR	0/59 (0%)

Abbreviations: PE, pulmonary embolism; DVT, deep venous thrombosis; NR, not reported.

using a rotational pigtail catheter. The procedure success rate was 70% with a 20% mortality rate, and no procedure related complications were reported (Table 1).

Combination Therapy

While the reports of using catheter fragmentation alone contain only a small number of patients, the combination of catheter fragmentation and adjunctive thrombolytic therapy has been more extensively studied. Early reviews, having five or fewer patients, reported excellent clinical outcomes with few, if any, complications (35,36). Fava et al. in 1997, presented a series of 16 cases in which patients with acute PE underwent catheter fragmentation of the embolus followed by intrapulmonary thrombolysis with urokinase (24). The procedure was successful in 14 patients giving a success rate of 88%. One patient required cessation of thrombolytic therapy secondary to a drop in the fibrinogen level. This patient required open pulmonary embolectomy.

The mortality rate was 6% from one patient with cardiac arrest during the procedure who was unable to be resuscitated. The other reported complications were hematomas at the venous puncture site (Table 1). Long-term follow up was not provided. The largest series to date using this endovascular technique was reported by De Gregorio et al. in 2002 (Fig. 2) (37). Fifty-nine patients with acute PE underwent an intrapulmonary bolus of thrombolytic agent, then catheter fragmentation, and finally regional thrombolytic therapy. Technical success, defined as completion of the procedure, occurred in all patients. Clinical success, defined as an improvement in the patients' symptoms, an improvement in oxygen saturation, and a decrease in pulmonary artery pressure, occurred in 56 of the 59 patients (95% success rate). The mortality rate was 5%. Two patients died immediately following the procedure and one within 24 hours; all failed to overcome their previous hemodynamic compromise.

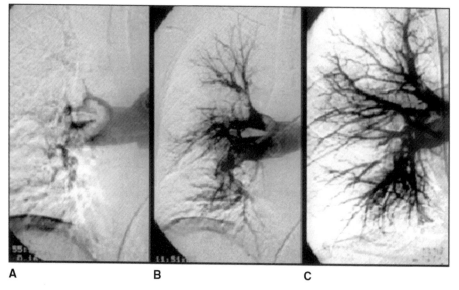

A   **B**   **C**

Figure 2   Serial radiographs from a patient presenting with a massive PE (**A**) who underwent catheter fragmentation (**B**) and subsequent thrombolysis (**C**).

Mechanical Thrombectomy

The use of mechanical thrombectomy devices to treat acute PE has been limited. The majority of publications are case reports or series with no more than five patients, making outcomes and complications analysis difficult (38–41). The major complications described in these reports are failure to completely clear the pulmonary artery of thrombus, dysrhythmias associated with the passage of the devices through the heart, hemoptysis, and death. The use of balloon angioplasty with and without stent placement to treat acute PE, particularly when complicated by cor pulmonale, likewise has been described only in case reports and no meaningful outcomes conclusions can be reached (23,42,43).

COMPLICATIONS

The series examining endovascular treatment of PE are generally small, making evaluation of their outcomes and analysis of the associated complications limited. The discussion in the ensuing paragraphs will be based mainly on the results from the larger series reported in Table 1.

Unsuccessful Thrombus Removal

The most common complication in percutaneous treatment of PE is failure of the specific procedure to remove the thromboembolus. Unsuccessful thromboembolectomy occurs in 5–39% of the cases. Most authors believe that success of endovascular thromboembolectomy is directly attributable to the age of the PE. Greenfield noted that embolectomy success was highest for major PE (100% success rate) and for massive PE (82% rate) and worst for those with chronic PE (56% success rate) (31). In most series, careful evaluation of the failures revealed that these patients had a history of previous PE, had elevated pulmonary artery pressures suggestive of chronic PE, or had chronic thrombus found at the time of surgical pulmonary embolectomy (25). In those studies with a higher success rate in which time from symptoms to treatment was reported, the majority of patients were treated within 24 hours of the onset of symptoms (24). It has been recommended that percutaneous treatment of PE is less effective beyond 72 hours of the initial event, and that it should ideally be performed on patients with a recent PE and a pulmonary artery pressure less than 50 mmHg (25,31). Only one case report has documented success in removing thrombus known to be between 10 and 15 days old (38). The majority of initial treatment failures require operative thromboembolectomy or they succumb to their hemodynamic compromise and die.

Mortality

Similar to treatment failure, mortality rates vary from 5% to 30% (Table 1). Initial problems with cardiac arrest were attributable to large volume bolus injections of contrast medium into the main PA (31). Selective pulmonary artery injections with smaller amounts of contrast medium have been better tolerated. The majority of short-term deaths were due to cardiovascular collapse secondary to irreversible right heart failure (24,25,31,37). Other causes of death included intracerebral hemorrhage, sepsis, and multisystem organ failure, most not directly attributable to the procedure.

Interestingly, the need for pre-procedural and intra-procedural cardiopulmonary resuscitation and use of vasopressors are not markers for increased mortality (31). Survival, however, has been shown to be directly attributable to the success of the procedure. In the Greenfield series, only 27% of the patients with an unsuccessful procedure survived short-term, and only 18% survived long-term as compared to 83% and 66%, respectively in the group that was successfully treated (31). A similar result was reported by Timsit in which only 57% survived short term in the treatment failure group as opposed to 82% in the treatment success group (25).

Hematoma

The development of a hematoma at the procedure site is not an infrequent event occurring in 0–28% of the cases (Table 1). The incidence does not appear to depend on whether the procedure was performed through a venous cut-down or percutaneous approach. The adjunctive use of thrombolytic therapy also does not appear to increase the incidence of hematoma formation. In most cases, patients were continued on anticoagulation therapy after thromboembolectomy, and this may be a contributing factor. Rarely did hematomas require more aggressive intervention than local compressive therapy, and there were no reported long-term sequelae.

Mechanical Trauma

Mechanical trauma to the heart or pulmonary vasculature appears to be a rare complication of percutaneous treatment of PE. Only one series in humans reports this complication (31). Greenfield et al. describes two patients in whom a perforation occurred. In one patient, the pulmonary artery balloon catheter used to measure pressures had lodged distally in the pulmonary artery resulting in a rupture of that vessel. Despite attempts at surgical control of the bleeding the patient died. A second perforation occurred in the right ventricle. The device used in this procedure had a metal-tipped suction cup, which subsequently was changed to plastic. No further episodes of perforation were noted.

Several animal studies examining alternative methods of endovascular therapy for PE, however, have reported trauma to the pulmonary artery. The use of a rotatable pigtail catheter in a canine experimental model of PE produced no macroscopic evidence of trauma, however, on microscopic evaluation there was evidence of perivascular hemorrhage (44). The experimental use of percutaneous mechanical thrombectomy devices to treat PE in animal models has also shown evidence of periadventitial bleeding and instances of vessel wall perforation (45,46). As the clinical use of these devices increases, the incidence of vessel-related trauma and perforation may increase.

Recurrent Thromboembolism

Recurrent DVT and PE occur infrequently. This complication has only been described in one series (31). The incidence of recurrent DVT was 4% and the incidence of recurrent PE was 4%. In the early experience of Greenfield, patients were taken to the operating room for clip application to the inferior vena cava following removal of pulmonary embolus. Episodes of fatal recurrent PE occurred in the time interval between treatment of the PE and the clip application. Since the development of vena caval filter devices, all patients in this series underwent placement of an inferior vena caval (IVC) filter following PE extraction. IVC filter placement following endovascular treatment of PE was reported in most series, but in one it was not routine (37). Clearly, its use as well as continued anticoagulation prevents the recurrence of PE, likely to be fatal.

Pulmonary Injury

Pulmonary injury, in the form of pulmonary infarction, hemoptysis, or pleural effusion, was reported in several series (31). Two smaller series reported incidences of hemoptysis following successful removal of PE by percutaneous mechanical thrombectomy devices (40,41). In both series, the episodes were self-limited and no intervention was required. No extravasation of contrast was seen on pulmonary angiography. It was hypothesized that the bleeding was due to a reperfusion syndrome with intrabronchial bleeding and focal edema due to an influx of blood into an area of infarcted tissue (41). None of the larger series have reported this complication. Greenfield et al. report an incidence of pulmonary infarction in 11% of their patients (31). The areas of infarction appeared to be in regions in which the pulmonary artery was not completely cleared by embolectomy. There were no reported long-term consequences of this. The series evaluating thrombus fragmentation, in which this incidence theoretically could be higher, did not report the occurrence of pulmonary infarction.

CONCLUSION

Initial results with endovascular therapy for the treatment of PE suggest it is a viable alternative to operative intervention in patients with an acute event and hemodynamic compromise or diminished right ventricular function. The morbidity and mortality rates, while never directly compared, appear to be equivalent if not better than those achieved with surgery. Few reports of complications directly attributable to these procedures exist. Barring failure to achieve successful thromboembolectomy, most complications have no long-term sequalae.

REFERENCES

1. Silverstein MD, Heit JA, Mohr DN, Petterson TM, O'Fallon WM, Melton LJI. Trends in the incidence of deep vein thrombosis and pulmonary embolism. Arch Intern Med 1998; 158:585–593.
2. Proctor MC, Greenfield LJ. Pulmonary embolism: diagnosis, incidence and implications. Cardiovasc Surg 1997; 5:77–81.
3. Goldhaber SZ, Visani L, De Rosa M. Acute pulmonary embolism: clinical outcomes in the International Cooperative Pulmonary Embolism Registry (ICOPER). Lancet 1999; 353:1165–1171.
4. Kasper W, Konstantinides S, Geibel A, Olschewski M, Heinrich F, Gosser GD, et al. Management strategies and determinants of outcome in acute major pulmonary embolism: results of a multicenter registry. J Am Coll Cardiol 1997; 30:1165–1171.
5. Wood KE. Major pulmonary embolism: review of a pathophysiologic approach to the golden hour of hemodynamically significant pulmonary embolism. Chest 2002; 121: 877–905.

6.   Goldhaber SZ, Haire WD, Feldstein ML, Miller M, Tltzis R, Smith JL, et al. Alteplase versus heparin in acute pulmonary embolism: randomized trial assessing right-ventricular function and pulmonary perfusion. Lancet 1993; 341(507):511.

7.   Kearon C. Initial treatment of venous thromboembolism. Thromb Haemost 1999; 82:887–891.

8.   Douketis JD, Kearon C, Bates S, Duku EK, Ginsberg JS. Risk of fatal pulmonary embolism in patients with treated venous thromboembolism. J Am Med Assoc 1998; 279: 458–462.

9.   Simonneau G, Sors H, Charbonnier B, Page Y, Laaban JP, Azarian R, et al. A comparison of low-molecular weight heparin with unfractionated heparin for acute pulmonary embolism. The THESEE Study Group. N Engl J Med 1997; 337:663–669.

10. Urokinase Pulmonary Embolism Study Group. Urokinase pulmonary embolism trial: phase I results. A cooperative study. J Am Med Assoc 1970; 214:2163–2172.

11. Sharma GVRK, Burleson VA, Sasahara AA. Effect of thrombolytic therapy on pulmonary-capillary blood volume in patietns with pulmonary embolism. N Engl J Med 1980; 303:842–845.

12. Sharma GV, Folland ED, McIntyre KM, Sasahara AA. Long-term benefit of thrombolytic therapy in patients with pulmonary embolism. Vasc Med 2000; 5:91–95.

13. Jerjes-Sanchez C, Ramires-Rivera A, de Lourdes GM, et al. Streptokinase and heparin versus heparin alone in massive pulmonary embolism: a randomized controlled trial. J Thromb Thrombol 1995; 2:227–229.

14. Konstantinides S, Geibel A, Olschewski M, Heinrich F, Grosser K, Rauber K, et al. Association between thrombolytic treatment and the prognosis of hemodynamically stable patients with major pulmonary embolism: the results of a multicenter registry. Circulation 1997; 96:882–888.

15. Arcasoy SM, Vachani A. Local and systemic thrombolytic therapy for acute venous thromboembolism. Clin Chest Med 2003; 24:73–91.

16. Mikkola KM, Patel SR, Parker JA, Grodstein F, Goldhaber SZ. Increasing age is a major risk factor for hemorrhagic complications after pulmonary embolism thrombolysis. Am Heart J 1997; 134:69–72.

17. Del Campo C. Pulmonary embolectomy: a review. Can J Surg 1985; 25:111–113.

18. Gulba DC, Schmid C, Borst HG, Lichtlen P, Dietz R, Luft FC. Medical compared with surgical treatment for massive pulmonary embolism. Lancet 1994; 343:576–577.

19. Aklog L, Williams CS, Byrne JG, Goldhaber SZ. Acute pulmonary embolectomy. A contemporary approach. Circulation 2002; 105:1416–1419.

20. Morgan R, Belli A-M. Percutaneous thrombectomy: a review. Eur Radiol 2002; 12: 205–217.

21. Brady AJB, Crake T, Oakley CM. Percutaneous catheter fragmentation and distal dispersion of proximal pulmonary embolus. Lancet 1991; 338:1186–1189.

22. Uflacker R. Interventional therapy for pulmonary embolism. J Vasc Interv Radiol 2001; 12:147–164.

23. Handa K, Sasaki Y, Kiyonaga A, Fujiano M, Hiroki T, Arakawa K. Acute pulmonary thromboembolism treated successfully by balloon angioplasty—a case report. Angiology 1988; 8:775–778.

24. Fava M, Loyola S, Flores P, Huete I. Mechanical fragmentation and pharmacologic thrombolysis in massive pulmonary embolism. J Vasc Interv Radiol 1997; 8:261–266.

25. Timsit F, Reynaud P, Meyer G, Sors H. Pulmonary embolectomy by catheter device in massive pulmonary embolism. Chest 1991; 100:655–658.

26. Greenfield LJ, Kimmell GO, McCurdy WC. Transvenous removal of pulmonary embolis by vacuum-cup catheter technique. J Surg Res 1969; 9:347–352.

27. Greenfield LJ, Bruce TA, Nichols NB. Transvenous pulmonary embolectomy by catheter device. Ann Surg 1971; 174:881–886.

28. Wakefield TW, Greenfield LJ. Diagnostic approaches and surgical treatment of deep venous thrombosis and pulmonary embolism. Hematol/Oncol Clin N Am 1993; 7: 1251–1267.

29. Lang EV, Barnhart WH, Walton DL, Raab SS. Percutaneous pulmonary thrombectomy. J Vasc Interv Radiol 1997; 8:427–432.

30. Moore JH, Koolpe HA, Carabasi RA, Yang S-L, Jarrell BE. Transvenous catheter pulmonary embolectomy. Arch Surg 1985; 120:1372–1375.

31. Greenfield LJ, Proctor MC, Williams DM, Wakefield TW. Long-term experience with transvenous catheter pulmonary embolectomy. J Vasc Surg 1993; 18:450–458.

32. Schmitz-Rode T, Gunther RW. New device for percutaneous fragmentation of pulmonary emboli. Radiology 1991; 180:135–137.

33. Brady AJB, Crake T, Oakley CM. Percutaneous fragmentation and dispersion versus pulmonary embolectomy by catheter device in massive pulmonary embolism. Chest 1992; 102:1305–1306.

34. Schmitz-Rode T, Janssens U, Schild HH, Basche S, Hanrath P, Gunther RW. Fragmentation of massive pulmonary embolism using a pigtail rotation catheter. Chest 1998; 114:1427–1436.

35. Essop MR, Middlemost S, Skoularigis J, Sareli P. Simultaneous mechanical clot fragmentation and pharmacologic thrombolysis in acute massive pulmonary embolism. Am J Cardiol 1992; 69:427–430.

36. Murphy JM, Mulvihill N, Mulcahy D, Foley B, Molloy MP. Percutaneous catheter and guidewire fragmentation with local administration of recombinant tissue plasminogen activator as a treatment for massive pulmonary embolism. Eur Radiol 1999; 9:959–964.

37. De Gregorio MA, Gimeno MJ, Mainar A, Herrera M, Tobio R, Alfonso R, et al. Mechanical and enzymatic thrombolysis for massive pulmonary embolism. J Vasc Interv Radiol 2002; 13:163–169.

38. Koning R, Cribier A, Gerber L, Eltchaninoff H, Tron C, Gupta V, et al. A new treatment for severe pulmonary embolism. Percutaneous rheolytic thrombectomy. Circulation 1997; 96:2498–2500.

39. Michalis LK, Tsetis DK, Rees MR. Case report: percutaneous removal of pulmonary artery thrombus in a patient with massive pulmonary embolism using the hydrolyser catheter: the first human experience. Clin Radiol 1997; 52:158–161.

40. Voigtlander T, Rupprecht H-J, Nowak B, Post F, Mayer E, Stahr P, et al. Clinical application of a new rheolytic thrombectomy catheter system for massive pulmonary embolism. Catheteriz Cardiovasc Interv 1999; 47:91–96.

41. Uflacker R, Strange C, Vujic I. Massive pulmonary embolism: preliminary results of treatment with the Amplatz thrombectomy device. J Vasc Interv Radiol 1996; 7:519–528.

42. Haskal ZJ, Soulen MC, Huettl EA, Palevsky HI, Cope C. Life-threatening pulmonary emboli and cor pulmonale: treatment with percutaneous pulmonary artery stent placement. Radiology 1994; 191:473–475.

43. Koizumi J, Kusano S, Akima T, Isoda K, Hikita H, Kurita A, et al. Emergent Z stent placement for treatment of cor pulmonale due to pulmonary emboli after failed lytic treatment: technical considerations. Cardiovasc Interv Radiol 1998; 21:254–257.

44. Schmitz-Rode T, Gunther RW, Pfeffer JG, Neuerburg JM, Geuting B, Biesterfeld S. Acute massive pulmonary embolism: use of a rotatable pigtail catheter for diagnosis and fragmentation therapy. Radiology 1995; 197:157–162.

45. Brown DB, Cardella JF, Wilson RP, Singh H, Waybill PN. Evaluation of a modified Arrow-Trerotola percutaneous thrombolytic device for treatment of acute pulmonary embolus in a canine model. J Vasc Interv Radiol 1999; 10:733–740.

46. Stein PD, Sabbah HN, Basha MA, Popovich J, Kensey KR, Nash JE. Mechanical disruption of pulmonary emboli in dogs with a flexible rotating-tip catheter (Kensey Catheter). Chest 1990; 98:994–998.

26

Complications Associated with Inferior Vena Caval Filter Insertion

Lazar J. Greenfield and Mary C. Proctor
Section of Vascular Surgery, University of Michigan,
Ann Arbor, Michigan, U.S.A.

The earliest mechanical approaches to prevent pulmonary thromboembolism were associated with significant complications when the techniques were limited to direct operative approaches to the vena cava for ligation, placation or external clip application. When endovascular techniques were developed for vena caval filter placement more than 30 years ago, morbidity was reduced significantly, since venous access could be achieved under local anesthesia. But a more significant change occurred in the 1980s, when percutaneous sheaths and dilators converted the procedure from surgical to radiological. With this change, a variety of innovative filters emerged, characterized by relative ease of insertion and smaller profile to minimize the size of the sheath for introduction. The focus of complications had shifted from the procedure to the actual placement and performance of the filter. Unfortunately, most efforts in recent years have been to further reduce the profile of the carrier systems, so current publications found in the radiological journals have more to do with techniques and ease of insertion than evaluation of device performance over time. In fact, there is very little information about the long-term performance and complications of most of the vena caval filters used today.

COMPLICATIONS OF INSERTION

Aside from the recognized complications of inadvertent arterial entry such as thrombosis, thromboembolism, and arteriovenous fistula, the characteristic complications of percutaneous filter insertion are insertion-site thrombosis and hemorrhage. Insertion site thrombosis has been variably reported in 0–33% of patients, with the major determinants being the underlying prothrombotic state, and duration of pressure on the site to control bleeding post-insertion (1,2). Since most punctures in the radiology suite are arterial, the tendency was to use more force for a longer duration than necessary for the venous system. Hemorrhage post-insertion is usually readily recognized by hematoma formation, which is rarely reported. It can be a more serious problem in the groin if the entry puncture is high, resulting in bleeding into the pelvis from the iliac vein, or in the mediastinum from a cervical puncture, which may not be appreciated until the patient is hypotensive.

If the presenting venous thrombosis involves the right iliofemoral veins, it is generally advisable to use the left femoral or the jugular vein for access. The left femoral can be more of a technical challenge since it enters the vena cava at a more obtuse angle and requires a more flexible carrier system. Concern regarding the difficulty of accessing the jugular vein can be addressed by the additional use of an ultrasound probe to identify and guide the access puncture. Experienced clinicians have been able to place filters through partially thrombosed iliofemoral veins without embolic detachment, but this is not advisable, particularly if the thrombus is of recent onset and not firmly adherent to the vein wall.

COMPLICATIONS OF FILTER POSITION

Once access is achieved, and a dilator/sheath is inserted over a guidewire, filter placement in the target zone of the vena cava becomes a matter of correct alignment and positioning of the sheath and carrier system. Filter misplacement was more common before current sheath techniques were available, but fortunately were of little clinical significance other than failing to provide appropriate protection from pulmonary embolism (PE). The one exception was intracardiac misplacement, where a misplaced filter could interfere with tricuspid valve function, or rarely, erode through the atrial wall producing cardiac tamponade.

Currently, filter misplacement is a rare occurrence, usually inadvertently into the right renal vein where it poses little risk to the kidney provided that it is a wire device that does not intrinsically promote thrombosis. This complication can be avoided by noting any deviation to the patient's right when the carrier system approach is from the jugular vein. The typical target zone of the vena cava is just below the renal veins at approximately the L2-3 level, but any placement between the renal veins and the bifurcation of the cava provides protection if it is a wire device that is non-thrombogenic. When the suprarenal vena cava is the target, placement at the T12-L1 level is recommended since the diaphragm and caudate lobe of the liver provide repetitive downward compression of the device, tending to push it caudad. For this reason, filter selection should be based on the filter's demonstrated ability to withstand these additional mechanical repetitive forces (3,4).

LATE COMPLICATIONS OF FILTER PLACEMENT

The most serious late complication of filter placement is occlusion of the device. This not only produces venous hypertension and stasis sequelae for the lower extremities, but also becomes a potential nidus for thrombus propagation into the proximal cava and major thromboembolism. Filter occlusion may occur on the basis of intrinsic thrombogenesis or the entrapment of a large amount of migrating thrombus. When a single massive thromboembolus produces acute filter occlusion, the consequences are equivalent to clamping the vena cava. The resultant hypotension can be misinterpreted as recurrent PE with devastating consequences if the patient is treated with vasopressor agents for the physiological hypovolemia. However, discrimination between filter occlusion and recurrent massive PE can be made at the bedside, since massive PE produces right heart overload and jugular venous distension. In contrast, there is no jugular prominence in filter occlusion and the central venous pressure is low. Rapid volume repletion will resuscitate the patient in this situation and a decision can be made whether or not the patient is a candidate for thrombolytic therapy to attempt to restore patency to the vena cava.

The efficacy of the filter with a smaller thromboembolus seems to depend on the design of the filter and the amount of metal comprising the filter (5). Cone-shaped filters that preserve flow around the trapped embolus facilitate subsequent thrombus resolution, preserving long-term patency. Therefore, this design has had the most favorable long-term results for the patient, combining long-term protection with no morbidity (6).

Over time, filters that exert sustained pressure on the wall of the vena cava can occasionally penetrate the wall without bleeding. When the extrusion is wire, it generally has little clinical significance in the retroperitoneum, but if it projects anteriorly into the peritoneum, it has been associated with small bowel obstruction. If this is encountered, the appropriate treatment is simply to use a wire cutter to remove the projecting wire. No attempt should be made to remove the filter that is embedded in the vena cava since the outcome is likely to require vena caval ligation and is unnecessary. Late wire breakage has also been observed in follow-up: 0.01% in Greenfield filters, but no rate is reported in other devices. This has not been associated with either impairment of filter function or complications for the patient.

Improved materials and manufacturing techniques have facilitated development of a new generation of vena caval filters that purport two advantages; reduced delivery system size and optional retrieval. The Food and Drug Administration (FDA) approved four new devices within the past three years. These include the Cordis Trapease filter from Johnson and Johnson; the Tulip filter from Cooke, the Recovery filter from Bard, and the LP filter from B. Braun. Each device is designed for delivery with a low profile system (6–8.5 French), and both the Tulip and Recovery devices are potentially removable.

It takes thousands of uses before the performance characteristics of a new medical device are fully known. Because approval of inferior vena caval (IVC) filters is obtained through the 510 K process, limited clinical data is available. In order to obtain regulatory approval, it is only necessary to demonstrate stable placement and resistance to vena caval penetration equivalent to some predicate filter device. A review of the literature in both Current Contents and Medline found no data on the Braun LP filter (7,8) with only two findings providing clinical outcomes. While there are several pre-clinical and case studies, Tulip filter data from the Canadian Registry provides the only comprehensive clinical experience with these devices (9).

The suggested clinical advantage of these devices is to facilitate placement by reducing the incidence of insertion problems, and in the case of removable filters, to prevent the longer-term complications reported with some permanent filters. While it is too early to evaluate long-term performance of the new filters, it is possible to determine whether the new designs have facilitated the insertion procedure.

To supplement the published data, adverse events listed by the FDA in their on-line Manufacturer and User Facility Device Experience (MAUDE) adverse event reporting system have been included. This registry contains structured reports on problems with controlled medical devices. The reporting is voluntary so the entries are subjective, however, this public registry does indicate clinical trends. Reports from a 15-month period ranging from December 2001 through March 2003 were included. There were 14 reports of the Braun LP filter, 28 for the Trapease, 18 for the Gunther Tulip, in addition to 33 for the Greenfield (17 for titanium and 16 for

Table 1 MAUDE Database of Adverse Event Reports for Each Filter/Total Reports

	Braun LP	Cooke Tulip	Cordis Trapease	BSC	
				SGF	TGF
Crossed legs	0	2/18	0	0	0
Fracture	1/14	0	2/28	0	0
Incomplete opening	4/14	4/18	4/28	7/17	11/16
Migration	10/14	8/18	3/28	3/17	1
Misplacement	2/14	2/18	0	5/17	2/16
Occlusion	0	1/18	14/28	0	0
Perforation	1/14	2/18	5/28	0	0
Asymmetry				0	3/16

Abbreviations: MAUDE, manufacturer and user facility device experience; BSC, boston scientific corporation; SGF, stainless steel greenfield filter; TGF, titanium greenfield filter.

the stainless steel). Tables 1 and 2 summarize the reports during the acute and long-term periods.

Insertion problems include inability to gain vascular access, device misplacement, incomplete filter opening and inadequate attachment (6). Problems with thrombosis at the insertion site are reported, as well as difficulties in performing other intravascular procedures. As a benchmark, we reference a report for insertion problems with the Greenfield percutaneous filters in a group of 133 trauma patients who had duplex ultrasound follow-up. The authors reported no intra-procedural or post-procedural adverse events (10).

Technical success was comparable among the devices. Asch et al. successfully placed 100% of filters in their sample of 32 patients using the Recovery device (11). There was only one misplacement of a Gunther Tulip filter in 90 cases (9); this filter has also been accurately placed in the superior vena cava without difficulty.

Table 2 MAUDE Database of Patient Outcomes/Interventions Associated with the Filter

	Braun LP	Cooke Tulip	Cordis Trapease	BSC	
				SGF	TGF
Embolized filter	9/14	4/18	2/28		1/16
Expired	1/14	1/18	4/28	0	1/16
Hemorrhage	0	2/18	3/28	0	0
Massive leg edema	0	2/18	3/28	0	0
PE	0	1/18	1/28	0	1/16
Removed	1/14	3/18	0	1/17	3/16
Renal failure	0	0	1/28	0	0
Unstable	6/14	9/18	9/28	1/17	4/16
Surgery	4/14	2/18	1/28	1/17	0
Thrombolysis	0	0	2/28	0	0

Abbreviations: MAUDE, manufacturer and user facility device experience; BSC, boston scientific corporation; SGF, stainless steel greenfield filter; TGF, titanium greenfield filter; PE, pulmonary embolism.

In a series of 65 patients, three Trapease filters were misplaced for a success rate of 95%; in a series of 189 placements, Schutzer had 100% technical success (7,8).

There are frequent MAUDE reports of devices failing to open completely. The clinical sequelae are variable. Among the four Tulip cases and the three Trapease, six patients were stable, however, one patient with an incompletely opened Trapease filter expired. Incomplete opening was reported with seven Braun LP filters and resulted in filter embolization in six cases. Incomplete opening occurred most frequently with the Greenfield filters (12), and the sequelae included one PE and one embolized filter.

Filter migration is important when it requires intervention to reposition or remove a misplaced filter, or place an additional device. Movement less than 2 cm in a caudal direction is not clinically important, but cephalad migration that results in an intracardiac position can have serious consequences.

Asch reported one significant cephalad migration of 4 cm when a Recovery filter trapped a large thrombus (11). The MAUDE registry listed eight migrations of the Tulip filter of which four embolized to the pulmonary artery; one had a recurrent PE, one died, and two required open-heart surgery (Table 1). Rosseau et al. found no migration of the Trapease filter among a group of 65 patients (8), however, in the MAUDE reports there were three cases, one of which resulted in renal failure requiring dialysis as a result of filter occlusion. Significant movement of 14 LP filters was reported in the MAUDE data, which required surgical procedures or cardiopulmonary bypass in four cases.

Attempted retrieval was successful in 100% of 24 Recovery filters that had been implanted between five and 134 days (12). In 90 Gunther Tulip patients, retrieval was successfully accomplished in 51 of 52 attempts. Four of these patients (8%) had filters replaced subsequently (9) (Fig. 1). Lorch reported placement of a permanent filter in 4.8% of cases in the temporary filter registry (13).

Early vena cava or filter thrombosis is a major adverse event. While a filter is designed to stop emboli, it is important that vena caval blood flow be preserved. Rousseau (8) reported two occluded Trapease filters in their series of 65 patients (3%) and in the larger series of 189 patients, there were three occlusions (7). Among 37 patients who had the Gunther Tulip filter left in place, 25 had follow-up, and two (8%) had vena caval occlusion. The small cone volume of this device may make it more prone to occlusion. In the MAUDE registry, there were 11 reports of occlusion with the Trapease filter in the review period. Three patients had massive lower extremity edema, two required lytic therapy, one suffered renal failure, and two expired. The double trapping surface adds increased turbulence and stasis of blood flow when a large thrombus is trapped so significant obstruction is observed. There were no MAUDE reports of occlusion with any of the other devices. The double trapping levels of these filters have been associated with higher rates of occlusion in animal and bench-top evaluations. The Lorch registry (13) of short-term results of the Antheor, Guenther, and Prolyser filters reported major filter occlusion in 16% of cases which required additional thrombolytic therapy, and placement of a second filter in 10%.

Symptomatic PE is rarely reported following vena caval filter placement as all of the devices effectively trap large emboli. In the literature, a single PE was reported among 189 placements of the Trapease filter (<1%) (7). In the MAUDE data, an additional PE was found in association with perforation of the IVC. Millward reported no symptomatic PE with the Tulip filter in the Canadian Registry (9). Likewise, Asch failed to find symptomatic PE in patients with the Recovery filter. In a registry of 188 patients with temporary filters, Lorch reported four deaths

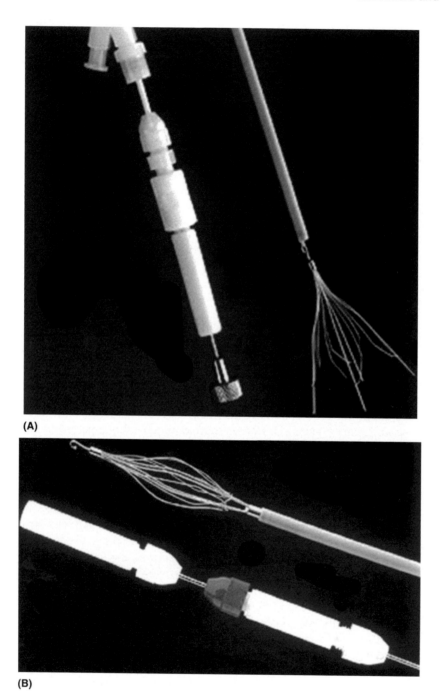

(A)

(B)

Figure 1 The Gunther Tulip venacaval filter has four legs with small hooks at each leg. There is a larger hook at the apex to facilitate retrieval. It can be placed from a jugular (**A**) or femoral (**B**) access.

due to PE despite the presence of a filter (19). A 2% PE-specific mortality is extremely high in a group of patients where 56% of devices were placed as prophylaxis during thrombolytic procedures.

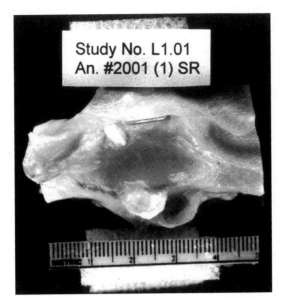

Figure 2 Necropsy specimen from a sheep obtained 60 days after placement of the Trapease filter. Note the extruded strut.

Major IVC perforations requiring intervention are a rare event in the filter literature. Rousseau found no perforations in 65 Trapease placements (8). However, in a larger series there was one retroperitoneal hemorrhage (7). The MAUDE registry has five cases of caval penetration within a 15-month period. Four of the five had serious hemorrhagic complications, one required surgical repair of the vena cava, and there was one death. This is significant because the device relies on radial force for attachment, which may result in caval perforation. This differs from previous filter designs that use hooks for attachment (Fig. 3). Two reports of perforation by a Tulip filter and by the Braun LP are found in the MAUDE data, both Tulip cases were associated with mortality while the Braun LP cases were stable. The characteristic features of the Tulip hook that enable retrieval may also make it subject to perforation. It is more difficult to understand perforation with the Braun LP stent design.

Fatigue fractures of vena caval filters have always been rare, occurring over an extended period of time. They may be the result of the design, the particular properties of the material or the manufacturing process. In our registry which records annual follow-up examinations, there has been only one fracture of a percutaneous Greenfield filter in 2600 placements over a 10-year period. In the MAUDE data, there have already been two Trapease and two Braun LP fractures reported, and while they did not occur at placement, they happened within 24 months. In our experience, metal fatigue rarely occurs in less than 60 months and is usually found in a filter placed above the renal vein where it faces longer excursion distances. The mechanism of failure for the new devices should be evaluated.

The limited number of published articles and the subjectivity involved with the MAUDE reporting system make it difficult to estimate rates of adverse events associated with the new vena caval filters. However, one thing is clear: these devices have not eliminated any of the problems that occurred with the previously marketed devices. Small profile and the option of retrieval have been achieved at the cost of

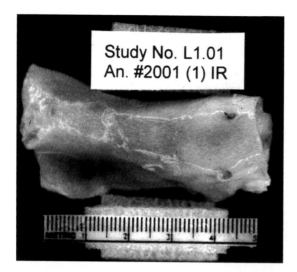

Study No. L1.01
An. #2001 (1) IR

Figure 3 This specimen also obtained 60 days post-placement of a Greenfield filter. The tip of one hook is visible while the others are contained within a fibrin cap.

clinically significant caval perforation, massive caval occlusion and life-threatening migration. Patient outcomes have not improved. The ideal combination of an effective and safe filter that can be inserted from a variety of sites and recovered when desired has not been achieved. Although the incidence of serious events is small relative to the number of filters placed, the significance of the complications is costly on both an individual and societal basis. Open-heart procedures, thrombolytic therapy, hemorrhage, renal failure, and death are tragic outcomes for a device intended to be life saving.

REFERENCES

1. Pieri S, Agresti P, Morucci M, de' ML. Optional vena cava filters: preliminary experience with a new vena cava filter. Radiol Med 2003; 105:56–62.
2. Tobin KD, Pais O, Austin CB. Femoral vein thrombosis following percutaneous placement of the Greenfield filter. Invest Radiol 1989; 24:442–445.
3. Greenfield LJ, Cho KJ, Proctor MC, Sobel M, Shah S, Wingo J. Late results of suprarenal Greenfield vena cava filter placement. Arch Surg 1992; 127:969–973.
4. Greenfield LJ, Proctor MC. Suprarenal filter placement. J Vasc Surg 1998; 28:432–438.
5. Couch GG, Kim H, Ojha M. In vitro assessment of the hemodynamic effects of a partial occlusion in a vena cava filter. J Vasc Surg 1997; 25:663–672.
6. Greenfield LJ, Proctor MC. Twenty-year clinical experience with the Greenfield filter. Cardiovasc Surg 1995; 3(2):199–205.
7. Schutzer R, Ascher E, Hingorani A, Jacob T, Kallakuri S. Preliminary results of the new 6F TrapEase inferior vena cava filter. Ann Vasc Surg 2003; 17:103–106.
8. Rousseau H, Perreault P, Otal P, et al. The 6-F Nitinol TrapEase inferior vena cava filter: results of a prospective multicenter trial. J Vasc Interv Radiol 2001; 12:299–304.
9. Millward SF, Oliva VL, Bell SD, et al. Gunther tulip retrievable vena cava filter: results from the registry of the Canadian interventional radiology association. J Vasc Interv Radiol 2001; 12:1053–1058.
10. Duperier T, Mosenthal A, Swan KG, Kaul S. Acute complications associated with Greenfield filter insertion in high-risk trauma patients. J Trauma-Injury Infect Crit Care 2003; 54:545–549.

11. Asch MR. Initial experience in humans with a new retrievable inferior vena cava filter. Radiology 2002; 225:835–844.
12. Murphy TP, Dorfman GS, Yedlicka JW, et al. LGM vena cava filter: objective evaluation of early results. J Vasc Interv Radiol 1991; 2:107–115.
13. Lorch H, Welger D, Wagner V, et al. Current practice of temporary vena cava filter insertion: a multicenter registry [comment]. J Vasc Interv Radiol 2000; 11:83–88.
14. Lorch H, Welger D, Wagner V, et al. Current practice of temporary vena cava filter insertion: a multicenter registry. J Vasc Interv Radiol 2000; 11:83–88.

27

Pre- and Post-Intervention Evaluation of Patients with Peripheral Vascular Disease

Michael R. Jaff

Vascular Medicine, Massachusetts General Hospital, Boston, Massachusetts, U.S.A.

INTRODUCTION

Despite the advances in endovascular techniques for the treatment of non-coronary vascular disease, complications exist which may limit the success of the intervention and result in significant harm and even death to the patient. In an effort to reduce the risk of complication, understanding the systemic nature of atherosclerosis, pre-intervention diagnostic methods must be accurate, safe, painless, and reproducible. Comprehensive testing promotes improved outcomes through appropriate patient selection. Once the procedure has been completed, post-procedure evaluation of potential complications will result in improved acute and long-term outcomes.

BASIC PREPROCEDURE EVALUATION STRATEGIES

Prior to any peripheral vascular intervention, basic historical review of all vascular systems must be performed. This includes questions regarding known or suspected coronary artery disease, particularly with reference to prior coronary revascularization and recent non-invasive cardiac testing. Evaluation of known extracranial carotid atherosclerosis must be part of the evaluation. Prior carotid revascularization, known carotid atherosclerotic disease, and symptoms of cerebral ischemia are elicited.

A thorough review of symptoms suggestive of intermittent claudication or exercise-induced limb discomfort is important, and may have a significant impact on access for endovascular procedures.

Physical examination findings will allow the physician to predict ideal access for endovascular procedures and lessen the risk of complications.

The most important complications of endovascular procedures include access site issues (pseudoaneurysm, hematoma, arteriovenous fistula), local or systemic atheroembolization, and target vessel trauma (dissection, rupture, thrombosis). The vascular diagnostic laboratory will aid in rapidly identifying many of these complications, so that appropriate and prompt therapy may be instituted (Table 1). Duplex ultrasonography

Table 1 Vascular Evaluation After Endovascular Intervention

Complication	Physical findings	Objective tests	Interpretation
Pseudoaneurysm	– Pulsatile groin mass – Audible bruit (Syst/Diast)	Duplex ultrasound	– Color evidence of extra-arterial flow – Classic "to-and-fro" Doppler waveform in neck
Access site vessel thrombosis	– Absent pulse – Ischemic foot (pain, pallor, paresthesias, motor deficit)	– ABI – Duplex ultrasound	– ABI$\leq$0.5 – Absent color flow and Doppler waveform in index artery
Atheroembolization	– Mottled "livido reticularis" appearance in feet, abdominal wall skin – Ischemic toes	– ABI – Laboratory studies (BUN, creatinine, ESR) – Duplex ultrasound of abdominal aorta/ peripheral arteries	– ABI variable (may be normal) – If renal atheroembolization, azotemia present – ESR>20 mm/hr – Abdominal aortic or peripheral arterial atherosclerosis/ mobile atheromata

Abbreviations: ABI, ankle-brachial index; ESR, erythrocyte sedimentation rate; BUN, blood urea nitrogen.

uses physics principals of the Doppler equation to correlate speeds of arterial blood flow with severity of stenosis (1). In addition, patterns of Doppler waveforms and real-time gray scale and color flow images will allow for prompt diagnosis of vascular complications.

LOWER EXTREMITY ARTERIAL VASCULAR TESTING

Preprocedure

The evaluation of patients with peripheral arterial disease (PAD) includes a historical review of patient symptoms and atherosclerotic risk factors, physical examination, and the use of non-invasive vascular tests. The first objective test is the ankle-brachial index (ABI). The ABI is a simple test that can be performed in a physician's office. This test compares the blood pressure obtained with a hand-held Doppler in the dorsalis pedis or posterior tibial artery (whichever is higher), to the blood pressure in the higher of the two brachial pressures. Generally, an ABI $\geq$ 0.9 is considered normal, >0.4 – <0.9 reflects mild to moderate PAD, and $\leq$0.4 suggests severe PAD. With exercise a challenge (classically constant speed, constant grade treadmill testing or active pedal plantarflexion), the arterial limb pressure decreases in association with symptoms of intermittent claudication.

Once the ABI has been performed, providing objective evidence of the overall severity of PAD in a limb, more specific non-invasive information may be obtained in the vascular laboratory (2). The use of segmental limb pressures can aid in localizing diseased arterial segments.

A series of limb pressure cuffs are placed on the thigh (some centers prefer high- and low-thigh cuffs), calf, ankle, transmetatarsal region of the foot, and digit. The ABI is calculated, and then the pressure is sequentially inflated in each cuff to approximately 20–30 mmHg above systolic pressure. Utilizing a continuous wave Doppler probe placed at one of the pedal arteries, the pressure in the cuff is gradually released, and the pressure at each segment is measured. If a decrease in pressure between two consecutive levels of >30 mmHg is identified, this suggests arterial disease of the arterial segments proximal to the cuff. In addition, comparing the two limbs, a 20–30 mmHg discrepancy from one limb to the other at the same cuff level also suggests a significant arterial stenosis or occlusion proximal to the cuff.

Pulse volume recordings (PVR) are plethysmographic tracings that detect the changes in the volume of blood flowing through a limb. Ankle-brachial indices, segmental pressures, and PVR are useful objective tests in patients with suspected lower extremity arterial occlusive disease, limb discomfort without an obvious cause, as a method of evaluating the success of an intervention, and as a method of follow-up. The test is inexpensive, painless, reproducible, and relatively easy to perform. The equipment required to perform these examinations is significantly less expensive than modern color-flow duplex ultrasound units.

Native vessel arterial duplex ultrasonography is also widely performed. This examination is generally accepted as a precise method of defining arterial stenoses or occlusions (3). The sensitivity of duplex ultrasonography in detecting occlusions and stenoses has been reported to be 95% and 92%, with specificities of 99% and 97%, respectively. Limitations have included tandem stenoses, tibial vessel imaging, and difficulty imaging the inflow arteries. Vessels are classified into one of five categories: normal, 1–19% stenosis, 20–49% stenosis, 50–99% stenosis, and occlusion (4). The categories are determined by alterations in the Doppler waveform, as well as increasing peak systolic velocities. For a stenosis to be classified as 50–99%, for example, the peak systolic velocity must increase by 100%, in comparison to the normal segment of artery proximal to the stenosis.

Arterial duplex ultrasonography has been used to guide the interventionist towards appropriate access to a lesion potentially amenable to endovascular therapy (5). This technology has also been used after endovascular therapy to determine technical success and durability of the procedure (6) (Fig. 1). Unfortunately, it appears that duplex ultrasonography soon after balloon angioplasty may overestimate residual stenosis, and may be a limitation of this technology after endovascular therapy.

Duplex ultrasonography is very helpful in identifying areas of vascular trauma, specifically iatrogenic. Pseudoaneurysms occur in up to 7.5% of femoral artery catheterizations, and can result in significant complications, including distal embolization into the native arterial system, expansion, extrinsic compression on neurovascular structures, rupture, and hemorrhage (7). Duplex ultrasonography can rapidly and accurately identify these lesions (Fig. 2). In addition, the use of direct ultrasound-guided compression or, more recently, ultrasound-guided thrombin

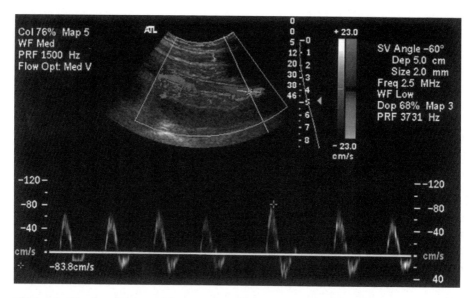

Figure 1 Duplex ultrasound image of an iliac artery stent. Note the laminar color flow (shown here in gray scale) and normal triphasic Doppler waveform with normal Doppler peak systolic velocity.

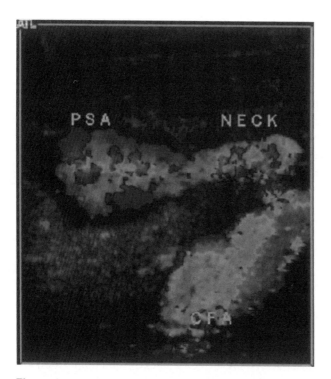

Figure 2 Color duplex ultrasound image (shown here in gray scale) of a CFA pseudoaneurysm. (*Neck*): Tract of arterial blood from CFA to sac of pseudoaneurysm. (*PSA*): Pseudoaneurysm sac. *Abbreviations*: CFA, common femoral artery.

injection can repair these lesions without the need for more invasive surgical procedures.

EXTRACRANIAL CAROTID ARTERY TESTING

Not only does significant internal carotid artery stenosis increase the risk for both transient and permanent neurologic events, but it also represents an increased risk for coronary atherosclerosis, myocardial infarction, and cardiovascular death. A safe and accurate method of identifying significant carotid stenosis is critical in the management of these patients.

Direct visualization of the extracranial carotid arteries with duplex ultrasonography has been shown to provide excellent accuracy and reproducibility. Because of the advances in endovascular treatment of extracranial carotid stenosis using balloon angioplasty and stent deployment, appropriate pre- and post-procedure evaluation of carotid disease is critical.

The carotid duplex ultrasound examination identifies plaque, stenoses, and occlusions in the common, internal, and external carotid arteries. The exam also identifies flow direction in the vertebral arteries. This examination is routinely performed for patients with a history of transient ischemic attacks, stroke, cervical bruits, after surgical or endovascular revascularization, and in patients deemed to be at high risk for the presence of carotid stenosis (Table 2).

Current data suggests the sensitivity of carotid duplex ultrasonography to be 85%, with a specificity of 90%. Duplex ultrasonography is highly accurate in identifying a carotid artery occlusion, with a positive predictive value of 92.5%, and is very useful in documenting results of revascularization. Many vascular laboratories use a combination of duplex ultrasonography and magnetic resonance arteriography to plan revascularization strategies (8).

Carotid duplex ultrasonography is useful in determining adequacy of carotid revascularization, either via endarterectomy (9) or stent-deployment. Using similar protocols to native vessel imaging, the site of revascularization is interrogated, and peak systolic and end-diastolic velocities are measured. Although imaging of carotid stents is straightforward, velocity criteria identifying restenosis have not been

Table 2 Diagnostic Criteria for ICA Stenosis

% Stenosis	PSV	EDV	Flow characteristics
0–19	<105 cm/sec	–	Normal
20–39	<105 cm/sec	–	Spectral broadening
40–59	105–150 cm/sec	–	Increased spectral broadening
60–79[a]	151–240	–	Marked spectral broadening
80–99	>240 cm/sec	>135 cm/sec	Marked spectral broadening
Occluded	N/A	N/A	No flow. Pre-occlusive "thump". "Externalized" CCA signal

Note: >4.0 Suggests >70% stenosis; <4.0 suggests <70% stenosis.
[a]PSV ICA/CCA.
Abbreviations: PSV, peak systolic velocity; ICA, internal carotid artery; CCA, common carotid artery; EDV, end-diastolic velocity.

determined. Most investigators compare post-procedural velocities to those in follow-up, determining significant increase over time.

RENAL ARTERY STENOSIS

Atherosclerotic renal artery stenosis (RAS) has become increasingly recognized as a contributing factor to resistant hypertension, deterioration in renal function, recurrent "flash pulmonary edema," and long-term ill effects of poorly controlled hypertension. Patients with severe bilateral renal artery stenosis, or stenosis to a solitary functioning kidney, are at risk for the development of end-stage renal disease. Long-term survival of patients with atherosclerotic renal artery stenosis requiring dialytic support is dismal.

Although a number of non-invasive methods of diagnosis in renal artery stenosis have been proposed, none have obviated the role of the "gold standard," renal arteriography. Each "screening" test has significant limitations that prevent widespread acceptance. Renal artery duplex ultrasonography has significant advantages that make it an excellent diagnostic test (10) (Fig. 3).

The advent of endoluminal technology to revascularize renal artery stenosis has caused intense interest in this disorder. Because of the limitations of percutaneous transluminal angioplasty in effectively treating ostial atherosclerotic RAS, endovascular stent placement has emerged as a revascularization procedure that prevents elastic recoil and may offer a more durable result. With simple evaluation of the renal resistive index using current duplex ultrasound techniques, physicians may predict the outcome of renal revascularization prior to the procedure (11).

Duplex ultrasonography is the ideal method of determining the adequacy of renal artery stent revascularization. The entire renal artery can be imaged, despite

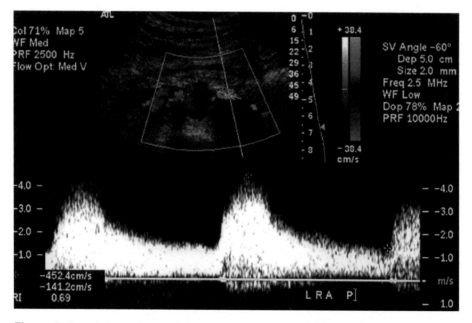

Figure 3 Renal artery duplex ultrasound image demonstrating significant increase in peak systolic and end diastolic velocities in the origin of the left renal artery, correlating with 60–99% left renal artery stenosis.

the presence of a metallic endoprosthesis. In addition, early or late restenosis is detected by an increase in the peak systolic velocity within the stented segment of the renal artery, as well as an increase in the renal:aortic ratio (RAR).

Duplex ultrasonography of the renal arteries, although technically challenging, is the optimal method of determining the presence and severity of a stenosis prior to intervention. Once revascularization has been performed, duplex ultrasonography is an effective and reliable method of documenting the adequacy of the revascularization, as well as noting the presence of early or late restenosis.

ABDOMINAL AORTIC DUPLEX ULTRASONOGRAPHY

Physicians have long understood the potential impact of abdominal aortic aneurysms (AAA). As the population ages, the incidence of death from AAA rupture is expected to rise. Approximately 6% of 70-year-old men develop AAA. The diagnosis of AAA is based predominantly in one of three scenarios: palpation of a pulsatile abdominal mass; a family history of AAA in a first-degree relative; or the incidental discovery of an AAA on an imaging study performed for alternate reasons. Management decisions are based on the transverse dimension of the aneurysm, the location (suprarenal versus infrarenal, for example), and the overall health of the patient (12). Many patients are instructed to have serial ultrasound examinations to follow progression in size of the AAA (13).

With the advance of endoluminal stent-grafts for AAA repair, the need for close surveillance for the development of endoleaks is critical (14). Although most recommend serial spiral computerized tomographic studies, this requires repeated radiation exposure and the use of intravenous contrast, which has potential risk. Current high-resolution color duplex ultrasonography has demonstrated utility especially in determining change in aneurysm size over time (15,16). Newer ultrasound contrast agents that have no serious side effects also seem to improve detection of endoleaks during a surveillance program (17).

REFERENCES

1. Stewart JH, Grubb M. Understanding vascular ultrasonography. Mayo Clin Proc 1992; 67:1186–1196.
2. Strandness DE. Noninvasive vascular laboratory and vascular imaging. In: Young JR, Olin JW, Bartholomew JR, eds. Peripheral Vascular Diseases. 2nd ed. New York: Mosby Publishing Company, 1996:33–64.
3. Whelan JF, Barry MH, Moir JD. Color flow Doppler ultrasonography: comparison with peripheral arteriography for the investigation of peripheral vascular disease. J Clin Ultrasound 1992; 20:369–374.
4. Bandyk DF. Ultrasonic duplex scanning in the evaluation of arterial grafts and dilatations. Echocardiography 1987; 4:251–264.
5. Elsman BHP, Legemate DA, van der Heyden FWHM, de Vos HJ, Mali WP, Eikelboom BC. The use of color-coded duplex scanning in the selection of patients with lower extremity arterial disease for percutaneous transluminal angioplasty: a prospective study. Cardiovasc Interv Radiol 1996; 19:313–316.
6. Mewissen MW, Kinney EV, Bandyk DF, Reifsnyder T, Seabrook GR, Lipchik EO, Towne JB. The role of duplex scanning versus angiography in predicting outcome after balloon angioplasty in the femoropopliteal artery. J Vasc Surg 1992; 15:860–866.

7. Kresowik TF, Khoury MD, Miller BV, Winniford MD, Shamma AR, Sharp WJ, Blecha MB, Corson JD. A prospective study of the incidence and natural history of femoral vascular complications after percutaneous transluminal coronary angioplasty. J Vasc Surg 1991; 13:328–335.

8. Borisch I, Horn M, Butz B, Zorger N, Draganski B, Hoelscher T, Bogdahn U, Feuerbach S, Kasprzak P. Preoperative evaluation of carotid artery stenosis: comparison of contrast-enhanced MR angiography and duplex sonography with digital subtraction angiography. Am J Neuroradiol 2003; 24:1117–1122.

9. Golledge J, Cuming R, Ellis M, Davies AH, Greenhalgh RM. Duplex imaging findings predict stenosis after carotid endarterectomy. J Vasc Surg 1997; 26:43–48.

10. Olin JW, Piedmonte MR, Young JR, DeAnna S, Grubb M, Childs MB. The utility of duplex ultrasound scanning of the renal arteries for diagnosing significant renal artery stenosis. Ann Intern Med 1995; 122:833–838.

11. Rademacher J, Chavan A, Bleck J, Vitzthum A, Stoess B, Jan Gebel M, Galanski M, Martin Kock K, Haller H. Use of Doppler ultrasonography to predict the outcome of therapy for renal-artery stenosis. N Engl J Med 2001; 334:410–417.

12. Ricci MA, Kleeman M, Case T, Pilcher DB. Normal aortic diameter by ultrasound. J Vasc Tech 1995; 19:17–19.

13. Reed WW, Hallett JW, Damiano MA, Ballard DJ. Learning from the last ultrasound: a population-based study of patients with abdominal aortic aneurysm. Arch Intern Med 1997; 157:2064–2068.

14. Seelig MH, Oldenburg A, Hakaim AG, Hallett JW, Chowla A, Andrews JC, Cherry KJ. Endovascular repair of abdominal aortic aneurysms: where do we stand? Mayo Clin Proc 1999; 74:999–1010.

15. Sato DT, Goff CD, Gregory RT, Robinson KD, Carter KA, Herts BR, Vilsack HB, Gayle RG, Parent FN, DeMasi RJ, Meier GH. Endoleak after aortic stent graft repair: diagnosis by color duplex ultrasound scan versus computed tomography scan. J Vasc Surg 1998; 28:657–663.

16. Raman KG, Missig-Carroll N, Richardson T, Muluk SG, Mararoun MS. Color-flow duplex ultrasound scan versus computed tomographic scan in the surveillance of endo-vascular aneurysm repair. J Vasc Surg 2003; 38:645–651.

17. Giannoni MF, Palombi G, Sbarigia E, Speziale F, Zaccaria A, Fiorani P. Contrast-enhanced ultrasound imaging for aortic stent-graft surveillance. J Endovasc Ther 2003; 10:208–217.

Index